Beating Lyme Disease
Using Alternative Medicine
And God-Designed Living

Written by
Dr. David A. Jernigan, D.C., B.S.
And
Dr. Sara J. Koch Jernigan, D.C., B.S.

Somerleyton Press
Benton, Kansas, USA

Somerleyton Press
13150 SW 41st
Benton, Kansas 67017
USA
www.jnutra.com

Edited by Charlie and Jean Brune
Dust Cover design by Jim Brune

Manufactured in the United States of America
Printed by Complete Printing Service, Decatur, Indiana
www.completeprintingservice.com

ISBN 0-9674623-1-2

Dedication

Dedicated to those doctors in the trenches who struggle to achieve lasting results in their Lyme patients; who fight a politically incorrect illness; who through sweat and tears fight stealth microbes; who struggle without any medical and insurance company agreement; who bravely reach beyond their conventional training for the betterment of their patients. This book is also dedicated to my patients, and the patients of other Lyme literate doctors who, often in desperation, stick with us while we continue to learn how to deal with this most dastardly of illnesses.

Special thanks also to:

Julie Taylor and family, who started me on this journey, fed me my first information about Lyme disease, and who patiently stayed with me as I struggled to put the pieces together that ultimately lead to the development of Borrelogen™.

Dr. Milton Dowty, D.C., my friend and mentor, and founder of Chiro-Plus Kinesiology, Inc.; who set my foundation on a higher mountain; and who taught me CPK, a tool which lead me to the development of Bio-Resonance Scanning™.

Dr. Lida Mattman, Ph.D., a Nobel-laureate, whose perseverance and dedication to truth and research is an inspiration; who survived years of political pressure, only to continue to debunk the popular monism of microbes with the truth of pleomorphism. And without whom none of my Lyme microbe research would have come to pass.

Dr. John Brimhall, D.C., whose intellect, wisdom and passion to teach doctors to become healers is unparalleled, whose love for God-designed healing through the latest technology inspires me to be a better doctor and a better person.

Disclaimer

This book is intended as an educational tool and guide for doctors and patients seeking alternative methods for addressing the human body suffering from chronic Lyme disease. All of the therapies and recommendations are designed to facilitate the restoration of the structure and function of the body's tissues, rather than "treating the disease." The recommendations, therapies, and methods described in this book are for the most part alternative, therefore, by definition, many of them have not been investigated and/or approved by any government or regulatory agency. Accordingly, it is recommended that one consults with his or her healthcare professional before using any therapy. Pregnant women are especially advised to consult with their healthcare professional before using any therapy.

Your health is important. Ultimately you must realize that it is your body, and it is your decision how to address any illness. You, the reader, must take full responsibility for your health and how you use this book.

Somerleyton Press and the authors expressly disclaim responsibility for any adverse effects resulting from your use of the information that is contained in this book. Check with your healthcare professional before starting any of the dietary supplements and therapies in this book.

Various chapters in this book describe the clinical practice of the authors as it exists at the time of publishing. As the researcher and developer of specialized dietary supplements, David A. Jernigan, D.C. and Sara J. Koch Jernigan, D.C. have financial interest in the products listed and marketed under the product label "Jernigan Nutraceuticals."

Table of Contents

Section 3: Changing Your Internal Environment So Lyme Microbes Won't Grow

Section 4: Stress and Lyme Disease

Section 5: Wellness Physicians of the 21st Century

Section 6: Important Therapies for Chronic Lyme Disease

Foreword

It would be very difficult to say how much Dr. David Jernigan means to my family. Basically, he gave us back our lives.

The journey back to a "normal" life is rewarding; however, it isn't always an easy task. It involves finding a path to follow and people who will encourage you along the way.

My family and I somehow all contracted Lyme disease. My wife, Jean, was the first who we noticed had something severely wrong. One symptom after another prompted visits to doctors of all types: five general practitioners, a rheumatologist, a hematologist, a cardiologist, three neurologists, three psychologists, an internist and an infectious disease specialist. Although most of these doctors meant well, none of them could direct a proper path of treatment for her.

The guessing games and pharmaceuticals that followed seemed hopeful at first but all ended in bewilderment. Even after a solid diagnosis of Lyme disease, most of these doctors told us that this illness was "all in her head," and that she or her family caused this breakdown of her body, mind and spirit. Other reasons were numerous: her husband expects too much; she is using this illness to escape from life's responsibilities; she needs more relaxation in her life, (yet at this point, all she was capable of was "relaxing"). The treatments from the Lyme Specialists were basically rounds of oral and intravenous antibiotics, which slightly relieved a few of the symptoms, but then Jean was told to "accept this disease and someday you will learn to live with it."

For any of you who have been ill for a long period of time, this probably sounds familiar. Well, we didn't accept it. We are very energetic people and we love life. What we were hearing didn't make sense.

Our path finally led us to Dr. Jernigan. We first heard about his product *Borrelogen* from a very nice, sympathetic Lyme disease specialist. The next day we found *Borrelogen* on the Internet, and called Dr. Jernigan's office to order. This is when we discovered that you could go to his clinic. This was the true beginning to a proper path of treatment for us.

Even though we now lead very "normal" lives, this path was not always an easy or a fast one as I mentioned before. I now view proper treatment and true healing as sort of a "slow food" trip to a fine restaurant. You must be patient. In today's world, most of us are used to an "I can have it now" type of attitude, similar to a fast food restaurant - we can go to our regular doctor and he or she will give us a prescription, and we'll feel better in a couple of days, right?

The truth about this "fast" approach is that the doctor is treating your symptoms only, not the true cause of your sickness. In some cases, the drug will make you feel better. What if it doesn't? More than likely, another prescription will be added, with perhaps others being added to deal with the side effects of the other prescriptions.

At some point **you** have got to stop the madness. You must realize that if your body has been "ill" for quite some time, it may take many months or a year to get you back to normal.

Our journey back to health seemed like a slow one, although in certain aspects, we saw "instant" results. At the time of our first visit to Dr. Jernigan, Jean could not hold her head up at all, but within 2 days of our first visit she could, and hasn't had that problem since. Dr. Jernigan showed us how her "circuits" were blown from the Lyme disease. After repairing them, she began to function normally. With our next visit 30 days later, she was able to walk properly. Within a few more months, Lyme wasn't a major factor in our lives.

You can greatly benefit from this book, and from the Jernigans' remedies and advice. But, **you** must want to do it. It can sometimes be a lonely journey. Your friends and even your family may tell you this is the wrong path, but that is not for them to decide. Look deep into yourself and ask if all of the tests, drugs, thousands of dollars spent, hours waiting in doctor's offices, trips to the emergency room, and countless hours filled with ineffective treatment are the proper path.

Hopefully this book will help you understand how your body needs to heal. God gave us all different bodies according to His will. Each body will require its own special treatment plan. Your body can heal itself given the proper support and care. Although prescription drugs can help in some cases, they can sometimes stand in the way of true healing.

The Jernigans also touch on several subjects in this book dealing with God. Most professionals are taught not to cross this line. However, Dr. Jernigan will explain to you why it is very important to put the example of Jesus Christ foremost in your life. This decision can be your most important step in healing.

Decide now to take a positive step toward beating Lyme disease. All of the drugs and guessing you have endured can't be right if you are still sick. The roller coaster ride will only end when you say stop.

- Charlie Brune, *editor*

Introduction

This book is intended to present a protocol for CHRONIC Lyme disease based on biological medicine, God-designed healing and God-designed living. It is intended for lay people and physicians who desire to learn to approach the illness from a whole-person perspective using non-toxic, natural methods, as well as following principles of healthy living from God's Word.

Some may question writing about Christian principles in a book on Lyme disease; however my clinical practice experience has shown that along with everything that can be done physically and medicinally, spiritual matters must also be addressed in order for lasting healing to occur. I definitely **do not** promote or represent "new-age"; however, Christians need to be empowered by all that God has promised. Christians must be liberated from the fear of using all that God has made available for His children. Everything in heaven and earth was made by Him for the benefit of His children. Christian Biological Medicine seeks to discover and utilize every natural, true, and good healing method God created for our benefit, whether it is by the coherent light of a therapeutic laser, a plant-based medicine, or the energy imprint of a substance in a homeopathic remedy.

One can easily pick up literature about a myriad of vitamins, minerals, botanical medicines, glandulars, homeopathic remedies, enzymes, and colloidal metals and minerals – all promising to "cure" what ails you. I see patients every day from all over the world who have been everywhere and tried everything (and many have the bags and sometimes suitcases full of remedies to prove it!). The point is, you may have Lyme disease, but when it is chronic the infection is well entrenched; the only way to rout it out is to change the environment of the body so that it is no longer a "happy home" environment for the bacteria. You must deal with all the areas of the body that are weak and out of balance. It is not enough to simply take an antibiotic: even intravenous antibiotics will only kill 85% of the bacteria at best, leaving 15% alive and now antibiotic-resistant.

The protocol presented in this book revolves around frequency-matched remedies and the principles of Circuit Healing™ and Euro-American Biological Medicine. Circuit Healing™ and Biological Medicine are, in my opinion, the most pure and advanced healing methods and philosophies. They do not rely on drugs to create the illusion of health but work to remove everything that interferes with the ability of your body to heal itself, while simultaneously providing the information and building blocks necessary for the body to truly become well.

It must be understood that the world's most celebrated and astute physicians cannot heal even the simplest paper cut, much less the major disease processes of the body. At all times, thoughtfully applied treatments and therapies must be utilized to enable the body to restore balance and health. Your body is the only one who can heal the paper cut, and it is your body that must heal you of Lyme disease. Every medicine should support the healing efforts of your body, not suppress them. It may surprise many of you to learn that your body can and does beat Lyme disease when balance is restored in every organ, system and tissue.

No one or two medicines or remedies can address all of the problems associated with a multi-system illness such as chronic Lyme disease. Each of the remedies, supplements, treatments and therapies presented in this book work to complement each other and have a strong synergistic effect on the entire body.

Most people with chronic Lyme disease have already used many antibiotics with limited success or may be intolerant and allergic to them.

I decided to write this book after seeing so many people suffering primarily using antibiotics. They all believed that "If my doctor can kill these bacteria, then I will be well." "Health in a bottle" is a myth! Health is the product of balanced living and thoughtfully applied treatments and therapies which enable the body to function perfectly... the way God designed it to.

I feel confident that at the very least this protocol will strengthen your body and give you the best fighting chance of conquering and reclaiming the quality of life you seek.

The concepts and protocol presented in this book are the result of my ongoing research to find and/or develop better remedies and therapies to help real people and alleviate real suffering in my clinic. Although we have trained many doctors in the practice of Circuit Healing™ and Euro-American Biological Medicine, most doctors are classically trained. It is my hope that more doctors will become interested in these practices upon reading this book and be liberated from the "germ theory" and "drug mentality" that is so pervasive in today's hospitals.

Not to be morbid, but keep in mind that we are all dying and coming closer to death with the passing of every second. The choices you make either add days to your life or take them away. Suppressive therapies used by themselves always take days away, since they weaken the tissues of the body. It is your body…it is also your choice.

I pray that you prosper and find good health all the days of your life.

Dr. David A. Jernigan, D.C, B.S.

Section 1

Understanding Lyme Disease

(Make sure you read the Introduction before reading on.)

Chapter 1

The *New* "Great Imitator"

The *new* "Great Imitator", Lyme disease (LD), is increasingly being confirmed in cases of misdiagnosed chronic illnesses. It is said to be the "great imitator" due to the fact that its symptoms are so diverse that it can mimic 200 illnesses. This fact, along with the fact that there have been no good laboratory tests available to positively confirm LD, has led to the polarization of the medical and scientific community. A good example of this can be seen in the following statement: I have seen people in my clinic who have been to many specialists who ran up to 700 different tests on the patient without finding anything conclusive. They would usually be labeled as "atypical Lupus" or "atypical MS" or some other symptom-based diagnosis. When I would check the person for Lyme bacteria I would often find it present in both the blood and urine. Upon returning to their other doctors with the news, many times the doctor would tell the patient, "We don't know what you have, but it isn't Lyme disease!" Even when faced with positive Lyme tests and symptoms that are known to be possible in Lyme disease, as Dr. Ed Masters, M.D., presented at the 1999 International Conference on Lyme disease, and even in the face of overwhelming evidence as he so eloquently demonstrated, Lyme disease is apparently a "politically incorrect" illness. Dr. Masters presented many photographs of the classic bull's-eye rash on his patients, a picture of the tick, the lab report verifying that the tick did indeed have the Lyme spirochetes in its stomach, the blood and urine lab tests of the patient that were positive, and the list of the patient's symptoms that are commonly found in Lyme disease. Even in the face of all of this, when he took his evidence to the Health Department of his state to get them to warn the public that they need to take precautions when doing outdoor activities, his state health department reportedly said something to the effect of, "With all due respect Dr. Masters, if we had Lyme disease in our state, more doctors than just you would be finding it."

Apparently ticks that attach to geese and other waterfowl in Connecticut fall off as the birds cross the state line, thus preventing the spread of infected ticks to every other state in the country – NOT! Another of my favorites is when I hear that only one type of tick is classically recognized as carrying Lyme spirochetes. Any other blood-sucking insect that drinks the blood of an infected deer mysteriously filters out the Lyme spirochete – NOT!

Some Lyme researchers have estimated that about 1% of mosquitoes, deer flies, black flies, horseflies and fleas have and could potentially transmit Lyme bacteria. It only makes sense that Lyme could be transmitted by just about any blood-sucking insect, especially when the Center for Disease Control in Atlanta estimates that every $1/20^{th}$ of a second someone contracts a mosquito-borne illness and that every 20 seconds someone dies from one!

Until recently, the lab tests could only detect the "shadow" or the "possibility" that your body has seen the Lyme bacteria, *Borrelia burgdorferi*, via serum antibody tests. Serum antibody testing, such as the Lyme Western Blot IgG/IgM, in reality does not confirm the actual presence of the Lyme bacteria. The presence of Lyme specific antibody seen in a Lyme Western Blot can arguably be said that your body has simply "seen" this type of bacteria before, but does not necessarily have an active infection.

If you had Strep throat, your doctor could perform a throat culture and definitively confirm the presence of the actual Strep bacteria. Also, the doctor could test and find that the white blood cell count and neutrophils were elevated, further confirming the strep bacterial infection. The Borrelia burgdorferi is a type of bacteria which can elude your body's immune system; therefore, the lab tests often show no elevated white blood cells, or neutrophils. The fact is your body's immune system apparently often cannot see these bacteria, leading some of the world's Lyme researchers to label the bacteria as a "*Stealth Pathogen*".

One can see why so many otherwise very intelligent doctors have a difficult time acknowledging Lyme disease as a possible diagnosis for their patients. The training that most doctors receive dictates that one must confirm facts with laboratory tests. If it does not show up on lab testing, if the patient does not fit the profile, or the greatest ignorance of all, that Lyme disease is seen only in the Connecticut area, then most doctors absolutely will not consider Lyme as a possible answer.

Thankfully, recent advances in laboratory testing have improved the detection of the actual microbe. The newer FDA-approved, Lyme PCR testing detects the genetic structure of Lyme in whole blood, serum, or cerebral spinal fluid. There is also ongoing research that has determined a culturing method that allows a laboratory to "culture" or grow the spirochete bacteria responsible for Lyme disease. This testing is still in its infancy, but has appeared in scientific peer-reviewed journals.

Keep in mind that NO bacteria or virus can replicate at will in a healthy body! Therefore, just testing positive with any test method does **not** mean you will definitely develop any symptoms…ever!

You are only as strong (and resistant to infectious disease) as your weakest link. If you have many weak tissues and organ systems, then you may manifest many of the following symptoms, therefore,

Lyme disease may express itself by the following symptoms (although this listing is certainly not all-inclusive):

Possible Lyme Disease Symptoms
- Rash at bite site or other sites
- Muscle twitching of the face or other areas
- Unexplained fevers, sweats, chills
- Headache
- Fatigue
- Neck creaks and cracks, neck stiffness
- Unexplained weight change (loss or gain)
- Tingling, numbness, burning, stabbing sensations
- Unexplained hair loss
- Facial paralysis
- Swollen glands
- Eyes/vision: loss of vision, double, blurry, pain, increased floaters
- Sore throat
- Ears/hearing: buzzing, ringing, ear pain
- Testicular pain/pelvic pain
- Dizziness, poor balance
- Increased motion sickness
- Unexplained menstrual irregularity
- Testicular pain/pelvic pain
- light-headedness, wooziness, difficulty walking
- Unexplained milk production (lactation)
- Tremors
- Irritable bladder or bladder dysfunction
- Disturbed sleep
- Sexual dysfunction or loss of libido
- Confusion, difficulty in thinking

- Upset stomach or change in bowel function
- Difficulty with concentration or reading
- Chest pain or rib soreness
- Forgetfulness, poor short term memory
- Shortness of breath, cough
- Difficulty with speech
- Heart palpitations, pulse skips, heart block
- Joint pain or swelling
- Mood swings, irritability, depression
- Stiffness of the joints, neck or back
- Heart murmur or valve prolapse
- Muscle pain or cramps
- Exaggerated or worse hangover from alcohol
- Rash at bite site or other site

Chapter 2

What is Lyme Disease?

In the United States, what came to be known as Lyme disease started in Lyme County, Connecticut in early 1975 with an epidemic of "juvenile rheumatoid arthritis." By 1983 Dr. William Burgdorfer, M.D., identified the cause of an illness sweeping the area as a spiral-shaped bacterium (spirochete) ultimately named Borrelia burgdorferi in 1984.

Of course, this type of bacteria has been with us throughout history. Historical records document what is now called Lyme disease as far back as 1882 in Europe.

The classic presentation was thought to be a tick bite and bulls-eye rash with joint pain and neurological symptoms. For years, it was thought to be confined to a few northeastern states, but as time passed it became apparent that surrounding states were also reporting the infection at an alarming rate.

Research now confirms that Lyme disease is rampant throughout much of the United States and Europe.

Many people with confirmed infection never remember being bitten by a tick. Some of my patients have told me that they have never personally seen a tick in their life. It was once thought that one must have the bulls-eye rash in order to have Lyme disease, but it is now known that only about 30% of individuals bitten by a Lyme infected tick even develop a bulls-eye rash, so having no rash does not rule out Lyme disease

Lyme spirochetes may lay dormant for weeks to years after initial infection. This dormancy is due to the fact that no bacteria or virus can replicate (reproduce) at will in a healthy body. This will be discussed in detail later. Suffice it to say, the Lyme spirochetes may lay dormant in a healthy body until the individual experiences a stress on the body that weakens the body's control mechanisms thereby allowing the spirochetes to replicate and spread out of control.

Deer are one of the primary carriers of Lyme bacteria, but in fact **no animal** has been found immune to the Lyme infection. Even farm animals have often been found infected with Lyme disease.

Let's look at how Lyme disease is spread. Lyme-infected ticks attach to and thereby infect a deer. The ticks fall off and have hundreds of baby ticks per tick, all of which will be infected from birth with Lyme spirochetes. The baby ticks can be smaller than the head of a pin. These hundreds of baby ticks climb onto blades of grass working their way up to the tip of the blade. From there the tick holds onto the blade of grass with a few legs and spreads its other legs wide to catch onto animals, birds, or people passing by. The tick burrows its head through the skin and injects stomach fluid and anesthetizing chemicals so that you don't feel the tick breaking the skin. This injection of fluids transmits the bacteria into your body.

This is just one way to get infected. Another might be that the deer is bitten by a tick, the tick falls off, has babies, and the babies attach to a goose which is infected. The goose then migrates all over the country where the ticks fall off later infecting other animals and people. Of course, our local ticks and mosquitoes could bite the infected goose resulting in an eventual plague of Lyme disease as those ticks and mosquitoes later bite other animals and people in the area. The truth of this scenario is evident today in the United States as the West Nile Virus is being identified in more states from the migration of infected crows; Lyme disease has crossed the borders of Connecticut.

I am not trying to scare anyone, although caution is warranted. What I am trying to do is help people and their physicians to wake up to the very real possibility of Lyme disease in their community. Until the proper diagnosis is determined, the proper treatment cannot be applied. And when Lyme disease looks like so many other illnesses one may be getting the absolute wrong treatment, such as steroid medicines. Steroid medicines and Lyme do not mix. Steroidal medicines are contraindicated in Lyme disease.

Many cases of Multiple Sclerosis and ALS are misdiagnosed and are actually what some call "Neuro-borreliosis." Recent research by Dr. Lida Mattman, Ph.D., et al., which is due to be published soon, has identified another strain of Borrelia spirochete to be found in every case of MS and a different strain as well in cases of ALS. This would explain the improvement often seen in treating these illness as "Lyme" disease. Both of these newly found strains react on blood testing to Lyme Borrelia antibody, which is why so many of these cases are called Lyme disease. They are in fact different species of Borrelia. The good thing is that these newly discovered strains will often respond to the same treatments as for the classic Borrelia burgdorferi of Lyme disease.

Improvement upon correct treatment also confirms the diagnosis. Compare this to typical MS treatments, which only work to slow down the progression of the illness. By the way, those of you with MS, ask any doctor what causes MS – good luck getting a straight answer. Why not a Borrelia type of cause?

Patients must understand that every doctor can only go as far as they have been taught. If they are taught that Lyme is only in Connecticut and the surrounding states, then they will not even consider Lyme or look for it.

The nice thing about the correct diagnosis of Lyme disease is that it is treatable, with a hope of permanent recovery. I have seen and heard so many people who have taken their positive Lyme lab tests to their M.D. who even in the absence of any other positive lab work identifying anything definitive would say, "I don't know what you've got, but it's not Lyme disease." I don't get this! It seems that some doctors would rather diagnose people with what I call a "non-diagnosis" such as unilateral cephalgia, Fibromyalgia, or Chronic Fatigue Syndrome, or atypical this or that. People, these are not a diagnosis! All the doctor is doing is turning what you told him into Latin or simply describing your symptoms. A good diagnosis should name the cause of the symptom. These other "non-diagnoses" are just fine if all you plan on doing is providing unending symptomatic relief. Unilateral cephalgia in the example above is really nothing more than "pain on one side of your head". With this diagnosis the doctor can do no more than prescribe pain killers.

Opponents of the diagnosis of Lyme disease, and there are many for some political or other bizarre reason that oppose the diagnosis of Lyme disease (even with positive lab tests) outside of New England, are afraid that one may arrive at the incorrect diagnosis of Lyme disease, mainly because the exact cause of the supposed autoimmune diseases is not known in most cases and they seem to be afraid that the patients would be not receiving their symptomatic treatments to slow the illness

I am not saying to treat every autoimmune disease as if it were Lyme. However in the absence of any labs identifying the *cause* of your condition and if you get a positive blood or urine test for Lyme disease *and* improve upon correct treatment, I say it confirms the diagnosis of Lyme and that is far better than most treatments for these autoimmune diseases, which seek only to slow down the progression of the disease.

Chapter 3

Pleomorphism of Lyme Spirochetes

A complication of successful diagnosis and treatment of Lyme disease can be appreciated by the fact that Borrelia burgdorferi (Bb) are *pleomorphic* organisms.[1] A pleomorphic organism takes on a different shape at different life stages, or in reaction to changes in its environment. A butterfly is said to be pleomorphic because it changes from a caterpillar to a cocoon to a butterfly. The Lyme bacteria are known to be pleomorphic. The different pleomorphic stages of Borrelia burgdorferi are unclear, but research suggests that it can definitely exist as *cell-walled bacterium or cell-wall deficient bacterium* depending on its lifecycle. Again, each stage of the cycle is relatively "stealthy", meaning they are basically invisible to the immune system.

Some antibiotics act by disrupting the mechanisms in the cell wall of the Bb in order to kill the bacteria. A cell wall is requisite in order for the spirochete Borrelia burgdorferi to achieve its spiral shape. It is suspected that the long-term antibiotic attack on the cell walls can cause the spirochete to revert into a *"cell-wall deficient"* form as a survival mechanism. The problem is that the Bb can revert back and forth between the classic spiral shape and the cell wall deficient shapes. To complicate matters more the Bb can exist simultaneously as both forms. Dr. Lida Mattman, Ph.D., a leading researcher in L-Form bacteria, has found that it is common to see three Lyme spirochetes for every seven Lyme L-Forms in a blood specimen. Also, it is not uncommon to see only L-Forms with no spirochetes to be found[1].

The cell wall deficient form is synonymously called *L-Forms* and *spheroplasts*. Many different bacteria and fungi can achieve this form. For unification purposes scientists now refer to the cell-wall deficient stage as L-Forms[2].

It may sound strange that any organism can exist at all without a cell wall. This term can be a little deceiving in that there is a membrane where the cell wall used to be. Without its cell wall, the Bb cannot hold its characteristic spiral shape. It has been speculated that Lyme infected ticks can also harbor the L-Form of the Bb, which may explain why not every infected person develops a bulls-eye rash or tests positive on initial blood tests[3]. It may be safely said that every chronically infected LD patient has both spirochetes and L-Forms.

Indications are that the Bb can be forced into remission for weeks to years with long-term aggressive use of antibiotics. During this remission there are usually no detectable Bb spirochetes, and titers go down to undetectable levels. The Bb could possibly be latent in its L-Form during this stage. Apparently when the conditions in the body are right the latent L-Form infection reverts back to the spirochete form, the symptoms return, and the titers go up, leaving one to wonder if they were bitten again by an infected tick.

Not only does the spirochete change from a cell-walled bacterium to an L-form bacterium but it is possible for each life stage to exist independently from the other stage[2]. Recent research has shown that laboratory animals injected with dead fragments of the classic spirochetal Borrelia burgdorferi contracted Lyme disease[3]. This is significant because bacteria do not replicate themselves from eggs, but from fision. Therefore, a possible explanation might be that the undetected cell-wall *deficient* life-stage actually was responsible for these laboratory-induced infections.

Bacterial pleomorphism is not unique to the Lyme bacteria. Treponema pallidum, also a spirochete, and the bacteria known to cause Syphilis, are also widely known to prefer different shapes depending on where they are found in the body[4].

Recently, scientists unlocked the genetic sequencing of the B. burgdorferi bacteria and found that 50% of its genetic make up is identical to that of the Syphilis bacteria[5]. Due to the homeopathic law of *similars*, or "likes cure likes", doctors should consider a single dose, or a few doses, of the homeopathic miasm remedy, Syphilinum 200c. Upon reading the homeopathic materia medica, one will see a great many similar symptoms of the chronic Lyme patient that may be corrected by this one homeopathic remedy. (Miasms are the tendencies and predisposition to certain physical and psychological problems either acquired or inherited due to illness or suppressive treatments[6]. Please refer to Chapter 26.)

The ability to change shape is thought to be the reason why the Lyme bacteria, once well established in the body, are able to survive even after long-term antibiotic therapies. It is possible that the Lyme bacteria flip-flop between several shapes to escape the antibiotics. People who receive antibiotic treatment soon after they were infected, often recover completely, since the organism has not had time to "dig-in" and cycle into the other pleomorphic shapes. The fact that most antibiotics only address the cell-walled spirochetal bacterial stage may also explain why many people under antibiotic therapy feel improvement while on the antibiotics only to relapse soon after discontinuing the antibiotics. The antibiotics may kill some of the spirochetal phase, but ultimately the bacteria get smart and shift to shapes that are resistant to the antibiotic, and these shapes may not be as pathological or cause as many symptoms.

Those placing their faith in antibiotics to "cure" them of ***chronic*** Lyme disease will, in most cases, be disappointed. Drug therapies such as antibiotics address only the offending bacteria in certain stages, but do nothing to heal the body as a whole.

Termites in Your House:

An analogy of the use of antibiotics as the sole treatment of Lyme disease might be seen in the following example: If you have termites eating their way through the wood of your house, you can call an exterminator to spray harsh chemicals into the wood, effectively killing the termites. You have now removed the cause of the problem, but the extermination did nothing to correct the damage already caused. To make matters worse, you now have a toxic substance soaked into the wood of your house. (Of course, this is over-simplified - understanding the fact of the pleomorphism of Lyme bacteria making complete extermination with antibiotics unlikely.)

Lyme disease is a systemic infection affecting your body on every level. Since every organ and tissue is totally integrated and reliant upon each other, any time one system is affected, it will ultimately create a chain-reaction of other organs and glands that become progressively dysfunctional the more time goes by. For example, anyone who has suffered with chronic Lyme disease will tell you that the mind and the body are affected over time.

As you can see, if you have chronic Lyme disease, you absolutely must take your healing very seriously. You must not rely on your doctor to "cure" you...he only sees you for a few minutes in his treatment room. It is up to you to walk out your healing minute by minute. If your doctor says to take a remedy four times per day, and you only take it two or three times per day, 'because it wasn't convenient to take it four times', or you 'keep forgetting to take it', you are prolonging your illness, and risk making the Lyme organism become drug-resistant. In this case, you will possibly be stuck with it for life. Lyme disease is a war that you fight 24 hours a day… as long as it takes.

If you have Lyme disease, your fight can be fought more intelligently now that you know the spirochete tends to be pleomorphic. Therefore, one must use a treatment protocol that addresses the many different shapes of this Lyme microbe.

As a doctor or patient reading this you must come to the realization that if you were to try to grow this Lyme spirochete in a laboratory you would need a very controlled environment, otherwise they would not grow at all! The growth medium, temperature, pH, oxygen levels, and polarity must all be correct in order for them to grow at all.

The same is true in an infected person. The treatments and indeed your diet, lifestyle, and mindset will either promote or prevent the microbe from replicating or growing. By restoring the body's ability to adapt to its internal and external environment you can absolutely eradicate Lyme bacteria.

Chapter 4

A Theory of
Intermicrobial Communication

In every epidemic there are those who walk through it unscathed. This immunity goes beyond simply having a healthy immune system, especially in the case of viruses. Once viruses become a problem, they are intracellular, using your cell's RNA to replicate. Therefore, while strengthening the body's immune system with thymus gland, mushroom extracts and antioxidants is a good idea, these interventions will likely not be enough to deal with rapidly progressing, highly virulent microbes. The following outlines a new and better understanding of how the body naturally controls the overgrowth of microbes.

Have you ever watched the futuristic television show "Star Trek, the Next Generation" and watched any of the "Borg" shows where the all-powerful Borg species function as a collective unit? Every Borg is part of the collective thought matrix of the entire Borg society. Or have you watched the children's show "The Magic School Bus" or the movie "Osmosis Jones"? Though child-oriented, these shows accurately describe bacteria, viruses, parasites and fungi functioning as a complete community inside the body. This community has a food chain of producers, predators, consumers and decomposers. They are all fighting and striving to survive. They all need each other in order to survive. On TV a Borg cannot survive outside of the collective. And any attack on the Borg ship may hurt them, but they immediately use their collective intelligence to adapt, repair, regenerate, change tactics, survive, and conquer.

To give your body an antibiotic or vitamin is like dropping a bomb on the microbial collective; it may hurt, but they work together to adapt. It is a war within your body. To win the war, one must stop bacteria, viruses, parasites and fungi from effectively communicating with each other. You must shut off all supplies and supporting materials they need and you must constantly change the body's environment so the microbes cannot adapt and survive.

I have developed a theory of intermicrobial communication as a method of microbial growth and survival in the human body. Research has determined all living tissue, whether the body's tissues or microbes, are made up of unique molecular crystalline structures. (Oschman JL 2001 Living Crystals. Energy Medicine, The Scientific Basis, p. 129) These crystalline structures are capable of creating laser-like bio-photons for the purpose of communication between tissues and molecules. In fact much of our understanding of how chemical molecules, such as hormones, function is now being recognized as a matter of proximity rather than actual physical contact of the hormone in the classic "lock and key" explanation we have used for years.

Instead of a "lock & key" mechanism, microbes, hormones or any pathology are communicating with laser-like bio-photons. It is through the unique molecular structure of hormones and indeed any pathology, including microbes, that gives it its own unique electro-energetic signature, often called a molecular signature. Understanding this concept one can begin to see how a radio station can also be likened to this communication link on a much larger scale. If the electrons of the radio station transmitter are oscillating at the same frequency as the setting on your radio, you can receive all of the songs and information embedded within the signal. This is known as co-resonance between the transmitter (radio station) and the receiver (your radio). All other radio stations in the area would be operating at a different frequency and would therefore not interfere with your ability to hear the selected radio station.

Now on a microscopic scale, microbes because of their unique molecular structure and oscillatory frequency can transmit and tune into each other across great distances within the human body via coherent laser-like biophoton emissions. Embedded within these microbial transmissions could be the information needed by other microbes "tuned" into the same frequency as to how they need to mutate in order to survive against an antibiotic, how to work together to change the host environment (your body) to one more conducive to their overall population, or just about any type of communication. (Popp, F.A., Gu Q., and Li, K. H. (1992) Recent advances in Biophoton Research and its Applications, Singapore: World Scientific) Millions of microbes can be communicating in this manner with signal velocities estimated at close to the speed of light.

Just like the radio station example, these microbial communications by their nature would not be restricted or impaired by illness-weakened human tissue. In fact, microbes most likely interface with the body's own crystalline matrix in order to communicate. It is also likely that this bacterial communication is cut off, making it impossible to communicate with each other, when health is restored in the human.

The first time a prescription antibiotic is introduced into the body, it is like a surprise attack, and there is not time to communicate with each other. As these bacteria die, the message is sent out via bacterial transmission of bio-photons and/or electromagnetic signals, like a distress call to all the rest of the microbes that were not affected by the antibiotic. This communication is what they need in order to mutate, thereby becoming antibiotic resistant. "Microfibers, including DNA within microbes, and cytoskeleton polymers, can function as biological antennae..." for receiving these intermicrobial communications. (Gitte S. Jenson, Ph.D., Lecture Dec. 2002 Second annual conference on applied neurobiology; Treating Lyme and Co-infections.) We now know for certain, mutation around the antibiotic occurs sometimes within 20 minutes of taking the first dose of an antibiotic.

Let's say the microbes did not communicate with each other. If this lack of communication were true, then as the antibiotic worked its way through the body, the drug would surprise each individual microbe and would effectively kill every microbe, but it is the arrogance of mankind that insists we are the only intelligent life on the planet.

In other words, it is believed that bacteria, viruses and other microbes can and do communicate with each other through their unique molecular crystalline matrix, and are transmitting and receiving vibrational resonance, laser-like coherent signals from each other. This communication is made possible by sending signals through the human body's own cellular matrix. (Vogel R. and Submuth, R. (1998). Bioelectrochemistry and Bioenergenetics, 45, 93-101) This molecular crystalline matrix concept is found in all living tissue, i.e. bone, muscle, tendon, ligament, all of which operate and respond in cooperation in order to adapt the body to the ever changing surrounding environment. We usually think of crystals as hard faceted minerals, however all living tissue is indeed composed of long, thin, pliable molecules that are soft and flexible, which are considered "liquid crystals." (Oschman JL 2001 Living Crystals. Energy Medicine, The Scientific Basis ch 9:129-136. Bouligand Y 1978 Liquid crystals and their analogs in biological systems. In: Liebert L (ed) Liquid crystals. Solid State Physics, Supplement 14:259-294) It is these "liquid crystals" that allow the internal living organisms to communicate.

Several scientific studies have identified that the molecules of the body interact with each other via crystalline vibrational coherent fields. Within this type of crystalline matrix, information/communication signals move through the tissues of the body at an astonishing rate, potentially up to half the speed of light or more. Now understand that when there is an overgrowth of microbes like Bb & L-forms, their molecular crystalline vibrational fields are integrated and imbedded within the matrix of the human body. (Allen HC, Cross PC 1963 Molecular Vib-rotors. John Wiley, New York), (Smith CW 1994 Biological effects of weak electromagnetic fields. In: Ho MW, Popp F-A, Warnke U (eds) Bioelectrodynamics and biocommunication. World Scientific, Singapore, Ch 3, pp 81-107) Can you visualize an array of Bb & L-forms embedded in your body, communicating with each other, preparing for an attack and attacking?

With only a few infectious microbes in the body's matrix they may be held in check forever by the energetic aspects of the healthy human body. Therefore, the infectious microbes may have little impact on the human and never develop into a disease. However, in an illness-weakened human, a few infectious microbes can multiply unimpeded. They now have a voice and can influence the form and function of the human, even influencing the mind and emotions, via their cooperative crystalline communication network. This can be seen as a computer virus overwriting the body's software in order to create a more hospitable environment for the bacterial collective.

Microbes need the human body to have a certain temperature in order to communicate efficiently. Too hot and their biophoton communications will overshoot their target, too cold and their signals will be too weak to communicate. (Slawinski, J., and Popp, F.A. (1987) J. Pl. Physiol., 130, 111-123.) Therefore, it is likely that one of the first things microbes work together to achieve in a new host is an optimizing of the host's temperature to suit their needs. Later in the chapter on "Low Body Temperature and Lyme Disease" you will read more on the importance of treatments for re-establishing a normal body temperature distribution throughout the body.

If we assign this form of intelligence to microbes one begins to wonder at the toxins these microbes produce, most of which are neurotoxins which function to impair the body's nervous system and organ systems from setting up energetic antimicrobial growth-restricting fields.

Along this same thought of inner microbial communications, the heart is a primary command post in the inner world of the body. First of all the heart is not just a pump. The heart is now known to be primarily an electromagnetic generator for the entire body, generating 1,000 times more electricity than the brain and nervous system. The electromagnetic energy from the heart is carried very well by the saline-rich blood, through 50,000 miles of blood vessels. Without the heart-generator, organ function, body chemistry/metabolism, and core temperature plummet. So, how better to weaken the human body's energetic "force fields" than by weakening its power generator? (Marinelli R, van der Furst, Zee H, McGinn A, Marinelli W 1995 The heart is not a pump: a refutation of the pressure propulsion premise of heart function. Frontier Perspectives 5:15-24), (Schwenk T 1996 Sensitive Chaos, Rudolf Steiner Press pp 90-93) This is probably why so many infections disturb the function of the heart.

The following explanation of cellular cascade and amplification by James Oschman may provide the scientific rationale of how microbes can work to alter the human organism, physically, mentally, and emotionally to promote a more hospitable environment:

"A single antigen (microbe), hormone, pheromone, growth factor or smell or taste or neurotransmitter molecule or single photon of electromagnetic energy can produce a cascade of intracellular signals that initiate, accelerate, or inhibit biological processes. This is possible because of enormous amplification – a single molecular event at the cell surface can trigger a huge influx of calcium ions, each of which can activate an enzyme. The enzymes, in turn, act as catalysts, greatly accelerating biochemical processes. The enzymes are not consumed by these reactions, and can therefore act repeatedly. Some of the reactions are sensitive to electromagnetic fields, some are not, and others have not yet been tested. Some frequencies enhance calcium entry, others diminish it. Steps in the cascade involving free radical formation are likely targets of magnetic fields. Some of the products of the cascade are returned back to the cell surface and into the surrounding extracellular space. Molecular events within cells set up electronic, photonic, and electromechanical waves (phonons) that propagate as solitons through the cellular and extracellular matrix. These feedbacks enable cells and tissues to form a functionally organized society. **The cells whisper to each other in a faint and private language. They can 'tune into' each other over long ranges**." (Oschman JL Energy Medicine, The Scientific Basis, 2001 pp 253)

This crystalline matrix theory could also help explain the psychological abnormalities individuals experience that seem to be unique to each type of microbial infection. Doctors the world over will attest to the fact that various types of infections seem to cause the infected person to be more prone to certain emotional patterns, such as depression, irritability, anxiety and frustration, as well as food cravings. Anyone suffering from yeast overgrowth can attest to the almost unreasonable craving for sugar, which just happens to be yeast's favorite food. In light of the molecular crystalline nature of microbes, and their potential to use your own tissues to control their environment, your thoughts may not be "your thoughts" at all, but may in fact be a superimposed thought pattern induced by the collective influence of microbes.

Microbial intercommunication is likely the reason why certain microbes seem to work in cooperation, such as the Borrelia burgdorferi of Lyme disease working synergistically with Babesia microti, Ehrlichia, Bartonella, and various viruses such as the Human Herpes virus-6, Cytomegalovirus, and Epstein-Barr virus.

It appears that many people accumulate several strains of herpes viruses and other microbes, which may interfere with normal body function. However, it seems that when Lyme bacteria come on the scene, they quickly assume a leadership position within the body. Lyme bacteria seem to organize the other microbes into a collective effort to work together to master their environment – your body.

All species of the world strive for survival. All attempt to control their environment or adapt to their environment in order to survive. Bacteria are no different. They work to change your body to suit their unique survival needs. However, no bacteria can overpower or alter a *healthy* body. They cannot get a foothold and replicate in large enough numbers to "have a voice" and alter the internal environment of the healthy human body. A healthy human body sets up energetic interference fields within the body to control the growth mechanisms of disease causing microbes. It is only when the body's own crystalline matrix becomes impaired that infection can set in. Understanding this can help doctors recognize infections such as Strep throat as a weakness or breakdown of the throat's electro-energetic crystalline matrix. This may be due to emotional distress, physical stress, or other cause, but is definitely not due to the invasion of Strep bacteria, which are now known to be present in everyone's throat.

How does the theory of "intermicrobial communication" change the way we treat people with infectious disease?

Understanding this crystalline-matrix network of the human body and microbes, I developed a method for tapping into this communication network of the human body, called Bio-Resonance Scanning™. Using Bio-Resonance Scanning™ I was able to create a completely new class of uniqu,e highly-effective, frequency matched, botanical formulas (Virogen™, Paragen™, Yeast Ease™, Borrelogen™, Neogen-4™,

Microbogen™...), to enhance and support the body's control mechanisms against virtually all microbes associated with infectious disease.

Recall that in every epidemic there are those people that walk through it unscathed. They likely had the virus in their body, but they never manifested the viral disease. The virus is held in check by the energetic aspects of their crystalline matrix. These new frequency-matched formulas enhance this same energetic aspect of "immunity" that is missing in the people who have developed the infectious disease or those who are susceptible to catching it.

To continue in the computer language of above, these formulas are frequency-matched to "overwrite" the microbial matrix and restore the original body programming. Each formula's complex molecular crystalline array matches those frequencies that the healthy human body uses to prevent specific types of microbes from being able to communicate and replicate, while guiding the body back to healthy coherence. In essence the desire in any infectious disease is that the treatments will help bring down the number of microbes and restore the body's ability to control the microbe's ability to live.

These formulas target the proper structure and function of the body rather than targeting the virus or microbe. In my opinion, this is the most pure form of intervention developed to date, in that it works *with* God's design of the human body. Antibiotics and high-power drug interventions take a sledgehammer to God's perfect design.

Of course the printed research on these high-power drugs is overwhelming in the scientist's optimism as to their drug's effect on the microbes; however, they leave the sledgehammer side-effects to the small print section of the article.

Keep in mind, sincerity is no guarantee of truth. Your doctor may sincerely believe antibiotics are the best. I too am very sincere in what I say, however, it is the truth as I see it, based on the best research and intuition we have to date.

All doctors and scientists attempt to explain the exact mechanism of illness based upon their area of expertise. Each describes illness from their unique perspective. It is like the story of the three blind men feeling an elephant, one at the trunk, one at the side, and one at the rear. Each may be absolutely correct, however each are simply describing the elephant from their perspective. So, while one scientist may focus on the microscopic, molecular and morphological properties of the microbe, others may focus on the autonomic changes in the body, and others may focus on the effect of antibiotic "cocktails". Still others may focus primarily on the electromagnetic properties. You see, doctors and scientists may all be correct in their assumptions, however, they may be way off in their treatment rationale.

Often there seems to be the assumption that the human body is dumb and needs drugs to help kill microbes. The truth is that the human body is highly intelligent and simply needs support. I heard one of the best examples of this truth while attending a lecture by Dr. Thomas Rau, M.D., of the world famous Paracelsus Clinic in Switzerland. He gave an example of the need to recognize the body's intelligence in a story about a dog that had swallowed a bone that was too large to pass through the stomach into the small intestines. The dog's normal stomach acid was unable to digest the bone; therefore, a stomach cancer began to grow. The stomach cancer created so much acid that the bone finally dissolved and passed on through. Once the bone passed out of the stomach the tumor rapidly disappeared – without treatment. You see, the cancerous tumor served a purpose, but most doctors' mentality and training is to diagnose the cancer and remove it, either by surgery or chemotherapy, which is really just a chemical scalpel.

In the same way, doctors should not give drugs such as antibiotics which basically tell the body to "Step aside! I'll kill these bacteria for you!" Instead, doctors should learn to facilitate the body's own natural ability to regain control over the bacteria. To do this the doctor must use frequency-matched nutraceuticals that enhance the energy already being created by the body to bring the bacteria under control, in combination with all protocols, other natural treatments, and therapies that work to optimize God's perfect design.

The doctor must facilitate the body's ability to heal itself by removing anything that is interfering with its ability to heal. Potential interferences are many; therefore, efforts must be made to remove anything and everything that ideally should not be there, such as detoxifying the body of heavy metals and organic toxins like pesticides, herbicides and petroleum-based toxins that jam up the machinery and crystalline matrix of the body. Scars can be primary sources of interference due to the fact that scars act as a dam to the flow of electrical information passing through the meridian system. Cold laser therapy can help reconnect these electro-energetic pathways through the scar thereby restoring the body's ability to communicate with itself unimpeded. These are but a few examples of the many ways your doctor should be working with the body to help facilitate healing on every office visit.

At the same time the doctor should be providing the information and building blocks needed by the body to repair the molecular matrix. This must occur in order to restore the body's healthy environment, making it non-conducive to microbial overgrowth.

Treatments and therapies should be applied with the goal of providing the body with the information it needs to heal itself. High-power prescription drugs are designed to provide you the illusion of health only. Does anyone really believe that aspirin is truly "fixing" the cause of your headache? The disturbance in your body is still there, you just can't feel it anymore. When your doctor gives you a medication for high blood pressure, does he ever say, "Take this medicine for six months and then you should be well and be able to stop taking it?" No, he says you must take the medicine until the day you die or until it quits working, because the medicine is not truly fixing anything. The underlying disturbance in your body's matrix remains untouched. The drug simply creates the illusion of a healthy nervous system or organ system. Antibiotics used in chronic infections also create the illusion of health; you may feel a little or a lot better while taking them, but they damage the body's healthy crystalline matrix further and simply push the microbes into a different shape. That is why if one stops taking the antibiotics the infection often returns within weeks to months, leading one to wonder if they were re-infected or if it is the same infection returning that never truly went away.

Many people defend their conventional medical doctor because he "also uses vitamins along with the antibiotics". This is great to incorporate vitamins, but not enough to effect permanent change and long-term restoration of true health. Remember, to give your body an antibiotic or vitamin is like dropping a bomb on the microbial collective; it may hurt, but they work together to adapt. It is a war within your body. To win the war, one must stop bacteria, viruses, parasites and fungi from effectively communicating with each other. You must shut off all supplies and supporting materials and you must constantly change the body's environment so the microbes cannot adapt and survive.

Of course, none of this new found understanding of microbes does away with the scientific facts of following good hygiene and using sanitary precautions. History is full of epidemics that killed millions that were caused by microbes due to unclean scalpels, unwashed hands and contaminated food. This research helps us understand how to get control of microbes, now that we know that antibiotics are not the "silver bullet –

cure-all" we originally thought they would be.

This book outlines many issues that must be addressed to provide the body with the information, energy, and building blocks needed to facilitate the body's natural ability to heal itself and stay healthy.

This book is not the all-inclusive compendium of treatment possibilities or even everything I do, as one would get lost in all of the nuances of being a doctor. You will see that we are not just another doctor trying to sell you vitamins and supplements. I am presenting what I feel works best, based upon the latest research and my clinical experience. Nor are doctors using these methods able to restore every patient to perfect health again, but we are definitely helping the majority and extending longevity.

I get calls from people from all over the world wanting to know if they can take my frequency matched formulas, and follow our protocols while taking antibiotics. The answer is yes, you can, but hopefully you see antibiotics and aggressive drug therapies are unnecessary in most cases.

Chapter 5

What Factors Lead to Illness from Microbes?

We have all heard the saying, "A chain is only as strong as its weakest link." This is so true in every aspect of the human body. I am talking about balanced living. Any area of your life that is out of healthy rhythm and balance becomes a weak point. The body's healthy crystalline matrix, discussed in the previous chapter, is compromised by its inability to adapt rapidly enough to prolonged imbalance and irritation, making it vulnerable to the collective crystalline matrix subsequently set up by microbes.

Weak links in a person's life can often be identified by where the focus of infection is located in the body. For instance, viruses much prefer nerve tissue, while bacteria prefer blood and metabolic tissues. Nerve tissues can become susceptible to viral infection from mental, emotional, or other sensory overload. Bacterial challenges often may be the result of nutritional deficiencies, toxin overload, weather extremes that weaken tissue resistance, and physical injuries such as cuts and abrasions. If your body is a "happy home" environment for microbes, then no medication will ever truly return you to the quality of life you seek. Anyone who has lived in Hawaii knows that it is a happy home environment for mold and fungus. The walls and shower stalls will rapidly turn green with mold. You can kill it with spray chemicals but it will always come back because Hawaii is warm and humid, a perfect environment for mold.

In the human body, all treatments and therapies should seek to change the environment inside the body back to one that is not a good environment for microbial overgrowth.

The factors that may lead to microbial illness through the upsetting of the body's healthy balance are numerous. The following is by no means complete:

- Imbalanced body pH (Too acidic or too alkaline)
- Prolonged or acute exposure to weather extremes
- Loss of the predominantly negative polarity of the tissues of the body.
- Lowered core body temperature

- Prolonged personal suppression from people in your environment
- Prolonged negative emotions
- Inherited predispositions and constitutional weaknesses
- Overuse of antibiotics, steroids, and other prescription medicines
- Vaccinations/immunizations
- Prolonged biomechanical stress
- Infection activated through auto-suggestion - normally news media
- Dietary imbalances/Food maladaptive syndrome
- Tissue toxin overload
- Poor function of the organs of elimination, i.e., colon, urinary tract, lungs, skin.
- Geopathic stress
- Overwork
- Over/under sleeping
- Excessive prolonged stress
- Spiritual distress
- Electromagnetic pollution
- Mental overexertion
- Depression/emotional imbalance
- Poor hygiene
- Lack of creative stimulation
- Loss of connection to the world around you
- Loss of direction and purpose
- Lost love and affection
- Hate

Basically, any influence that leads to an over or under stimulation of any aspect of life can adversely alter your receptivity to infection. Lyme spirochetes may lay dormant in the body for years only to erupt into a major problem when the environment changes within the body.

The type of symptoms and the areas affected are determined by the factors involved. Sometimes several of the above listed factors are involved in creating the illness. The point is that an effective treatment strategy must include therapies that will correct any and all factors leading to the receptivity.

Most people have taken antibiotics at some point in this day and age. Once the symptoms are gone, most people don't give it another thought. Yet the best antibiotic in the world only kills about 85% of the bacteria at the very most. **Remember, some bacteria have already mutated or**

changed shape within the first 20 minutes of taking the antibiotics!
Taking more of the antibiotic or switching from a pill form to intravenous
won't matter. Taking the antibiotic for six months won't matter!

Can you see now that the antibiotic didn't kill all of the bacteria, and
yet you may never have to take another dose? In the same way, when you
balance all aspects of your body and life, and your healthcare team using
Circuit Healing™ and Biological Medicine has restored the integrity of
the environment within your body, the bacteria and the symptoms will
disappear, never to return as long as you stay in balance.

Antibiotics undoubtedly have saved lives and suffering in early stage,
early diagnosed Lyme. At times antibiotics may have been used with some
success in some chronic cases.

I personally have had five family members test positive for Lyme, one
severely affected. My own children have tested positive on several
occasions. I have treated hundreds, maybe up to close to a thousand people
who tested positive to Lyme, either through resonance, blood, and/or urine
testing. I have seen and heard the horror stories of patients at the hands of
doctors, telling many that in the absence of blood tests findings that the
person is basically a psychiatric case, it's all in their head, and so on. I
have heard of the severe Herxheimer reactions or toxic effects of the strong
antibiotics creating more problems than they fixed.

There will always be those who insist antibiotics, and lots of them, is
the only way to address chronic Lyme. I have just not seen this to be true.
I was at a recent Lyme conference with about 50 M.D.s in attendance;
every doctor there acknowledged that antibiotics provided only limited
relief at best. I was pleased to see that these brave few M.D.s were seeking
new ways of helping Lyme patients! So for those of you out there with no
hope, here is real hope: a small but growing number of health professionals
not only acknowledging the widespread existence of Lyme, but also seeking
more effective and natural methods of treating people with Lyme!

I have not been able to help bring every patient back to perfect health,
but the vast majority has been greatly improved.

Chronic Lyme disease is serious and just like there are very few Lyme
literate medical doctors, there are very few doctors practicing natural
medicine that are Lyme literate. It is my hope that this book will help both
types of doctors as well as every person suffering with Lyme.

Chapter 6

A Better Way to "Fight" Infectious Disease–
Balanced Living

Prior to becoming ill, a person often senses that something is "out of balance" or "out of order"– simple but appropriate expressions since every illness provides its own unique signs of impending illness, sometimes hours, days or weeks before the full-blown illness is made manifest. Paying attention to the changes in your body, mind, emotions and spirit is the best way to recognize the preamble of infectious diseases.

Most people miss these early signs because our society has trained us from birth to live either in the past or the future. Rarely do people live in the exact moment they are in, therefore missing the earliest signs of imbalance and impending illness. We must all strive to live only in the moment we are in, no matter how busy our life. In truth, the busier you are, the more disciplined you must be to stay focused in the moment you are in to complete the tasks that lay before you. This does not mean that you "live in the moment" at the expense of your body, the so called "burning the candle at both ends".

Living in the moment is a way of life; it is not a matter of time. It is focusing on whatever task needs doing at the moment, while remaining centered and alert to every change in your internal and external environment. The past is road kill so don't go there. It is okay to plan for the future while living in the moment, but do not be worried or anxious about it. We will go into this topic in greater detail later.

The first symptoms of infectious processes arise once the population of microbes gets beyond the control of the body's growth-regulating mechanisms. Remember earlier we discussed that the only difference in a healthy person and a person experiencing symptoms of infectious disease is the increased number of the microbes in the sick person. It may seem that the obvious treatment is to take a prescription antibiotic and bring down the population of microbes, but is it truly?

What is the goal in the treatment of any infectious disease? This one question should be paramount in your mind when dealing with any symptoms of bacterial, fungal, mycoplasmal or viral infection. If you understand the goal then the treatment selection becomes more logical.

If a perfectly balanced and healthy body is impervious to any infectious disease, then restoring the loss of balance from whatever cause should be the primary goal of treatment. Secondary to this is assisting the body in bringing down the populations of infectious microbes.

Often modern medicine spends a disproportionate emphasis on laboratory findings and diagnosis as compared to treatment. Objective findings, such as the numerical values of blood tests, perfectly support the prevalent symptom-based treatment style found in most hospitals and clinics in America. Critics speak of a "number-credulous laboratory medicine," estimating that 88% of all medications are of a symptomatic nature; moreover, their therapeutic value is asserted to be smaller than "we had assumed in the tumult of medicine's great and unquestioned victories." (Schaefer, H. *Plaedoyer fuer eine "neue Medizin"*.

The majority of antibiotic usage in the United States falls within this 88% of symptomatic treatments. **If the microbes are not the cause of the illness then they too are a symptom!** The cause is whatever caused the body to lose its ability to inhibit the unchecked growth of the microbes.

Many people will read all of this and still choose antibiotics as their primary treatment of choice because they may feel that the cost of balanced living is too high. These people live the way they do, and make the choices they do, because it fits their self-sabotaging goals, and most accurately fits the adaptation of their lives to their imbalanced choices. Balanced, healthy living requires one to want and do the right thing, to be self-disciplined, self-observant and patient. Balanced life is a learned process. It requires lifelong effort to unlearn the past imbalanced living patterns and learn from the present moment challenges. One must learn to not be so disconnected from one's internal and external environment.

Most of us do not even remotely live a balanced life. Thankfully, God designed our bodies to function very well within a range of relatively balanced living. Given half a chance, the body will be able to restore the semblance of normal symptom-free life. This said, supplementation with nontoxic medicines must be used to help the body halt the unchecked replication of microbes. This can be achieved by restoring the integrity of the body's energetic and crystalline-matrix properties, boosting the immune system, by using frequency-matched natural medicines that work with the body's own energy to bring the microbe population back under control.

The foremost question in your mind should still be, "What changed in your life recently that weakened the body to the point of losing growth control of the microbes?" Go through the previous list of potential causes of breaking down the body's defenses. Find the likely changes in your life that set you up for this infectious disease. Make changes to correct the situation.

Keep in mind that once you have allowed infectious disease of any kind to get a foothold in your body, the damaged tissues will take time to heal. In strep throat, once the membranes of the throat have been damaged, the throat will be scratchy, irritated and sore. It is just like a blister on your hand – the damage is done and it is simply going to take time for the tissues to heal and stop hurting. When people experience pain as in strep throat – I've seen it a hundred times – they run to an antibiotic, not with the goal of killing all of the bacteria, but for what boils down simply to be pain relief. The event of painful strep throat is interfering with their life, and instead of looking at it as a sign of imbalance, a message, and a chance to learn, they miss the entire point of the illness. Trust that your body will take control over the strep bacteria again with appropriate life-choice modifications and natural, nontoxic support. The pain can be eased through other natural methods and time. Learn to observe what changed just previous to the earliest signs of illness. You should be able to identify and modify, thereby averting illness altogether.

No matter what the plague, epidemic, or infectious disease, some people always survive unscathed in the midst of it all. It matters not that you are bitten by a mosquito, tick, or are sneezed on by a sick person and have the infectious microbes injected into your body from the bite or breathe into your lungs the sick person's microbes! If your body is balanced and therefore healthy your body will respond correctly and you will stay healthy. **If you realized just how many potentially disease causing microbes you breathe in, eat, or drink every single day of your life without getting sick, you would never worry about infectious disease again.**

Municipal water departments around the United States are warning people with specific illnesses not to drink the tap water because of the various microbes they cannot filter out and the chlorine cannot kill. Why do you think they don't warn everyone not to drink the water? They too understand that while these microbes in the drinking water can cause disease, a generally healthy person will be able to drink it without harm.

This book will guide you through some of the processes of living a balance life in body, mind and spirit. You will learn to "sour the milk" and change the internal environment of your body so that disease from infectious overgrowth of Lyme spirochetes cannot continue to replicate at will. You will have no spirochete overgrowth when your body is no longer a happy home environment for growing these bacteria!

Chapter 7

Borrelia burgdorferi & Mycoplasmal Infections

When the Bb are in their L-Form phase, the morphology, or appearance, cannot be distinguished from that of Mycoplasma organisms. In fact, there is only one primary difference between the two organisms; mycoplasma by definition cannot generate a cell wall.[1]

For those of you who are unfamiliar with the term mycoplasma, do not feel bad. It is only recently that the pathogenic nature of these organisms has come into the forefront of the medical mindset. A mycoplasma is larger than a virus and smaller than bacteria. Mycoplasma are more closely akin to bacteria than viruses. They are said to be the smallest self-replicating life form.[2] Like Bb these mycoplasma can infect deep tissues and create almost all of the same symptoms as Lyme Disease (LD).[3] A plethora of research has connected mycoplasmal infections to many of today's most prevalent illnesses such as Lyme Disease, Chronic Fatigue Syndrome (CFS), Fibromyalgia Syndrome (FMS), and even the Gulf War Syndrome (GWS).[4]

How does this impact you?

Any person suffering with chronic LD knows that it is affecting multiple systems of the body. This fact causes a weakened and susceptible immune system. Sufferers of chronic LD/CFS/FMS/GWS become microbe collectors. The body's resistance to foreign invaders such as mycoplasma is greatly reduced. When considering the effects of having multiple pathogenic infections at the same time, it is no wonder that so many people undergo years of treatment without complete resolution of their symptoms. Each of these microbes is part of a community in your body and are either a producer, predator, consumer or decomposer. With the knowledge of intermicrobial communication, via their crystalline matrix hotwired into the body's normal crystalline matrix, one can see that they are all working together to survive. Successful treatment can only be realized by addressing the entire body to restore the body's own control mechanisms of all microbes.

It is well recognized that people suffering from LD may also have other infections going on at the same time, such as Babesia microti,

Ehrlichiosis, viruses (EBV, CMV and HHV-6) and Candidiasis. To make matters worse we are now realizing that mycoplasmal infections can be detected in the blood of 60-70% of all LD/CFS/FMS sufferers. According to Dr. Nicholson, Ph.D., "Systemic mycoplasmal infections are a major source of morbidity in CFS, FMS, and Gulf War Illness patients, and they need to be treated with antibiotics...and nutritional support".[5] Of course, antibiotics were anticipated in the development of this biological warfare microbe, so it is unlikely antibiotics are a good treatment.

When considering the fact that the Bb can also revert to a mycoplasmal look-alike L-Form when antibiotics are introduced, one can begin to grasp the true difficulties of determining an effective treatment protocol. But do not get disheartened – all of this is treatable! I am simply attempting to educate you so that you can know what you are up against and understand your enemy. Your body is well equipped to deal with any microbe if given the proper support – and I don't mean antibiotics. Anyone who would tell you otherwise is stuck in a medical model of drug interventions on a statistically sick, dysfunctional, and otherwise imbalanced population.

If you have been treated for Lyme disease, and have reached the point where all of the lab tests indicate that you no longer have any Borrelia burgdorferi yet you are still feeling very sick, then your doctor needs to do a mycoplasma PCR test on you. Also have him test for the other common co-infections – Babesia microti, Ehrlichia, Human Herpes Virus-6, Epstein-Barr Virus, Cytomegalo-virus, Adeno-virus, and systemic Candida. If you have never tested positive to having Lyme disease, then definitely get your doctor to test for mycoplasmal infections.

Chapter 8

Borrelia burgdorferi Toxins...

The Cause of Your Symptoms!

Research and clinical studies have determined that there are neuro-toxins released by the Borrelia burgdorferi (Bb) spirochete.[1] Neurotoxins are nerve poisons. These toxins according to research are the cause of most if not all of the symptoms of Lyme disease. It is also believed that tissue damage is not caused by Lyme bacteria directly; in other words the bacteria are not "eating" your tissues. It is the accumulation of Bb toxins in a body, that is most likely responsible for the symptoms experienced by Lyme sufferers. Another astonishing new finding was just released by John Travis in the July, 2003, Volume 164 of the Science News. He reported that research performed by John F. Prescott found that certain antibiotics, such as the fluoroquinolones, the class of antibiotics that includes Cipro, actually trigger a type of virus called bacteriophages (viruses that normally eat bacteria) to cause the bacterium they have infected to start producing toxins[2]. These viruses can act as genetic delivery vans, invading bacteria, such as spirochetes, often lying dormant, until activated by a change in the host environment. Once activated these viruses insert their toxin generating genes into the bacterial chromosomes. These viruses turn basically harmless bacterium into killers through this genetic sequencing of toxins[3].

So now we see that not only are these toxins released through the die-off of bacteria, and not only can antibiotics actually increase the production of the toxins, but theses viruses can cause the bacteria to rupture, spilling their toxins into your body[4].

When a doctor uses an antibiotic and kills some Lyme spirochetes, there is a resultant Jarish-Herxheimer reaction…a worsening of the patient's symptoms in response to the increased release of bacterial die-off toxins. The toxins are dumped into the blood stream and are circulated throughout the body until they can either be eliminated by the body or become lodged in areas of weakened tissues. As neurotoxins they are preferentially taken up by nerve tissue. These lodged toxins are one of the reasons that symptoms can persist even after the actual Bb infection is gone because the toxins can remain as an irritant in the tissues for years.

Chronic Lyme sufferers do not have adequate detoxification mechanisms to detoxify these Bb toxins. Our newly developed, patent pending products should assist in the elimination of these specific Lyme-related toxins, which should to a large degree eliminate many of the Lyme symptoms, and the worsening of symptoms from effective treatment. But remember, symptoms will not completely disappear just with the elimination of Lyme toxins, simply because health and healing entails more than the absence of toxins.

There is a very good test for detecting the presence of neurotoxins in the brain called the VCS test, which stands for Visual Contrast Sensitivity Test. (It is sometimes called the F.A.C.T. test.) The VCS test has been successfully used in medical diagnosis and subclinical neurotoxicity detection. The VCS, produced by the Stereo Optical Company, is simple to use, and can be used indefinitely without ever wearing out. If your doctor does not use this test, let him know about it, because it is well researched, and for once you can track your progress on a daily basis if you so desire. As neurotoxin levels go down your test should improve. To perform the test you simply hold the apparatus in front of you, as directed on the instructional sheet, and the degree that you can visually see certain images on a card determines the level of neurotoxins. See the back of this book for ordering information. Another option we are working on is to enable you to actually perform the VCS test anytime you like over the internet via our website: www.jnutra.com. This would be a great way for you to track your progress.

General body detoxification nutritional and botanical supplements are plentiful on the nutraceutical market. These products are designed to be general detoxifiers of the liver and intestines. While these products are a very good idea for almost everyone, they are not designed to handle Lyme neurotoxins. That is why I have developed a line of four targeted supplements using Bio-Resonance Scanning™, which are frequency-matched to the specific neurotoxins of Lyme spirochetes and the other Lyme-related microbes. Each of the following formulas are bottled with 240 capsules, which should last about a month at a general recommended adult dosage of three capsules, three times per day, or as directed by your healthcare professional. This dosage recommendation should be doubled, two to three days prior to any mercury amalgam dental filling removal, as well as four days following the removal.

1. **Neuro-Antitox Cardio™** - for those suffering primarily from heart problems from Lyme toxins and heavy metals. Indications: angina, palpitations, hypertension, arrhythmia, valve problems, shoulder and arm pain, shortness of breath, chronic fatigue.
   - Ingredients – Silphium lac. 100mg, beta-sitosterol 100mg, chlorella 250mg, molybdenum 100mcg, as well as the sarcobioenergetic potencies in P6, 12, and 30 of cardiac plexus, cardia, myocardium, endocardium, mitral valve, tricuspid valve and aorta.

2. **Neuro-Antitox Musculo-Skeletal™** - for those suffering primarily from muscle and joint problems from Lyme toxins and heavy metals. Indications: Muscle and joint pain and weakness, sensations in the extremities of burning, tingling, radiating pain, swelling, arthritic and rheumatic conditions.
   - Ingredients – Silphium lac. 100mg, beta-sitosterol 100mg, chlorella 250mg, molybdenum 100mcg, as well as the sarcobioenergetic potencies in P-6, 12, and 30 of connective issue/fascia, cartilage, Intervertibral joints (cervical, thoracic, and lumbar), humoral joint, elbow joint, intercarpal joints, knee joint, interphalangeal joint, bamboo, rhus toxicodendron.

3. **Neuro-Antitox CNS/PNS™** - for those suffering primarily from problems in the brain, meninges and peripheral nerves from Lyme toxins and heavy metals. Indications include, but are not limited to – cognitive disturbances, dizziness and vertigo, disturbances in vision, neuritis, neuralgia, numbness, palsies and headaches.
   - Ingredients – Silphium lac. 100mg, beta-sitosterol 100mg, chlorella 250mg, molybdenum 100mcg, as well as the sarcobioenergetic potencies in P6, 12, and 30 of cerebrospinal fluid, dura mater, cerebellum, optic nerve, substantia nigra, cerebral cortex, cranial nerve VIII (vestibulocochlear n.), myelencephalon, temporal lobe, occipital lobe, quadrigeminal plate, lumbar plexus, brachial plexus, periodontium.

4. **Neuro-Antitox Basic™** - good for global detoxification of the Lyme toxins, heavy metals, and for those who are unsure which specific Neuro-Antitox to take. This formula does not contain any sarcobioenergetic potencies added. Ingredients – Silphium lac. 100mg, beta-sitosterol 100mg, chlorella 250mg, molybdenum 100mcg.

The chief ingredient in all of these formulas is a novel-use botanical, Silphium laciniatum. Out of 5000 different natural substances tested using Bio-Resonance Scanning™, Silphium tested superior for detoxifying the Lyme-specific neurotoxins. The Neuro-Antitox formulas also contain the next best substances identified as synergistic, or supportive along with the

Silphium… chlorella, beta-sitosterol, and the trace mineral molybdenum. The only difference between the Cardio, Musculo-Skeletal, and CNS/PNS formulas is the use of Sarcobioenergetic Potencies™ which may act as driving agents or in other words act to direct the Silphium and other key ingredients to the specific tissues where they are needed, instead of just circulating around the body randomly. These are not homeopathic potencies, rather energetic imprints of tissues of rabbit, porcine, or bovine origin, depending upon which animal's tissue most closely matches human tissue. In that they are only energetic imprints, there is no potential for viral contaminants, such as Mad-Cow virus. The "Basic" formula does not have any of these Sacrobioenergetic Potencies and is therefore good when you are not sure which formula you need, or for more global symptoms.

The combined effect of these key ingredients makes the Neuro-Antitox formulas an absolute must in any well-rounded treatment plan. I would recommend that Neuro-Antitox dietary supplement be taken for at least one week before beginning any antibiotic or other medical or alternative treatment to minimize any Herxheimer reaction. Remember, Herxheimer reactions are caused by toxins; the Neuro-Antitox formulas are designed to "mop up", bind-up, and breakdown these Lyme-related toxins to hopefully eliminate any adverse reactions to the Lyme bacteria die offs.

Besides Silphium laciniatum being an awesome anti-neurotoxin, it was successfully used in times long passed to treat various cancers, all forms of asthma, bronchitis, and was effective in breaking down mucus in the tissues. Resonance testing reveals that Silphium may also bind heavy metals, and breakdown isopropyl alcohol, and benzene accumulations, adding to its phenomenal arsenal of beneficial effects[5].

Molybdenum is a trace mineral that can dramatically aid in the detoxification of the toxins caused by the dysfunction of multiple tissues in chronic illness. Molybdenum is very useful for detoxifying the toxin aldehyde from the die-off of Candida-type yeast. This is important to Lyme sufferers due to the fact that aldehydes are also considered neurotoxins, or nerve poisons. Aldehydes are also the toxins responsible for the hangover experienced by drinking excessive amounts of alcohol. I know of many Lymies who complain of this hung-over feeling without having drunk any alcohol. (However, it is our experience that it will not completely detoxify the specific Bb toxin.) Taking molybdenum will help slow the degeneration of tissues and related symptoms from the toxic overload[6].

Another detoxification nutrient in this formula, beta-sitosterol has been shown to perform well in the role of breaking down the Lyme toxins. At a 2003 Lyme conference, the medical doctors reported that it is one of the best nutrients they had found for helping the body to eliminate the Lyme toxins. For those of you familiar with the prescription Cholestyramine®, which has been used as an anti-neurotoxin, beta-sitosterol and chlorella are reported as being as effective without any of the problems common with Cholestyramine®.

Last but not least is chlorella. Chlorella was reported at the 2003 Lyme Disease Conference, put on by the Academy of Neural Therapy, as a preeminent antitoxin for Lyme toxins. It also enjoys a great reputation as an excellent detoxifier of heavy metals, such as mercury and lead, both of which also target nerve tissues. As a matter of fact, chlorella is said to bind more toxic metals than any other natural substance. Components of chlorella actually help repair the body's detoxification systems, dramatically increases reduced glutathione production, kills viruses, and even binds environmental toxins such as dioxin and benzene[7].

Even though I feel every Lyme sufferer should take a Neuro-Antitoxin formula, one also needs to read and combine many of the detoxification therapies outlined in this book.

Overall detoxification can be supported by simply drinking 8 ounces of purified water, Kaiki™, Penta-Water™, Young-Living™ Purified water, or ozonated water every hour to keep the everyday metabolic toxins flushed out of the tissues. We have some patients that have a hard time drinking water, so we learned that if the patient will put fresh lemon juice, or Berry Young juice™, in cool, but not cold water, it will be easier to drink more water per day.

In truth, a severe Herxheimer reaction is a sign of poor elimination pathway drainage, poor organ support and poor treatment! The body of most chronic Lyme sufferers is a toxic dump to start with. Therefore, if the doctor does not get the pathways of elimination open and working, then the body gets even more toxic when the bacteria begin to die and their toxins dump, or when the antibiotics activate the viral genetic sequencing to cause the bacteria to start manufacturing and releasing more toxins.

Many doctors think good treatment is indicated by the fact that you feel like crap, which seems to confirm they selected an effective antibiotic. With the politics of Lyme disease some think it is good that one has a "herx" after antibiotics are taken, so at least it gives the doctor and the patient hope that they are finally on the right track, but it is better to eliminate the "herx" reaction if possible. Most of my chronically ill patients cannot afford to feel worse just from the treatment! The person with Lyme disease has already suffered enough that they don't need to go through a "herx" just to prove they have Lyme disease.

References:

1. Klinghardt D, *The Klinghardt Neurotoxin Elimination Protocol*, 2nd Annual Conference of Applied Neurobiology; Treating Lyme and Co-infections, Bellevue, WA, Dec. 2002.

2. Prescott J., *Journal of Infection and Immunity,* June, 2003.

3. Travis J., *Phages Behaving Badly; Viruses can Control how Dangerous Some Bacteria are*, Science News, July 12, Vol. 164, 2003.

4. Waldor M., *Molecular Microbiology*, May, 2002.

5. Foster S., Duke J., *Medicinal Plants and Herbs,* Eastern/Central, Peterson Field Guides, New York, 2000.

6. Balch J., and Balch P., *Prescription for Nutritional Healing,* 2nd Ed., New York, Avery, 1997.

7. The Burton Goldberg Group, *Alternative Medicine, The Definitive Guide*, Fife, Washington, Future Medicine Publishing, Inc., 1995.

Chapter 9

Beating Chronic Lyme Disease is More Than Killing Bacteria

I cannot stress enough the need for your doctor to be addressing all the systems of the body on every visit. The body is totally integrated, and should perform like an orchestra, with every organ and tissue keeping rhythm with all the rest of the body. Taking an antibiotic, multi-vitamin/ mineral or even Borrelogen™ only addresses a part of what is required by your body to restore its ability to heal.

If one organ becomes dysfunctional due to illness or trauma, it ceases to move with correct rhythm in relation to the three dimensional movement of the other organs. When this happens it throws off the natural rhythm of the entire body. Eventually no tissue is able to maintain the proper rhythm. It is inevitable that this chain reaction will occur progressively over time if left uncorrected. Proper rhythm is part of what is necessary to maintain the integrity of the communication throughout the entire human organism.

While it is true that there is usually one offending issue that starts the whole chain-reaction, if left undiagnosed and untreated for very long, the problem will become complicated by the after effects of the original cause. Weakened tissues lose their natural crystalline-matrix resistance to and control of things such as parasitic infection, toxin overload, dysregulated chemistry, and fungal and microbial infection.

Let us take the example of Lyme disease. A person gets bitten by an infected tick and becomes infected with the bacteria known as Borrelia burgdorferi. The bacteria migrate through the tissues making their way to the muscles, joints, connective tissues, organs, the brain and nervous tissues. The bacteria wreak havoc on your body. To let you know that there is something wrong, your body responds with a multitude of symptoms.

If treated early in the infection, all is well, but if the infection is not detected and treated immediately, then the body's resistance is weakened and the chain reaction begins. Like every organism, the Lyme bacteria live a certain life span and then die. This means that even without treatment you will have a certain number of Borrelia burgdorferi bacteria dying off every few weeks. These dying bacteria end up causing you trouble since they release toxins upon dying (also known as the cause of a Jarish-Herxheimer reaction). These toxins lodge in the tissues of the body causing a worsening of the symptoms you feel. Research has shown that there is no direct tissue damage from the spirochetes. The damage to tissues is primarily due to the spirochete toxins which increase the inflammatory and immune responses.[1] Here is where the chain reaction begins to be most pronounced.

To examine how this happens let us start with a hypothetical example. Let us say the toxins are primarily affecting the elasticity of your muscles for argument's sake. The muscles perhaps of your right leg become tight and cramp, with wandering pains. You begin to favor that leg, walking with a limp. You are not designed to walk in this manner, so structural integrity is compromised. Your body's structural components are now exceeding their design limitations. The knee and hip joints begin to swell in response to the strain. The pelvis becomes unlevel, throwing the entire spine into fits attempting to compensate for the tilted pelvis. The pelvis and intervertebral discs of the spine become inflamed from the changes in weight distribution, which in turn irritate the spinal nerves. The spinal nerves are important in carrying the brain's messages for regulating every organ's function. With the spinal nerve irritation comes radiating pains in different areas of the body, along with tingling, numbness, and loss of muscular control. The organs begin to reflect the spinal problems and cannot get a clear signal from the brain; therefore, the chemistry and hormones become dysregulated. Any area of inflammation and weakness in the tissues, such as the spinal nerves, becomes susceptible to viral and bacterial infection. Beating chronic Lyme Disease is more than killing bacteria. For instance, what happens when a chain reaction has damaged an organ?

Every organ is on its own dedicated electrical circuit with at least one set of muscles. When there is a problem anywhere in an organ circuit, it causes the entire circuit to become, for all intents and purposes, short-circuited. The damaged organ circuit will only work at about 40% of its normal electrical and functional capacity. This is one of the body's protective mechanisms. The body will "turn down" the available electricity to a damaged area so that you cannot damage it further by still being able to exert 100% energy into an area that needs to be repaired. It is like when one breaks a bone in the leg; upon breaking the bone, special nerve fibers in the muscles send a signal to the brain to shut down the muscles. In an instant, the brain shuts down the circuit containing those muscles. Otherwise having 100% energy in the muscles might allow them to break the bone further.

Decreased energy in one circuit disrupts the rhythm of the organs which, one by one, respond by going into compensation mode and eventually into complete dysfunction. By now, you hurt all over. You have tender spots in the muscles. Your joints take turns aching and hurting. Your brain won't seem to work right, and you can't seem to sleep even though you are completely worn out all day long. It seems like nothing in your body is working correctly. You go to the doctor, who may not believe that Lyme is a problem in your state, but runs other tests, which are "inconclusive", since there is no "real" disease process, only the compensation of tired organs. And the Lyme disease goes on.

Finally, you have found a doctor who determines you have Lyme disease. "Not a problem", he may say. "Just take this antibiotic and you should be better in six weeks". At the end of six weeks he proclaims you cured; only you don't feel any better or you feel like you are still not well. Did he address everything? Usually all he has addressed is just the infection. That's great, but what about the structural imbalances that have now been there for months or years? Even if he recommends vitamins it is not enough. How about the organ circuits which didn't magically come back "online"? Did he address the opportunistic parasites, yeast and viruses that found a home in your body while your resistance was down? How about the toxins stored in the tissues? What about building up the nutrients and jump-starting the glands of the body so that the body can begin the work of healing itself?

Folks, can you begin to see how difficult it can be to achieve total wellness after a long fight with something terrible such as Lyme disease? If your doctor is simply giving you antibiotics with the hope that everything will go back to normal as soon as the bacteria is gone, then you need to find a new doctor, one who will cover all the other areas needing healing, even if you must go outside of your PPO or HMO insurance network. Addressing the totality of the human body is impossible without a technique like Bio-Resonance Scanning™ or other diagnostic and treatment technique like electro-dermal screening, Voll-testing, CPK, AK, Computerized Regulation Thermography (CRT), and other regulatory techniques like Neural Therapy. All of these techniques have been developed by scientists and doctors in order to eliminate much of the "educated" guesswork, or "cookbook" doctoring that has dominated the last hundred and fifty years. Without these techniques, doctors are just guessing at what is needed, and hoping you won't be allergic to the medicines, and hoping the combination of medicines won't conflict or create adverse effects in the body.

Getting rid of the bacteria in a disease such as Lyme disease can many times be just the beginning of the fight. You now must rebuild every tissue of your body. This takes time. A general rule of thumb in chronic illness is to expect three months of doing everything right for every year you have had the problem. This doesn't mean that you won't feel better sooner. It simply means that *feeling good and being healthy are two different things.* Most people diagnosed with cancer or heart disease say they 'never felt better'– their doctor just found the problem in a routine examination. So, be patient with yourself.

Beating chronic Lyme disease is much more than killing bacteria. Beating Lyme disease requires your complete attention and cooperation. You cannot simply take the medicines and hope for the best.

Keep a journal so you can see improvement over long periods of time. Rejoice in small triumphs. Control your thinking…don't allow yourself to become depressed. Don't talk about the different symptoms…talk about the things that are better. See yourself *half-well instead of half-sick.* Cooperate with the different doctors and therapists who are trying to help you. Don't be lazy in your mind, rejoice and actively participate in the healing of your body. You cannot afford to just take the pills and live a dark, dismal life, waiting for the pills to work. Change your routines. Strive to be vital in rebuilding your body. You are not a victim; you are simply living life like everyone else…all have problems to deal with. You cannot afford to allow yourself to "become an illness"; this just leads to a rapid decline. The illness is not who you are. Become one with God and one with yourself, not one with the illness. Get outside in the sunshine and close to nature and simplify life so that your priorities are correct. The decisions you make today will determine your tomorrow. Above all control your thinking – it's the one thing God gave you total control over. It's your free-will choice to accept or reject the illusions and lies that come to your mind. You can reclaim your quality of life and the journey is the prize.

Chapter 10

What to Expect with Biological Medicine

If you are suffering from any chronic illness it is almost a given that you have had "suppressive" therapies used on you. For example: if you went to your doctor for headaches, what would the doctor usually give you? A painkiller most likely. After all, you are having a headache due to the fact that your body is deficient in aspirin, right? Wrong answer! The headaches continue to worsen until the aspirin no longer works, so your doctor puts you on something stronger. The cause of the headache remains untouched. You just can't feel it. All you are doing is buying yourself time. You will have to "pay the piper" eventually when all of the different painkillers don't even faze the headaches anymore. Always remember that true healing cannot occur by simply masking the symptoms.

Doctors practicing the principles of Biological Medicine attempt to address the cause of the headaches by restoring the integrity of the body as a whole: structurally, chemically, energetically, bio-electrically, and by addressing lifestyle, stress issues and spiritual problems. The resulting relief is sometimes as quick as or quicker than prescription drug painkillers. Sometimes, as the body begins to truly heal from a chronic illness, you may feel worse before you feel better as your body is now dealing with the many issues that it had to "put on the back burner" for so long. This is good in most cases, because it means that the causes of your symptoms, instead of the symptoms only, are finally being addressed. Some people call this a "healing crisis", but a thoughtful planning of treatment by your physician can limit the severity of these problems. Over-aggressive treatment will undoubtedly cause more severe healing crises.

In the treatment of chronic Lyme disease one may experience something called a Herxheimer reaction. This is a medical term for an anticipated worsening of your symptoms in reaction to the die-off toxins from bacteria breaking apart. To most conventional doctors this is good sign and their way to know that the drug is working. In truth, a Herxheimer reaction is a sign of poor elimination pathway drainage, poor organ support, and poor treatment! The body of most chronic Lyme sufferers is a toxic dump to start with, and if the doctor does not get the pathways of elimination open and working then the body gets even more toxic when the bacteria begin to die and their toxins dump. Many doctors think good treatment is indicated by the fact that you feel like crap, which seems to confirm they selected an effective antibiotic. The "herx" most often indicates a poorly designed treatment program.

Feeling worse during the natural treatments of alternative and Biological Medicine happens sometimes, because so much of what is wrong in your body are things that your body has adapted to over a long period. If you do not get the appropriate treatment at the initial stages when something goes wrong, the body is forced to adapt to things being out of place and out of balance. When your doctor begins to correct these issues, the body will bring all of these problems "off the back burner" to be finally dealt with. Often you will find that you retrace your symptoms chronologically, the most recent problem will be the first to go, while the first or initial problem to show up will be the last to go. Once you realize that this is what is happening you can rejoice because you know where you are in your healing. If you stop treatment halfway through this chronological retracing you can already know much of what you have to look forward to in the upcoming months and years, since you have already been there. This said, none of the worsening here is a true Herxheimer reaction, and most patients do not experience a worsening of their condition. Some of the more severely affected Lyme patients I have seen could not tolerate feeling any worse!

Much thought was given in developing the treatment protocol outlined in this book in order to limit or eliminate any "healing crisis" by effectively addressing the needs of the body in states of chronic illness.

Do not be afraid. It took a long time to get to this point, and it is going to take time to heal as well. Remember, as a general rule, you should allow three months of doing things right, balanced lifestyle and proper treatment, for every year you have had your condition. Every single atom of your body is replaced at least one time per year. It takes about six weeks for the bottom layer of skin to become the top layer. Old skin cells are constantly dying and being replaced by new ones. You get a new liver, however, every four months. The goal is to remove the problems that are causing the perpetuation of dysfunctional cells so that when the body replaces cells it is able to replace them with good, healthy cells. Nerve tissue takes the longest to regenerate. When considering that the body's structure and function is driven primarily by its energetic and vibrational properties, any interference with the body's normal crystalline laser-like coherent matrix will result in altered structure and function. So, do not look at this illness as a possible quick-fix situation. It is going to take good therapies that do not harm the body plus a whole lot of time.

Keep in mind that so many symptoms are blamed on Lyme disease when the fact of the matter is that it may be a mix of Lyme and something entirely different causing some of your symptoms. Parasites, non-related bacterial and viral infections, systemic yeast infections, toxic overload, and poor lifestyle choices can be the cause of some of your symptoms. This is one of the strengths of our treatment protocol outlined here; it addresses many of these common problems.

The true skill of the doctor of Biological Medicine can be seen in his understanding of the interconnectedness of every tissue of the body. The majority of doctors are trained to treat based upon the numbers on a lab test, and have only basic training in reacting to symptoms with symptomatic treatments. For example, a conventional doctor will address frequent and burning urination with an antibiotic, an inflamed joint with an anti-inflammatory, or treat a skin rash with cortisone cream or antihistamines. This is not determining cause and effect; it is effect and anti-effect medicine.

The doctor trained in Biological Medicine has learned to "read" the signs and decipher the clues the body is revealing to form a working set of functional diagnostic conclusions. If the point is to facilitate the body's ability to heal itself, instead of simply providing medicines that will counteract the symptoms, then the doctor must learn how to determine where the primary problem is to be found. The doctor's job then becomes one where he works to remove whatever is interfering the body's ability to heal itself, and to provide the information and building blocks the body needs for optimal function. The beauty of Biological Medicine can be seen in the following patient stories. But before we get too far along, I want you to realize that many times abnormal findings on blood tests still do not tell the doctor why that aspect of the blood is outside of normal limits, and are therefore simply more clues that should be integrated into the global view of the patient. Blood tests are still a good way to track progress.

Selected cases from the Somerleyton Center:

Mr. B., a big man at over 6'4", had been a good patient for almost a year, and although practicing some poor lifestyle choices, such as smoking, presented consistently in good health overall. Recently, Mr. B. came in complaining of excessive weakness, pain, and decreased range of motion in the right arm and shoulder that had been bothering him for the last four weeks. He stated that it was so weak that he couldn't lift his lunch box.

He had no idea what caused his problem. With my training as a Doctor of Chiropractic, I would have focused in on the subluxations and the musculo-skeleton system but instead I examined the shoulder using Bio-Resonance Scanning. This exam revealed emotional upset as the primary cause of the problem. The pain in the shoulder was not coming from the shoulder but instead it was referred pain from the liver. Upon questioning Mr. B. whether he had been under any excessive stress he revealed that he was in danger of losing his job of 20 years if a company merger took place. He had found out about it six weeks earlier and even though his job had been threatened this way before, it was definitely bothering him more this time than ever before. He went on to describe his feelings as frustration, irritability and resentment – all emotions that specifically affect the liver.

Further testing identified that the problem could be addressed by applying a specific essential oil blend over the liver. This was one of those moments when I wish there were a video camera in the treatment room. As soon as the oil blend was applied and he tried his arm and shoulder, all of the pain and weakness was gone, and he had complete restoration of his range of motion! His eyes wide, he exclaimed, "Even if I tell the guys at work about this, they will never believe it!"

Understand, without Bio-Resonance Scanning to identify not only the primary cause, but the corrective remedy, one would be left ultimately treating the symptoms. Four weeks of suffering had been remedied in less than five minutes, possibly avoiding months and years of chronic arm and shoulder problems. Before ending the office visit, I told Mr. B. that he could put the problem back again by continuing to carry negative emotions forward day after day. By controlling his thinking and living only in the moment he has remained symptom-free, without any further treatments.

Question: How does the essential oil get rid of an emotional problem in this case?

It is scientific fact that our thoughts are extra-low frequency waves found within the electromagnetic spectrum. When one allows a negative thought process to be perpetuated overnight, and in Mr. B.'s case, for weeks, the frequency will get stuck in the crystalline matrix of the body, causing a physical disturbance. The essential oils all have their own electromagnetic frequency, based upon their unique molecular structure. These oils have some of the highest frequency of any substance on the planet. The Bio-Resonance Scanning identified the specific oil blend in this case that had a combined frequency that would push out or dissipate the stuck negative emotional frequencies in the liver (irritability, frustration and resentment).

Mr. M., a 68-year-old man suffering from heart arrhythmia, a condition where the heart does not beat with the correct rhythm. Although he took fistfuls of vitamins for years and prescription medicine for the condition, nothing was working. During our Bio-Resonance Scanning portion of his physical, the testing showed that the primary cause of his heart arrhythmia was heavy metals coming from his mouth. He laughed, thinking that he would show this form of testing to be bogus, stating that he wore dentures top and bottom with no metal!

As it turns out, his dentures were hardened and colored with various metals. I had Mr. M. take out his dentures, which I set aside. I then checked his heart rhythm… It was perfect! Knowing his wife would never believe it, I called her to the room and placed a blood pressure cuff on Mr. M. so that she could watch the needle on the cuff jump crazily when his dentures were in his mouth. Then I had him take out the dentures again. Upon inflating the pressure cuff again, the needle reflected the perfect rhythmical beating of his heart!

I can tell you, dentures affecting the heart are not listed in medical pathology textbooks, nor had I ever heard of it before.

I then recommended that Mr. M. get a new set of dentures, ones specifically made without any metals. He smiled and said, "These are not expensive dentures, but they are the first ones that feel good." "I'll just wear them when I eat, and for social occasions." That may sound good enough to some, but I informed him that it was unacceptable. Every organ circuit in the body has its time of highest energy. Each organ has two hours in every 24 hours during which it gets the most energy to heal. The heart's time is between 11 a.m. and 1 p.m., lunch time. Mr. M. would be putting his dentures back in at lunch time, the time of highest stress on that organ, and interestingly the time, according to some, when most heart attacks occur.

No matter what I said, he insisted on keeping his dentures. He continued to not experience arrhythmia when he didn't have the dentures in, however he would put them in to eat. Sadly, Mr. M. died of a heart attack at 12:30 p.m. a few months later, which was just a few weeks after he passed an electro-cardiogram test with flying colors without his dentures in his mouth.

Mr. W., a 65-year-old, three-time kidney transplant recipient presented with excessive pain, weakness, and occasional numbness in both shoulders, arms and hands, threatening his ability to do his job. The case was complicated by the fact that he must remain on immune-suppressive drugs so that the transplanted kidneys would not be rejected. This complicates things since there is virtually nothing Biological Medicine could do that would not cause at least a secondary improvement in immune function. However, it was agreed that doing nothing would leave Mr. W. to degenerate further and lose his livelihood and career.

The agreed upon treatment plan was to address the many large and long scars on his abdomen, which was crisscrossed with scars from the kidney transplants, gallbladder and appendix removal.

Biological Medicine recognizes that scar tissue acts as a dam to the flow of electricity through the meridian system and indeed a dam to the communication through the crystalline matrix of the body.

Keep in mind, if a doctor truly cannot heal a simple paper cut, then if true healing is to occur, the doctor must work to remedy anything interfering with the body's ability to heal itself. Scar tissue is a definite interference!

Corrective scar therapy using a frequency-modulated, low-level laser, a non-cutting type of therapeutic laser, was used to reconnect and redirect the flow of bioenergetic information through the many scars. This procedure took about 45 minutes, after which Mr. W.'s individual arm muscles were strength tested. The before and after strength testing was remarkable! The previously weak muscles were absolutely strong and firm when challenged, the numbness was gone, and the previous pain was gone with the exception of one specific movement!

Subsequent visits showed that the correction remained, much to the delight of Mr. W. Keep in mind, this is far from resolving all of Mr. W.'s health problems, but up to that point nothing had helped this problem that had been worsening gradually over the last 10 years.

Mrs. P., a 39-year-old, had been suffering from viral-induced ulcers coating her tongue, gums, and inner cheeks. In this case I want to show the logical path that training in Biological Medicine provided. With virtually no more information to go on as this was an initial phone consultation, I was able to determine the following predictable findings. Over the phone I asked her if her tongue was thin, red overall, but with a redder tip, and tooth marks on the sides – she said it was. I asked her to gently put the tip of her tongue on the roof of her mouth and observe if there were big blackish-purple veins visible – there were. I told her that it was likely that she was a "chronic thinker", one who never relaxed her brain. She said she even dreamed that she was solving problems at work. I said, "It is likely that you are cold natured." She said all her friends even knew that her hands and feet were always "ice cold." I said it was likely that it hurt too much to get a massage, and difficult to stretch her muscles. She said "My friends want to rub my shoulders just to be nice, but I can't even stand the pain." I then said that she is likely tired all the time, even after a good night's sleep. On the affirmative, I replied that it is also likely that she had taken a lot of antibiotics. She replied that she had been on many years of antibiotics and was sickly as a child. "How do you know all this," she cried! "No one has ever been able to tell me anything about my condition. "I've gargled with every essential oil and concoction friends have suggested, and the prescription drugs don't work either."

I knew these findings should be present, because a chronic viral infection of this nature requires a certain internal environment… a cold body temperature, which as you may read more about in the chapter on "Low Body Temperature and Lyme." The cold body leads to a devitalization of the blood, decreasing its ability to carry oxygen and nutrients, and leads to an acidic condition throughout the body. The cold, sluggish, devitalized blood is reflected in the swollen black-purple sublingual veins of the tongue.

Years of antibiotics often damage the fluid transformation and transportation of the body leading to the tooth marks on the tongue from the resulting systemic dehydration. She may drink a gallon of water every day, but she just urinates it out as the result of this fluid regulation problem. The tooth marks often also reflect a person who never relaxes the mind, a condition that mirrors a person who is so physically tired all the time that they basically must live in their head; the body for all intent and purposes is just "along for the ride."

The dehydration further results in a hardening of the tissues and an overheating of the organs. The red tongue body reveals a condition of overheating throughout the body. The redder tip of the tongue reflects excessive heat in the heart circuit from a deficiency of fluids. This overheating of the body must be seen as a relatively descriptive term only, as the body's core temperature even during this "overheating" remains low and completely dysregulated.

The heart is the body's electromagnetic generator, supplying the energy and vitality throughout. With the heart's energy production compromised, her energy levels were low; making her tired all the time.

She states that she cannot tolerate meats or cheeses, high sources of protein. This is a given since protein must be carried by the lymph fluid, which in her is too congested to perform this task efficiently. Upon testing, Mrs. P. has a very poor response to color stimulation and cannot generate any complementary (after-image) color. Excess protein disturbs the light metabolism of the body and can result in disturbances in the body's warmth organization. (We will talk much more about light/photons as a nutrient in the chapter on "Biophysics of Color Therapy.") The protein intolerance here simply verifies the overall condition of collapse of the body's crystalline matrix. All of these problems must be reversed before the viral condition can be eliminated. All of these problems create a "happy home" environment for the viruses. This is why she got no relief from some really good treatments from some big name hospitals and specialists. They all focused upon the virus, instead of the body as a whole.

There is a happy ending to this story. The ulcers went away for good after these and many more problems were identified and corrected from the perspective of Biological Medicine and Bio-Resonance Scanning. The types of treatment used here were too numerous to list, as the entire body had to be restored. No one treatment can be pointed to as "the" treatment that did the job.

Chapter 11

Introduction to Body Circuits and Circuit Healing™

The body is set up on electrical circuits much like your own house. In your house you have a circuit breaker box. Each circuit switch has a label that tells you basically what is on each circuit, i.e. "Water heater, refrigerator, and kitchen lights." The electrical circuits of the body always have one organ, specific teeth, a specific set of muscles, specific joints, and a specific gland on one circuit.

The human body was created this way because, from an electrical perspective, we have very low electrical energy. The body has circuits because if all of the body got all of the energy all of the time, there would not be enough electrical energy to go around. God made it so that each circuit of the body has its own time of highest energy directed to it for 3 hours only per day.

In a house, if something on a circuit has a problem it knocks the entire circuit "offline". So, if the refrigerator from the above example has a problem, it will cause the water heater and kitchen lights to not work either. Houses were designed this way so that if anything along the electrical circuits is having a problem, the problem would not get so bad that it would cause a fire, burning the entire house down.

Similarly, in the human body, if something on a circuit has a problem it can knock the entire circuit "offline" as well. While we don't have a switch that gets turned off as in your house circuit breaker box, God designed our bodies with secondary "wiring" as a backup system in case you blow out the primary "wiring". This secondary wiring will carry only about 40% of the normal amount of energy. So, if the organ becomes diseased, it will cause the teeth, muscles, joints, and gland on that circuit to also only function at 40% of their normal capacity. God designed the body this way so that if anything along the electrical circuits is having a problem, the problem would not get so bad that the problem would worsen out of control.

By the age of 20, most people have blown out all of the body's circuits and are living on secondary wiring. One can live a long life on secondary wiring, even reaching over 100 years of age, but the quality of life is less than half what it should have been if all circuits of the body had been maintained correctly.

Treating the Body Circuits

The concept of the human body being set up on electrical circuits is not a metaphor. The circuits of the body have been recognized as fact for thousands of years before western scientific thought decided that the microscopic view of the inner workings of the body was more important than the macroscopic or larger view, such as the body's circuits.

Conventional medicine truly relies heavily upon a microscopic view of the various body components, blood cells, immune cells, tissues, and fluids. While a doctor cannot throw out medical advancements that have stood the test of time, he must be humble to the realization of where true healing comes from in the first place. Only the human body can heal itself. Doctors do not heal. On the best of days they can only facilitate the body's own God-designed ability to heal. If you cut yourself I hope you have a band-aid, because I cannot heal that cut. At best, I can provide your body with remedies to speed the healing.

Biological Medicine combines the best of microscopic view with the best macroscopic circuit view of healing. In other words, Biological Medicine seeks to find where on the circuit the primary problem is coming from. Finding the primary problem is complicated by the fact that 85% of the time, where you feel the pain is not where it is coming from. So, do you understand now that looking at the body fluids through a microscope may tell you that something is wrong, but it will not tell you from where the primary problem is coming? This is why 88% of all conventional medicine is treating the symptoms only! Conventional medicine could treat the cause if it could identify it. It would only be able to identify it if it would view the body in its entirety, a system of interrelated and interdependent circuits.

The doctor specializing in Biological Medicine is trained to identify where within each circuit the primary problem lies. Once the problem is identified and corrected, the entire circuit goes back to 100% or maximum electrical capacity. Optimal health is achieved and maintained by keeping all of the body circuits functioning as close to 100% as possible.

Circuit Healing™ and the Swiss Watch

If you were to take the back off of a Swiss watch, you would see an incredibly complex system of gears. The precision that has made these watches famous is created by many gears meshing together. Each of the gears is a separate piece, but each gear is interconnected with the rest of the gears through a complex system to ultimately achieve perfect time keeping.

Remove or damage one gear and the precision will be lost and the watch is completely useless. Not one gear out of the dozens of gears in a Swiss watch can perform its function if even one gear is missing or damaged.

The human body is much more complex than the most intricately designed Swiss watch. Similarities can be made however. The circuits of the body can be likened to the various gears in the watch. Each circuit in the body must work in unison with all of the other circuits of the body. The precision of the watch is determined by the perfect timing and rhythm of every single gear. The precision of the body is determined by the perfect function and rhythm of every single circuit.

Imagine if you will, that the circuits of the body were simply gears that fit together and all had to be turning at the same time in order to function. Can you see that if all of the gears were stuck, then repairing one gear will never get the body functioning correctly? This is the way most medicine is practiced today. The "Specialist" doctor attempts to get his "gear" unstuck. He can't tell that the gear is stuck because of something gone wrong far removed from his stuck gear because he is focusing only on his specialty…that one gear.

Each of the body's circuits is self-contained but interconnected with the other circuits. Problems in one circuit will then necessarily create a chain reaction of the other circuits progressively becoming dysfunctional.

The doctor specializing in Biological Medicine is trained to identify where within each circuit the primary problem lies. Once the problem is identified and corrected the entire circuit goes back to 100% or maximum electrical capacity. Optimal health is achieved and maintained by keeping all of the body circuits functioning as close to 100% as possible.

The Role of Teeth in Circuit Healing™

Certain teeth are on each organ circuit in the body, and can therefore cause dysfunction throughout the entire circuit. It must be realized that teeth are alive. They are not bones in your jawbone. Each tooth has up to two miles of micro-dental tubules, small tubes within the tooth which in a healthy tooth maintain the nutrient and energetic flow within the tooth.

Conventional dentists are primarily concerned with the appearance of your teeth and in repairing cavities and fighting infection. However, a new type of dentist is emerging known as a Biological Dentist. These dentists recognize that tooth problems will ultimately cause dysfunction in the rest of the circuit.

While the tooth may not kill you directly, it can cause a major problem to arise in the organ or gland that shares its electrical circuit, ultimately causing your untimely and premature death.

Most of the problems in teeth arise from the efforts of dentists, either by placing toxic heavy metals such as mercury in the fillings, or by multiple metals in your mouth creating random charges of electrical currents in a battery effect, or through direct toxic waste leaching out of decaying and dead root canals.

In one study in Europe, dental problems were the primary cause of breast cancer in 96% of the cases. Amazing as it may seem, there are at least 8 teeth that have direct electrical connections via the body circuits to the mammary glands. Interestingly, 80% of all breast cancer arises in the mammary glands. Another interesting finding was that the tumors had up to 80 times more mercury metal than the surrounding healthy tissue. Your primary source of mercury (which is 1000x more toxic than lead) is from your silver/mercury amalgams in your teeth. Experts feel mercury is leached out of the teeth throughout its entire electrical circuit, potentially ending up in joints, muscles, glands, and organs.

Doctors specializing in Biological Medicine are trained to identify problems anywhere in the body's circuits, even the teeth. If the problem is coming from a tooth, then no treatment will work completely until the tooth problem is resolved.

The Role of Joints in Circuit Healing™

A joint is where two bones meet. All of the joints of the body share specific electrical circuits with an organ, specific muscles, teeth, and glands. As a part of the circuit, a problem in the joint can and will cause a problem throughout the circuit. So, a problem in a joint can potentially cause a circuit to blow, reducing the available energy in the circuit to about 40% of what it normally should have. Not only does the joint become dysfunctional, but the organ sharing the same circuit will become dysfunctional as well.

Any joint can lead to circuit problems, but the primary joints are the inter-vertebral joints in the spine, pelvis, knees, feet, and the many joints of the skull.

Doctors specializing in Biological Medicine are trained to identify and address joint problems. Problems in joints usually arise from misalignments, where the bones are slightly out of normal position; fixations, where the bones of the joint are stuck and not moving through their correct range of motion; toxic accumulations in the joints, where chemical and/or biological poisons have been trapped in the joints; and other joint problems such as bone spurring and other degenerative conditions.

Remember, in order to heal completely, every aspect of the body must be functioning as close to 100% as possible. So, in any type of disease it makes sense that the integrity of the joints must be addressed. That is why the adjusting of the spine and other joints of the body, by a trained Doctor of Chiropractic, is included as a part of Circuit Healing™.

No other doctor in the world is as well trained to address the various bio-mechanical problems of the body than a Doctor of Chiropractic. Nor is there a branch of medicine so well suited to practice Biological Medicine, since they are now trained almost identically to Medical Doctors, with the exception that Doctors of Chiropractic must work with natural means to facilitate healing to occur. Biological Medicine recognizes the body's interconnectedness and focuses on true healing through natural methods and recognizes the body's ability to heal if given the chance.

The Role of Organs in Circuit Healing™

I have seen patients who had always had perfect teeth until they got very sick and their teeth began to go like light bulbs. This unfortunate event beautifully demonstrates the truth of body Circuit Healing™. As organs malfunction due to disease, the entire sequence of electrical circuits is affected.

Remember, the circuits of the body are electrical pathways that are shared by an organ, a specific set of muscles, glands, teeth, and joints. So, in actuality, the heart circuit is shared with the subscapularis muscle, the wisdom teeth and the anterior pituitary…etc.

Of all of the components in a circuit in the body, the organs are the most critical, since major problems arise when organs malfunction, compared to muscles and joints which cause a progressive problem to arise with the end result being the ultimate disruption of the normal function of the organ.

Imbalance in organs is most often noticed in lab tests, but is most often felt in the dysfunction of joints and muscles. If an organ is rigid, stiff, and generally dysfunctional, the muscles and joints on the same circuit will be rigid, stiff, and generally dysfunctional. It really is that easy. The entire circuit will be affected in much the same way.

Doctors specializing in Biological Medicine are trained to recognize and address organ dysfunction from all causes.

Organs can malfunction from many different causes such as toxic substances, parasites, microbial overgrowth, hormonal, nutritional, and enzymatic imbalances, not to mention electrical circuit problems.

As unfair as it may seem, we are not all born equal. All of us are born with problems that predispose us to organ problems. This is why it is so important to have your children treated using Biological Medicine principles. It will start them on the road to a long and functional life. The longer the organ problem has been there, the longer it may take to resolve.

The Role of Symptoms in Circuit Healing™

Symptoms are the problems you feel when circuits are not functioning correctly. Pain is a symptom; it is your body's way of saying "Don't do that or it will cause more damage." A tumor in a cancer patient is a symptom! Joint swelling, neuritis, depression all are common symptoms in people with Lyme. They are not the cause, but are the result and symptoms of the underlying problems. We know indisputably this to be true. If you surgically remove the tumor the body will generate a new tumor. If you take a pain medication, it will wear off.

Symptoms are good for alerting us that something is wrong. Symptoms also provide us with a way to learn what not to do that creates pain. Symptoms can also be a way to track your progress while under a treatment program. We want to see your symptoms going away, since that is what brought you to us in the first place.

Doctors specializing in Biological Medicine are trained NOT to treat symptoms. The symptoms will improve, sometimes remarkably fast, when the cause has been addressed.

I can guarantee that you are never having a headache due to a deficiency in Tylenol and aspirin. Taking Tylenol treats the symptoms, but does nothing to correct the underlying cause of the headache. You may not feel the pain anymore, but whatever was causing the pain grows bigger and worse and eventually the pain medicine will no longer work. Now you are faced with the question of finding a stronger pain medicine, or finding a doctor specializing in Biological Medicine who can finally address the cause. You must trust that the symptoms will go away as the result of the body healing itself.

A simple blister on your foot may arise from wearing a new pair of shoes. I can "cure" you for all intents and purposes by having you not wear those shoes. I removed the cause. The blister should not get worse unless you aggravate it while it is healing. No doctor can heal that blister. It will just take time…about 4 weeks for the body to completely heal the skin so that you can't see where it was. In the same way all healing takes time to be fully appreciated. Be patient with your body; the older it is, the longer it may take. And be patient with your team of healthcare professionals.

The Role of Muscles in Circuit Healing™

The muscles are the most obvious way to detect circuit problems. All muscles are controlled electrically. We know this from observing Multiple Sclerosis (MS) and Lou Gherig's Disease (ALS), which damage the electrical pathways, nerves, much like cutting the power cord to your T.V.

No muscle will work without electricity. Muscle problems are very common in Lyme patients. When a circuit in the body is "blown" from whatever reason (teeth, organ, joint, gland, muscle), the muscle will immediately weaken and stay weak until the cause is addressed. For example, if a tooth is rotten and leaking toxic waste into the circuit, the entire circuit will "blow", reducing the available energy down to 40% of its normal energy. When this happens, the muscle will weaken, and due to its decreased energy it will also begin to cool down temperature-wise. Now it is weak and due to the coldness, it will begin to stiffen. As it stiffens it develops a hard knot in its core that is tender to touch. This hardened core is called a trigger point.

Having many trigger points is what conventional doctors use to diagnose Fibromyalgia Syndrome (FS). These trigger points are a symptom of multiple organ circuits that are chronically blown.

Muscles serve two primary purposes in the body. They move bones, and they move fluids through the body. The joints must have proper muscle control in order for the joint to function without pain. Muscles also provide a pumping mechanism to move toxins out of the tissues, and to move nutrients into the tissues. So in Circuit Healing™, the muscles need to be addressed in order to bring the circuits online again.

Doctors specializing in Biological Medicine are trained to use muscles in testing the integrity of the various organ circuits.

Muscles may need to be addressed directly through the use of Therapeutic Massage, and/or through the use of essential oils and exercises. However, the muscles reflect the integrity of the entire circuit, so they may not fully release until the rest of the circuit is repaired.

Any healing protocol for chronic Lyme sufferers must recognize the full scope of potential problems in the muscle circuits.

The Role of Glands in Circuit Healing™

Glands produce hormones. Hormones are chemical messengers to specific organs. Hormones trigger an organ to perform a certain function depending upon the type of hormone.

In Circuit Healing™, any time a circuit is "blown" the gland on that circuit will be affected along with each tissue on that circuit (i.e., organ, gland, joint, muscle, tooth).

To say that there is an imbalance in the hormones simply means that there is imbalance in that gland's electrical circuit. Hormones normally are produced or are not produced as dictated by the demands of the body. There are really many types of hormones. Most people are only familiar with estrogen, progesterone, and testosterone because doctors like to supplement with these.

Doctors specializing in Biological Medicine are trained to recognize that glands will respond correctly when the circuits have been corrected. Since glands produce hormones that regulate the proper functioning of organs, one can see why this area of the circuits cannot be left out of a successful treatment protocol.

Glands and their hormones can be affected by outside influences, especially the estrogens, which are truly a class of many chemicals with "estrogenic" actions. For example, most petroleum based cosmetics, shampoos, and personal care products have estrogenic actions on the body. This means that the chemicals from your personal care products are "turning on" or "turning off" the function of some of your estrogen receptive organs. This normally should only happen when the glands are directed to produce estrogen by the brain.

We, at the Somerleyton Center will instruct you in ways to avoid substances that may interfere with the glands of the body. After all, how can we get the organs turned back on electrically if the glands are turning them off due to chemical interferences?

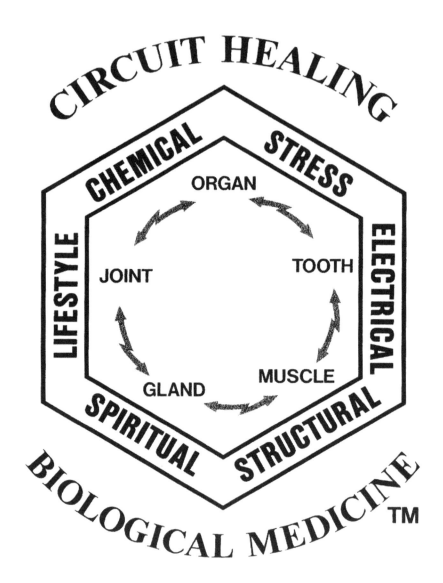

Section 2

Treatment Protocol for Chronic Lyme Disease

Chapter 12

Healing at Home

Through the years, many people have called me wanting to know what they should do at home to heal, since they cannot find a doctor in their area that is able to address all of their needs. While no two people are exactly the same and therefore cannot be treated exactly the same, there are many things that I have found to be almost universally needed in every Lyme sufferer.

The following recommendations are just that...my recommendations, not a prescription...and in an ideal world you would always either find a doctor who already practices all the techniques outlined in this book, or you would come to our clinic, or give a copy of this book to your local doctor so that he or she can help you implement as many of the items as possible.

If you cannot find a good doctor in your area, and wish to be proactive in taking responsibility for your own health at home, and I say this as a worst case scenario… the following protocol is what I have found works the best.

First of all, do not get into the trap of taking fistfuls of every nutritional supplement that sounds like it may help. The goal here is not to get you to take supplements for the rest of your life, but to provide your body with those specific things that will restore the body's ability to completely heal. If you are truly correcting the bottom-line problems with any supplement, then eventually the problem would be corrected and you would no longer need to take them.

Second, you must know in your heart that God truly did design the human body to heal itself of virtually any illness. I have seen miraculous recoveries from seemingly permanent damage. Just two months ago a lady came to us from Alaska who had not had the use of her entire right leg and foot for over a year from the effects of Lyme disease. Within 10 seconds of treatment with a specific technique using the Magnetic Resonance Bio-Oxidative Therapy, she was able to lift her knee up to her chest, walk on her toes and heels, and climb stairs! She and her husband were just amazed and ecstatic, as was I! The correction has remained without further treatment of that specific problem ever since. (This was achieved because of the restoration of the body's normal crystalline matrix, which is necessary for nerve conduction and subsequent muscle control. Remember how we discussed the crystalline matrix nature of the body in the chapter called, "A Theory of Intermicrobial Communication"? See also the "Color Therapy" chapter for a more detailed explanation of this phenomenon.) So, the point I am trying to make is this: provide the body with the *specific* information and building blocks it needs and the body will do the rest. Don't just take some of everything in the health food store; find a doctor who can determine what your body primarily needs. In the Alaska lady's case, it was not a nutritional supplement that her body needed to restore the normal function of her leg; it simply needed the stimulation that the Magnetic Resonance therapy provided.

It is not expected that Lyme microbes and your symptoms will miraculously go away within a short period of a week or month of doing this protocol, although it is often reported. So, don't let the absence of immediate apparent benefit disappoint you. It took your body a long time to get into this condition, and it may take months to years of doing the right things to fully restore the quality of life you seek. Feeling good or feeling bad during your journey does not indicate that you should stop doing the right things.

The Healing at Home Protocol

For your convenience ordering information is provided in the back of this book.

(Follow this protocol for 3-4 months beyond the disappearance of your symptoms.)

Nutraceutical Product Recommendations:

• **Borrelogen**™ ....1 to 2-droppers under the tongue, then swish it around the teeth and swallow, 3-times per day with or without food. As we talked about in the chapter on "Intermicrobial Communication" no matter what treatment is done it is a given that the microbes will immediately strive to survive. They will either attempt to morph or change their shape to survive, and/or they will attempt to change your internal environment. Borrelogen has been clinically tested for over 6 years and from that experience we know that even as good as we believe it to be, some of the microbes will eventually be able to become resistant to the changes it makes in your body's energy. Therefore, we must employ a better strategy. The most effective strategy we have come up with is to rotate remedies in the following manner. Take Borrelogen for 2 months, then switch to Microbojen for 2 months, and then take the Borrelogen and Microbojen at the same time for 3 months. By this time, all the while employing as much of the rest of this book, you should be well on you way towards the quality of life you seek. Even if you feel dramatically better soon after beginning this protocol, it is not wise to discontinue this plan of attack, since history has shown us that most people who feel better early on, and quit the treatments, experience a reoccurrence of their symptoms and blood tests show positive still. Borrelogen contains the following botanical ingredients, each of which is added to the formula based upon Bio-Resonance testing as opposed to the selecting plants based upon their known actions or historical uses. Phragmites communis rhizome, Morus alba leaf, Baptisia bractiata, Fiddle-leaf fig folium, Chrysanthemum moritolium flower, Platycodon grandiflorum root, Prunum armeniaca kernel, Glycerrhiza uralensis root, Baptisia australis, Mentha hapocalyx, Ophiopogon tuber, Una-de-gato, Morus rubra fruit, Cuscuta, Scindapsis aureus, Ipomoea quamoclit, Dracaena dermensis, distilled water and 20% grain alcohol. Sensitive individuals may want to work up this amount, starting with only a few drops and see how your body reacts before increasing the amount. If you feel worse, then your organs of elimination likely are not working well and need to be supported. In this case follow the recommendations outlined in the chapter on "Detoxification Therapies." If you are feeling worse upon starting any Lyme treatment, it is likely due to the increased movement of Lyme toxins. This problem is often remedied by significantly increasing your dosage of Neuro-Antitox Formula™ listed below, in order to breakdown and bind up more of these toxins. In other words, the less Lyme toxins, the fewer symptoms.

- **Microbojen™**............ 1-2 droppers, 2-3 times per day in water, with or without food. Like all of the Jernigan Nutraceutical formulas, Microbojen is frequency matched to provide the body with the information and building blocks it needs to overcome and control specific problems. Neither Borrelogen nor Microbojen treat disease in the classic sense of the term. They are not an "antibiotic" although they provide the body with the specific informational frequencies needed to overcome and control microbes. They are therefore designed to work with God's design of the human body, instead of, "doing for the body what the body should do for itself" as in the case of most prescription drugs. Microbojen was initially developed in an effort to prepare for the worst-case scenario of biological warfare. Bio-Resonance Scanning was used to simulate the worst condition we could think of. We simulated that "if" a person had, all at the same time, the following microbes, what corrective frequencies would the body need to overcome them. We simulated a person having smallpox, anthrax, HIV, hepatitis B and C, West Nile Virus, Epstein-Barr Virus (EBV), Cytomegalovirus (CMV), Mycoplasma fermentans incognitus, and Bubonic plaque all at the same time. Obviously, this is an unlikely event, however by formatting the test for such a condition it is likely that the resulting botanical formula, Microbojen, will be highly effective against a wide range of the world's worst "designer microbes." The end result of this research, Microbojen, just so happen to test amazingly well against the just as evil microbe...Lyme spirochetes and their partners, Babesia microti, Ehrlichia and the many viruses found in chronic sufferers. Microbojen contains the following botanical ingredients: Tragopogon (aerial), Isatis root, Lasiosphaera fungus, Scrophularia root, Oldenlandia herb, Moutan peony bark, Phellodendron bark, Poria cocos sclerotium, Glycerrhiza uralensis.

- **Neuro-Antitox Formula**...... 1 to 3 capsules, 2 to 3 times per day, with or without food. This product was developed to detoxify the body of the Lyme-related toxin. This is a must for any type of treatment to limit feeling worse from the bacterial die-off, called a Herxheimer reaction. It is needed in the body for detoxification and in various enzymatic functions. It is good also for various aches and pains and even helps normalize blood sugar levels. You may select the specific formula you need based upon where your worst symptoms are, i.e., nerves, brain (CNS/PNS Formula), muscle and joint pain (Musculo-skeletal/Joint Formula), heart problems (Heart Formula), or if you are not sure then there is the Basic Formula. It may be that you have to use more than one formula as in someone with problems in the muscles and the nerves, in which case one or two capsules from each of the CNS/PNS Formula and one or two from the Musculo-skeletal/Joint Formula can be taken. Refer back to Chapter 8 for more information about the Neuro-Antitox Formulas.

- **Wobenzym-N**............Take 8 to 11 of these smooth, coated pills (they are about the size of an aspirin and go down easily) 3 times per day, on an empty stomach. Take them at least two hours after eating and at least 45 minutes before you eat something. These are systemic enzymes, so we don't want them to be used up simply coming in contact with food in your small intestines. Wobenzym-N should be continued for the duration of treatment until full restoration of quality of life is restored. Wobenzym-N is a very effective anti-inflammatory product as well as a potent immune system booster. In that most pain involves inflammation, improvement in even stubborn pain can be expected often within 24-48 hours. Improvement is often cumulative improving gradually the longer one uses Wobenzym-N.

Research performed in Europe showed that Wobenzym-N helped various antibiotics penetrate the tissues up to 40% better. Bio-Resonance Testing has so often demonstrated complementary/synergistic effects when used with Borrelogen and Microbojen, that it has become a foregone conclusion in many doctor's clinics that it is needed in virtually everyone needing these remedies. Wobenzym-N is second only to aspirin in over the counter sales, with one-hundred million people taking them every day, including many European Olympic athletes.

Wobenzym-N seems to help remove interference in the tissues to the movement of healing energy and medicines. Volumes of research over many years and millions of people bring strong confidence in this well-known systemic enzyme. Its many benefits include immune system support, anti-inflammatory activity, and acceleration of the rate of healing. Wobenzym-N in my experience also helps restore the body's warmth organization through breaking up the accumulation of antigen/antibody complexes and by freeing the metabolic processes from their cold, sclerotic, low output. It seems that in Lyme disease, as in many cold/sclerotic illnesses, the body's chemical reactions (metabolism) are being held captive and the energy producing mechanisms of the cellular factories have wrenches in all of their gears. Wobenzym-N seems to remove these wrenches over time by directly and indirectly breaking up excessive protein accumulations in the intracellular spaces. Excessive protein, as we have said, promotes darkness and cold, therefore Wobenzym-N should break up the darkness allowing the light and warmth metabolism to be restored by the other treatments specifically designed to do so. Dosage is large due to the fact that these enzymes are used up as they work their way through to the farthest reaches of the body. This is not a digestive enzyme, it is a systemic enzyme. This dosage should be maintained for 1 month, then reduced to 6-8 pills, 2-3 times per day thereafter for six months to a year, or as directed by your doctor.

Side-effects: With overwhelming research, and millions of people using this product every day, there is virtually no safer product on the market. An expected effect of Wobenzym-N is the healthy thinning of the blood. This is one of its healthy effects; however caution is warranted in those using prescription blood thinners, anti-coagulants, or those suffering from bleeding disorders. It is generally recommended that Wobenzym-N be discontinued 2-3 days prior to any surgery, or dental work due to its blood thinning properties.

- **Pleo-Alkala** ....This product is a powder that comes with its own measuring spoon and a packet of urine pH strips for determining how much powder you need to take. Simply wet a pH strip during urination and match the color of the strip to the color code provided.

- **Molybdenum** .... 1 to 3 capsules, 2 to 3 times per day, with or without food. This mineral is one of my absolute favorites. It is needed in the body for detoxification and in various enzymatic functions. It is good also for various aches and pains.

- **Beyond Chelation™** .... 1 packet, taken 2 times per day, with or without food, taken for 6 months to a year, or indefinitely. This product will support the nutritional needs of the body while it is being stressed by the detoxification process. Beyond Chelation provides the highest quality essential fatty acids, botanicals, minerals, and nutrition needed for optimal function of the brain and nervous system, heart and circulatory system, and virtually every other tissue in the body. Beyond Chelation also contains Calcium EDTA which will help remove many of the toxins and heavy metals jamming up the machinery of your body. It also contains high-allicin garlic, which is a favorite antimicrobial of some of the world's leading medical doctors who treat Lyme disease naturally.

- Add to the above recommendations any products from the "Adjunctive Therapies For Lyme-Related Symptoms" to address your specific symptoms.

Essential Oil Support

- Clarity oil blend
- Joy oil blend
- RC oil blend
- Sacred Mountain oil blend
- Thieves oil blend
- White Angelica oil blend
- Aconite Nerve oil
- Solum Uliginosum Oil

Rub 1 to 4 drops of each of these oils in the following areas, 2 to 3 times per day. These oils are very aromatic, but are usually well-tolerated by even the most chemically sensitive individuals, most likely due to the fact that they are pure plant oils, with no solvents, and no synthetic or petroleum-based additives. You may want to delay putting on these oils on days that you have meetings and such to attend. Even though they smell good, everyone around you will smell them as well. Daily use is best, but it is not "written in stone" or an absolutely must-do before going out. Definitely use before bedtime. If you feel itching or experience redness of the skin after applying an oil then simply rub olive oil on the area which should soothe the skin. From then on dilute a drop of the oil you were sensitive to with a drop or two of extra-virgin olive oil or extra-virgin grapeseed oil, then apply it. If skin sensitivity persists, discontinue the oil that is causing it, but continue with the other oils.

- Clarity oil blend on the back of the ears
- Joy oil blend rubbed over the heart
- RC oil blend rubbed on the chest and inhale
- Sacred Mountain oil blend rubbed on the back of the neck
- Thieves oil blend rubbed on the feet and over the thymus
- White Angelica oil blend rubbed on the forehead
- Aconite Nerve Oil (Wala/Raphael) on any area experiencing neuropathy, such as numbness, tingling, or nerve pain.
- Solum Uliginosum oil can be rubbed all over the body nightly, on

top of the other oils or by itself. It can also be added to and whisked into bath water in order to coat the entire body, a very helpful way to get it all over the body when there is no one around to rub you down all over. Soaking for 20 minutes in this warm water and oil bath is best.

Magnetic Resonance Bio-Oxidative Therapy - Comfort Covered Ceramic Bio-Oxidative Magnets

- 4" x 6" x 1/2" Magnet......... strap one of these large ceramic magnets with the black (Negative polarity only) vertically over the heart especially during sleep although it is perfectly okay to wear it 24 hours a day over the heart, while your body heals. This can be used with the bed unit listed below.
- 1 1/2" x 1/2" Bitemporal Soother Magnets.... These smaller ceramic magnets have Velcro backing so that the negative polarity side can be held by a strap over the temporal region of the head (In line with the top of the ear and just forward of the ear on both sides of the head). These have been used with great success in stopping mood swings, depression, panic and anxiety attacks, but also increase the oxygen levels in the brain, so that the brain can function at maximum efficiency, and because Lyme spirochetes are primarily anaerobic organisms, their growth may be inhibited. Use daily as much as possible, especially around the house or in the car where you will not be so conspicuous.
- Super Head Unit......... a must for anyone suffering from neurological Lyme in the brain. Some of the latest research efforts are working to verify benefit in eliminating plaquing in the brain, often seen in M.S. and Lyme. There are no contraindications to using this device and this unit's deep penetration of the brain may allow it to reach deeply imbedded spirochetes and viruses affecting the brain. This unit is still used even if you have the Super Magnetic Bed unit.
- Super Magnetic Bed (400 lbs.)...... Sleeping on this bed unit saturates the entire body with only the beneficial negative polarity needed to facilitate healing of those people with multiple problem areas that cannot be efficiently dealt with using smaller magnets. (It is likely best not to use this bed unit during pregnancy. Definitely do not use it if you have a pacemaker or other medical electrical device)

- If your body temperature is too low, follow all recommendations in the section of the book for correcting a low core body temperature.

Eliminative Organ Support:

The liver, kidneys, intestines, lungs, and skin are usually very overloaded in Lyme disease. I would recommend you use all of the various Detox Baths in this book. My favorite is Detox Bath #1 for overall daily use, however listen to your own body to determine which one seems to work the best for you. Ideally, use the Strengthening/Nutritive Bath after every 4-5 detox baths. You may want to skip the detox baths for a few nights and add the Solum Uliginosum Oil or Rosemary oil to the water to revitalize your body, since detoxifying can be tiring to the body. Constipation and poor elimination is usually at the heart of the many symptoms related to toxins associated with Lyme disease. Laxative tea combined with coffee enemas, and skin brushing (see Detoxification Therapies section) will greatly relieve this toxic condition. Remember, you were not okay prior to being bit by whatever gave you Borrelia burgdorferi. Prior total body problems had to be present in order for one to manifest infectious disease. Do the ilio-cecal Valve / Valve of Houston Reactivation 2-3 times per day. (See therapies section)

Color Therapy

Please refer to Chapter 34 on "Color Therapy". Color therapy is inexpensive to do at home and is beneficial in restoring your overall health.

Balanced Living

Practice all of the principles in this book for balanced living in regards to the body, mind, and spirit. I would recommend that you read this book several times and keep reading it until you know it inside and out and can apply all of the balanced living on a daily basis.

Chapter 13

Euro-American Biological
Adjunctive Therapies for Lyme-related Symptoms

The following are general treatment considerations based upon clinical experience. The assumption is that one is already doing the standard Lyme protocol recommended in this book. These remedy recommendations are generally recognized as safe for the layperson to apply, unless otherwise noted with * which indicates it requires a health professional to provide it to you. You should be doing the recommended protocols for Lyme and Low-body Temperature (if indicated). For your convenience, all **bolded** products are available by ordering through Jernigan Nutraceuticals and are listed in the back of this book for your convenience.

1. Unexplained fevers

Gradual Onset Fever:

• At the early onset of fever such as at 99.0° F, one should support the fever process with a general goal of reaching about 102.0° F. Initial treatment of 6-10 drops or pellets of homeopathic **Belladonna 6x** should be given every half hour. The belladonna supports and directs the efforts of the body without allowing the fever reaction to progress out of control. The head and torso will be warm and dry to the touch, while the arms and legs will remain cool during this stage due to the fact that the body is focusing its healing efforts where it is most needed. Do not attempt to bring the fever down with compresses or baths during this phase, as the fever should continue to rise...which is a good thing. (There are some people who advocate the use of saunas and hot baths early in the beginning stages of illness, to "bypass" the need for the fever entirely...do not do this! In light of the prevalent low core body temperatures experienced by most children and adults today, it is of great importance to support and allow the body's own efforts to go through the process of generating the heat necessary for the condition.

- If the fever continues to progress beyond 102.5° F, then homeopathic **silver 30x (Argentum)** should be used to restrain the excessive fever process. Use 6-10 drops or pellets every fifteen minutes until fever breaks or stops rising. Although fevers much higher than this present no great danger in children they generally indicate that the organizational and restructuring efforts of the body are somewhat in need of greater control of the situation. (Homeopathic silver is not the same as colloidal silver; the latter will not achieve the same results, nor is the homeopathic silver being used to "kill" bacteria in this situation.)   In this excessive fever condition, measures to assist in bringing down the body temperature can be used. Lemon-water compresses on the abdomen and calves, as well as tepid water enemas can help to disperse excessive heat.

- If the fever is only weakly manifested, around 99.0° to 100.5° F then one should support and strengthen the body's efforts, yes actually promote a stronger fever response, so that the goal of the inflammation is reached. Support the weak fever by using 6-10 drops or pellets of homeopathic **Sulphur 6x** or **Hepar sulphuris 6x** at the same time as adding external warmth through warm baths (no warmer than 100° F). Ensure that the sick room is warm. It can be comforting and warming to the spirit to have the room lit with candlelight. Rub the body with Peat-based oils, such as **Solum Uliginosum oil** (Wala/Raphael) and wrap the body warmly in peat/ wool blend bedding.

- When the fever breaks and begins to fall it is time to support the formative forces working with the purpose of the rebuilding and restructuring of the body. It is at this stage that the heat of the fever will be felt in the arms and legs and one may break out in perspiration as the heat is no longer needed and the body is attempting to vent it in the extremities. Lemon-water compresses can be used on the abdomen and calves to help the cooling process. Herbal extract of **Echinacea augustafolia** along with homeopathic **Quartz 3x** are beneficial for supporting the formative process well beyond the end of the illness event. Refer to specific illness protocols for how to proceed after the fever breaks. Remember the fever is just the first stage of the body dealing with the problem.

The Sudden onset Fever: (see protocols for individual illnesses for more specific treatment recommendations.)

- When dealing with a sudden onset rapidly increasing fever, as opposed to a gradual onset fever, it usually indicates virus-associated inflammation. In that it is likely viral the initial supporting measures will be different than for bacterial infections.

- Viruses can cause a sudden and rapidly rising fever and no remedy is more indicated than homeopathic Aconite napellus. The optimum dosage is **Aconite 6c to 30c** potency, 6 to 10 drops every 15-30 minutes increasing time between doses as fever begins to slow its incline. Aconite has strong anti-viral actions, but is used all the way to the breaking of the fever. Aconite puts a restraining action on the rapidly progressing fever process of the body. Remember viruses do not replicate well in a hot body, so once again the point of this remedy is not to bring the fever down but to harness the fever and drive its attack. Be patient; do not use anti-viral medicines until the fever begins to fall. We want the body to achieve the degree of fever it needs and trust its wisdom.

- If the fever continues to progress beyond 102.5° F, then homeopathic **silver 30x (Argentum)** should be used to restrain the excessive fever process. Although fevers much higher than this present no great danger in children they generally indicate that the organizational and restructuring efforts of the body are somewhat in need of greater control of the situation. (Homeopathic silver is not the same as colloidal silver, the latter will not achieve the same results, nor is the homeopathic silver being used to "kill" viruses in this situation.) In this excessive fever condition, measures to assist in bringing down the body temperature can be used. Lemon-water compresses on the abdomen and calves, as well as tepid water enemas to disperse excessive heat.

- When the fever breaks and begins to fall discontinue the homeopathic aconite. It is time to support the formative forces working with the purpose of the rebuilding and restructuring of the body. It is at this stage that the heat of the fever will be felt in the arms and legs and the patient will break out in perspiration as the heat is no longer needed and the body is attempting to vent it in the extremities. Lemon-water compresses can be used on the abdomen and calves to help the cooling process. Herbal extract of **Echinacea augustafolia** along with homeopathic **Quartz 3x** are beneficial for supporting the formative process well beyond the end of the illness event.

• **Febrile Convulsions in Children:** The possibility of a convulsion is remote and is not necessarily due to an excessively high temperature. The convulsion might manifest as shaking of the whole body, biting the tongue, wild, rolling eyes, and may even include loss of consciousness. Dr. Otto Wolf, M.D. says it best in his book, *"Home Remedies,"* "In rare instances there can be febrile convulsions. While this looks dramatic, in most cases they have passed by the time medical help has been sought. Such convulsions can happen during the time of the increase of the fever, but not at the time of its maximum. For this reason anti-fever drugs are inappropriate. However, if the convulsions last for longer periods, or are repeated, the doctor should be consulted." Wolf, O. Home Remedies, Herbal and homeopathic treatment for use at home. Anthroposophical Press 1991

2. Unexplained weight change—(loss or gain)

• Digestive Enzymes will help take the strain off of the pancreas and digestive system. Digestive enzymes, such as protease, lipase, amylase, cellulase, and peptidase work to break down your food into smaller, more easily digestible molecules, releasing the nutrients. They help eliminate food allergies from foods passing into the colon incompletely digested. By improving digestion weight loss and gain should be improved. **Total Enzymes** by NutraWest, Inc. are strongly supported by clinical evidence of improvement seen in darkfield live-blood analysis as well as the improved digestion.

• Never eat the same food more than two times in a four day period. This will help eliminate maladaption and poor digestion of foods. This will also speed the utilization of your food into energy instead of it being stored as fat.

• While Lyme disease can cause unexplained weight loss, so can cancer. Have your doctor rule out the possibility before assuming it is due to Lyme infection. In the case of "Cell-Replication Problems" our favorite remedy is **Neogen-4,** a nutraceutical we developed. This works phenomenally in combination with **Wobenzym™-N** and **Iscar*** to help restore the body's control and regulation of any cell-replication problems.

- In the case of weight gain, as the body begins to heal as a result of the protocols and God-designed living, one should see that the body has a cellular memory of its optimal weight and move in that direction as balance is restored and activity level is increased.

3. Fatigue, tiredness, poor stamina

- Fatigue plagues almost every Lyme sufferer. The Magnetic Resonance Bio-Oxidative therapy combined with the Low-Body Temperature Protocol will go a long way to restoring the mitochondria, which are the energy factories of every cell in the body. A **4"x 6" x 1/2" ceramic magnet** over the heart 24 hours a day can help recharge the electromagnetic energy of the blood and heart. Many people can be said to have "lost heart". This is a term describing an actual physiological event of weakening of the heart muscle. The "tired heart syndrome" can be aggravated by elevated homocystiene, an amino-acid that is a normal breakdown product of protein. The newest and possible best nutraceutical for helping restore normal processing of homocystiene is **Silphium lac Capsules** created by Somerleyton Healing Products. Silphium, according to BRS testing, also helps eliminate heavy metals, and breaks up mucus/phlegm in the chest. Normal dosage is 1-2 capsules, 3 times a day. Direct heart support is best supplied by Dr. John Brimhall, D.C.'s perfectly formulated product, **Total Heart** by NutraWest, Inc.

- Adrenal gland fatigue is almost universal in chronic illness and people under chronic stress. Alexis Carol won the Nobel Prize in Medicine demonstrating that a person given a glandular product from bovine or other source would stimulate vitality in the corresponding gland in the human body. There are many different adrenal support products on the market. A beautiful product, developed by Dr. John Brimhall, D.C., called **DSF – Formula**, produced by NutraWest, Inc., is my first line product which I have used for years with outstanding results, while being safe enough to be used by just about anyone. A normal dose would be from 1 tablet split in half, 2 times per day, up to 1 tablet three times a day. I would not recommend taking DSF near bedtime as you may find yourself too alert, even though there are no stimulants, such as caffeine in this product.

- Mitochondria fatigue is made evident by the progressive weakening of muscles as they are used in repetitive activities. Mitochondria are the energy factories that produce adenosine triphosphate (ATP), the fuel of every cell. ATP is needed for muscles to work and not fatigue. Body builders with large muscles actually do not have more muscle fibers than the next guy, they have just pumped up their fibers with more mitochondria. Another product formulated by Dr. John Brimhall, D.C., who is a genius at formulating highly bio-available and highly active nutritional products based upon sound research, is a product called **Total Mitochondria** by NutraWest, Inc. A normal dose would be 1 tablet, 2-3 times per day.

4. **Exhaustion upon awakening, disturbed sleep—too much, too little, early awakening**

- Definitely use the MRBT... **Magnetic Resonance Bio-Oxidative Therapy bed or the Super Magnetic Head Uni**t, or at the very least one of the **4" x 6" x 1/2" ceramic magnets** under your pillow and another over the heart. Super Magnetic Head unit is placed on the pillow you sleep on and provides great sleep, while focusing high gauss strength negative polarity to the deepest tissues of the brain. Remember, the negative polarity is antibacterial, antiviral, anti-cancer, and has many other benefits. Ideally, the entire head would be covered in negative polarity. The head unit, therefore, provides more hours of treatment per day with unparalleled benefits and no side-effects. It also does not require a doctor's prescription. The MRBT stimulates the pineal gland in the brain to secrete melatonin, the hormone responsible for sound sleep and waking you up rested.

- Get rid of all electrical clocks, radios, computers, electric blankets, and such from your bedroom. Don't use laptop computers on your lap, or laying in bed without using a peat-fabric apron or blanket covering your body to protect you from the emitted electromagnetic energies! The motors of all electrical devices emit 60 cycle alternating frequencies, which interferes with the normal functioning of your nervous system and therefore alters the secretion of brain chemicals. You should hit various sleep stages, such as REM sleep. If you are being awakened to go to the bathroom or other things it will interrupt the sleep chemicals of the brain, especially if you turn a light on or there is a street-light, night light or other light source used while getting up. The light tells the pineal gland to reduce the levels of melatonin to almost zero, which will not return to sleep levels for up to hours later, therefore impairing sleep and making it almost impossible to awaken rested. Supplemental **Melatonin** can be used before bedtime to help reset the body clock to realize it is time to go to bed. About 10 mg before bedtime is the usual dosage. If melatonin causes aggravation, and you find it difficult to fall asleep, the body's clock may be completely set wrong. In this case take the melatonin in the morning for a week or so then try it closer to bedtime again until you are sleeping well.

• Keep your bedroom as dark as possible, but still be able to wake up to the sunrise. The sunlight will be detected by your pineal gland even with your eyes closed, which will then awaken you through the release of waking chemicals. If you wake with a start from an alarm clock, the pineal does not have time to secrete "waking up" chemicals, so that you will wake rested and refreshed feeling.

• Showering with a hot shower often causes increased fatigue due to the fact that the chlorinated water of most cities, when super-heated in the water heater comes out in the steam of the shower as chloroform gas! A **Shower Head filter** or better yet, a whole house filter system to remove the chlorine will eliminate this source of exhaustion and grogginess in the morning.

• For men and women, **Progesterone Cream** applied one to two times per day can be a God-send for balancing the emotional reactions. For menstruating women, a general dose is 20 mg, morning and evening.

- High dose **Vitamin B-6** can improve sleep patterns. One way to tell if you need B-6 is if you don't remember your dreams, or feel you don't dream. This has nothing to do with interpreting dreams, only if you don't dream it indicates a B-6 deficiency. B-6 is also needed for proper hormone function and energy production in the body. A good starting dosage is one 200 mg pill, 1-3 times per day. Discontinue or cut back if you experience tingling sensations, which would indicate you are getting too much.

5. **Very nervous, laughs or weeps without cause, mood swings, depression**

- Using the bi-temporal ceramic MRBT magnets during periods of emotional upsets will normally calm and restore balance.

- The homeopathic Bach flower remedy, "**Rescue Remedy**" is a tried and true remedy for balancing your emotions in stressful situations. It is absolutely safe and can be used as often as needed without fear of addiction or toxicity.

- Homeopathic **Palladium Cord** is most indicated for depression, where one holds up brightly in public and crashes when alone. Palladium is a metal that is a component in catalytic converters of cars. It is being sprayed out in the car exhaust… you breathe it in. Palladium is known as "the depressive metal." Is it any wonder the world is suffering from epidemic depression? Homeopathic Palladium cord will cause the stored palladium in your body to be released and also calm the depression.

- For men and women, **Progesterone Cream** applied one to two times per day can be a God-send for balancing the emotional reactions. For menstruating women, a general dose is 20 mg, morning and evening, skipping the week of your period. Men and menopausal women can benefit from 20 mg applied one to two times per day. My favorite Progesterone creams are those with pump bottles that meter out exactly 20 mg per pump and last a month or so.

- Often when one can't seem to respond to stress or stimuli appropriately, causing laughter at the wrong time, or weeping at every trifle, the first thing to come to mind may be adrenal fatigue, which many times is a result of the prolonged stress of Lyme disease and life in general. **DSF–Formula**, produced by NutraWest, Inc., is my first line product which I have used for years with outstanding results, while being safe enough to be used by just about anyone. A normal dose would be from 1 tablet split in half, 2 times per day, up to 1 tablet three times a day. I would not recommend taking DSF near bedtime as you may find yourself too alert, even though there are no stimulants, such as caffeine, in this product.

• For adrenal fatigue your doctor can advise you to place the **4" x 6" X 1/2" ceramic magnet** with the Positive polarity over the adrenal glands for ONLY 30 minutes maximum. Almost every beneficial use of MRBT is found using exclusively Negative polarity, however minimal positive polarity is stimulating to the weak adrenals. This should be limited to two sessions a day.

6.   Unexplained hair loss

• Hair loss may be aggravated by poor thyroid function, however the thyroid may be hypo-functioning as a result of adrenal gland fatigue. So, **DSF-Formula** by NutraWest is always a first line supplement in hair loss.

• **Liquid Iodine** provides the thyroid with the needed iodine to create thyroid hormones.

• **Total Thyroid**, is a Dr. John Brimhall, D.C., NutraWest, glandular/ nutritional formulation that provides glandular thyroid, along with all of the associated supporting glands and all of the nutritional synergistic support needed for optimal thyroid function.

• Stop using potentially toxic shampoo. If you can't pronounce what is on the label, it is likely not too good for you. My favorite shampoos are made by Weleda of Germany, Dr. Hauschka, of Germany, and the shampoos of Young Living Oils, of the USA. See personal care products list for types and prices.

• **Endoflex Oil** blend by Young Living Oil, is an inspired blend of Spearmint, Sage, Geranium, Myrtle, Nutmeg, and German Chamomile essential oils, which tests well with Bio-Resonance Scanning™ for balancing the endocrine system and hormone balance.

7.   **Swollen glands**

- **Thyme oil** and **Eucalyptus oil** from Wala of Germany rubbed over the swollen glands using a stroking and gliding motion towards the heart.

- If you have the **4" x 6"x 1/2" MRBT magnets**, you may lay the negative polarity over the swollen node. (You should always use a large enough magnet to completely cover the swollen node.) Keep the magnet over the swollen node as many hours as possible until resolved.   The negative polarity increases the lifespan of the antibodies, phagocytes and lymphocytes, and functions as an antibiotic against viruses, bacteria, fungi, mycoplasma, and parasites.

- **Pleo-Reb** capsules are a homeopathic remedy produced by Sanum-Kehlbeck of Germany and distributed by Pleomorphic Sales, Inc. of Glendale AZ, USA... open one capsule three times per day and pour the capsule out onto each tonsil. This product is made from homeopathic peyer's patches, which are very immune-stimulating. These capsules are one of my favorite immune boosters, safe enough for children and the very old, non-toxic, and they don't compromise any of the other treatments you may be using.

8.   **Sore throat**

- **Eucalyptus oil** from Wala of Germany rubbed over the sore throat using a stroking and gliding motion starting at the back and base of the ears moving towards the heart.

- Gargle with about 3 drops of pure **Melaleuca oil (Tea tree oil)** in a mouthful of water.

- **Lemon Wheel Throat Wrap**... this unusual treatment is one I picked up from the Medical doctors in Germany. It sounds odd, but works like a charm, and the best thing about it for you is that it doesn't cost much and you can get the supplies from the grocery.

- Another tried and true remedy is a hot tea you can buy in just about every healthfood store and grocery, called Throat Coat tea, by Traditional Medicinals, Inc.

- Low level "cold" laser therapy for 5 minutes can completely take the pain away. Clinical research seems to show it also may "kill" viruses and bacteria… it most definitely promotes healing and restores balance to the tissues.

9. Neuralgia / Neuritis

- The **Super Magnetic Bed Unit** is the treatment that provides the most correction for the greatest number of problems. Neuralgia and neuritis mean nerve pain and nerve irritation. These conditions are due to the Lyme toxins as well as other exogenous toxins and structural aggravations. The strong negative polarity of this bed penetrates with high-gauss strength up to 18" while you lay on the bed. This provides correction and treatment all through the night. Many of my patients return to the bed four times a day in the acute phases of illness for an hour each time.

- **Aconite Nerve Oil** is useful rubbed into all neuralgia pains and neuritis symptoms. It has been beneficial in herpes-related nerve problems as well as rheumatic joint diseases. It can be rubbed on as needed, the effect is somewhat cumulative, so keep with it, and don't just stop if the first application doesn't do much.

- Homeopathic **Rhus Toxicodendron Cord** is actually Latin for Poison Ivy. Don't be alarmed; it contains no actual poison ivy, just the homeopathic dilution/potentization of poison ivy. It has been used for over 100 years for easing nerve and joint pains.

10. Upset stomach

- Upset stomach in Lyme disease can often be associated with lowered acidity of the stomach. A favorite of mine is a product by Thorne Research, Inc. called **SF-734** which contains, among other ingredients, betaine hydrochloride, bentonite, bismuth, and deglycerinized licorice, all of which is regulating and normalizing to the stomach.

- Antibiotic usage is almost always shown to have damaged the stomach's ability to transform and transport fluids out to the tissues. The only way your tissues get fluid is through what you drink. Many Lyme patients have "beef jerky" for muscles due to chronic dehydration of the tissues. This damage to the stomach leads to what the Chinese call a Spleen Qi deficiency and ultimately a state of dehydration of the blood and tissues. This can be seen on the tongue as tooth marks along the edges from basically a dehydrated tongue. Being over-mental, or otherwise too much mental stimulation – never turning off the brain activity, will also cause this stomach/spleen problem leading often to upset stomach. For this condition, a product by K'an Herb Company called **Gather Vitality** is my favorite for stopping the continued progression.

- An often overlooked "cure" for stomach pain is simply to drink purified water, not juice, coffee, or other liquids, but just water…8-10 glasses a day. See product list for my favorite water purifier.

- You may also have a hiatal hernia where the stomach herniates up through the hole in the diaphragm where the esophagus comes through. This can cause terrible stomach pain, no pain, heart burn, and acid reflux, not to mention the fact that it can lead to chronic "walking pneumonia" or recurrent bronchitis from the aspiration of stomach gases into the lungs. This does not require surgery! Your doctor of Chiropractic can usually correct this in 2 minutes! It can be almost miraculous how this correction by your doctor of Chiropractic can instantly end the pain and acid, and heartburn and chronic pneumonia through simply pulling the stomach back down and resetting the muscular tone of the diaphragm and correcting the fascia restrictions usually aggravating it!

11. Heart palpitations, pulse skips, heart block, heart murmur or valve prolapse

- A **4"x 6" x 1/2" ceramic magnet** over the heart 24 hours a day can help recharge the electromagnetic energy of the blood and heart. Since the 1970's scientists and medicine has known that cholesterol was not the enemy! It is a symptom of poor liver/gallbladder function as well as poor digestion. Even though this has been known, the cholesterol industry that has been built cannot just be shut down. It is becoming widely known that elevated Homocystiene is the primary cause of heart disease. Homocystiene, an amino-acid, is a normal breakdown product of protein from your diet. The problem lies in the inability to break down homocystiene into other amino acids, so it builds up in your body, wreaking havoc. If you were to inject the tiniest amount of homocystiene into a lab animal, the blood vessels would become inflamed, sticky, and clog up with plaque. The newest and possible best nutraceutical for helping restore normal processing of homocystiene is **Silphium lac. Capsules** created by Somerleyton Healing Products. Silphium, also according to BRS testing also helps eliminate heavy metals, and break up mucus/phlegm in the chest. Normal dosage is 1-2 capsules, 3 times a day. Nutrititional support for breaking down homocystiene is found in the product **Homocystiene Redux.**, by NutriWest. Direct heart support is best supplied by Dr. John Brimhall, D.C.'s perfectly formulated product, **Total Heart** also by NutriWest.

12. Joint pain or swelling

- Homeopathic **Rhus Toxicodendron Cord** is actually Latin for Poison Ivy. Don't be alarmed, it contains no actual poison ivy, just the homeopathic dilution/potentization of poison ivy. It has been used for over 100 years for easing nerve and joint pains. It is my absolute silver-bullet for carpal-tunnel type wrist pain and unstable joints.

- **Rheuma Comp Oil** is a blend of oils from the German company Wala. It is very good for rheumatic aches, pains, and neuralgias. Inflamed joints are often greatly relieved by rubbing this soothing oil. This oil is both soothing and curative. Another great oil blend from Germany is the **Solum Uliginosum oil and bath essence**, which is possibly the best remedy for those whose joints hurt due to changes in the barometric pressure, associated with weather changes and storm fronts moving in. I feel like I have used gallons of this oil on my patients. You see, whenever you have swelling in the tissues and joints of your body it hurts. However, when the barometric pressure outside falls, there is not as much atmospheric pressure on the outside of your cells, so the already swollen cells in your muscles and joints will swell even more, causing you to know it is going to rain before the weatherman. No other remedy treats this better. It also treats joint pain associated with reactions to being around chemicals, perfumes, exhaust fumes, etc. **Homeopathic Solum Uliginosum** is also available for those seeking extra benefit.

- The Soother **Bi-temporal Ceramic Magnets** can be strapped over joints, providing ongoing relief to painful joints. With the magnetic field therapy, the joint inflammation is reduced, the joint is oxygenated, the painful accumulation of acid in the joint is eliminated, and the toxins are broken down and eliminated. The **Super Magnetic Bed** is a must for anyone suffering with multiple joint pain.

- From the nutraceutical perspective the product **Joint-Aide**, by Ancient Formulas, Inc., has been a best results winner with my patients. It contains Glucosamine hydrochloride (the best form of glucosamine), which is one of the first known substances to actually repair and regenerate the worn out cartilage of joints! It also contains high-yield bromelain, an enzyme from pineapples, which research shows goes right to any area of inflammation in the body, instead of just circulating around aimlessly in your bloodstream. Bromelain stimulates increased healing, it is anti-inflammatory, and pain-relieving. If that were not enough, Joint-Aide contains Boswellia, Sea Cucumber, and a whole bunch of synergistic joint support nutrients and minerals.

13. Muscle pain or cramps

- **Marjoram oil** rubbed into painful muscles is warming to the body and has been used for all types of muscle problems for centuries. Interestingly, it is known to be anti-bacterial and while it works on your muscles it is very calming to the nervous system; it helps with constipation, asthma, bronchitis, insomnia, neuralgias, migraine headaches, and it is anti-viral.

14. Dyslexia

- See next protocol.

15. Difficulty processing auditory or visual information.

- In any Central Nervous System disturbance all efforts must be made to oxygenate the brain, control the brain waves, stimulate normal communication between the right and left hemispheres, and eliminate irritations to the brain and nervous system. There are no better ways to hyper-oxygenate the brain than through Hyperbaric Oxygen Therapy and the MRBT, **Super Magnetic Head Unit**! Almost 90-95% of all brain disturbances are caused by irritation, low oxygen and the Cytomegalovirus, Epstein-Barr virus, and the Human Herpes virus-6. To date there are very few safe medicines that will cross the blood-brain barrier. So, the HBOT and MRBT are the safest and most restorative therapies of the brain known to man. Both will increase the levels of oxygen all the way to the core of the brain, both will kill viruses, both will stimulate regeneration of the neurons. HBOT is a one hour treatment several times per week, while the Super Magnetic Head unit is placed on the pillow you sleep on and provides great sleep while focusing high gauss strength negative polarity to the deepest tissues of the brain. The head unit, therefore provides more hours of treatment per day with unparalleled benefits and no side-effects. It also does not require a doctor's prescription.

- From a nutritional perspective, the product **Neuro-Plus** by Thorne Research, Inc. is beneficial in supporting normal brain function, and contains Bacopa, an herb from India which is known to increase one's ability to learn new information.

- The frequency modulated, low-level "cold" lasers are being used with remarkable results in restoring cognitive disturbances. Many Doctors of Chiropractic as well as Neurologists are using this high-tech device. When it comes to the nervous system these doctors handle it best.

- **Eyelights**™ are some of the most amazing brain treatments to come along in years. These are specially designed glasses with four small red lights that can be selected to flash with different intensities in the various fields of vision. They are easy to use and work by stimulating specific parts of the nerves of the eye, which will thereby stimulate the part of the brain responsible for various tasks. They can be used to re-educate and strengthen the muscles of the entire body, improve coordination, improve reading comprehension, improve learning time and more. I have done timed mathematics tests on my on children, before and after using the eyelights…the results are phenomenal. My children were able to cut the amount of time to do the tests in almost half! This is a must for anyone with cognitive difficulties, and should be used in rehabilitating the brain and musculo-skeletal system.

16. Difficulty with speech or writing

- Same as protocol above #15.

17. Symptoms worse from alcohol

- The byproduct of alcohol is aldehyde. It is the aldehyde that gives you the hangover; it is a neurotoxin. Many Lyme sufferers are creating alcohol in their gut from yeast overgrowth from the excessive antibiotics killing off good friendly bacteria that would normally keep yeast under control. Supplementing the diet with the mineral **Molybdenum** will decrease the symptoms by deactivating and detoxifying these aldehydes. Molybdenum is safe, non-toxic, and has no known side effects when taken in normal dosages. A general recommendation is 300 micrograms 2-3 times per day.

- When yeast is overgrowing in the gut, any sugar you consume or anything that breaks down into sugar is digested by the yeast into alcohol. Even fructose, the sugar from fruits – remember grapes plus yeast equals champagne, so gas, belching, and bloating are good indicators that you have your own brewery going on in your gut! To bring the yeast back under control my favorite product is **Yeast Ease**. It is frequency-matched using Bio Resonance Scanning to be active on just about every strain of candida-type yeast. It has also been shown in independent laboratory testing to be very effective even if diluted 1:3200 for some types of yeast.

- Probiotics is a term used for the friendly bacteria of the gut. This is acidophilus and many other types of good bacteria used to reinocculate your gut after you killed 400 different strains of friendly bacteria with the first round of antibiotics. So you can see why it is a good idea to put some back! Especially since they keep the yeast under control once the Yeast Ease has helped the body bring down the overgrowth. One of the best probiotics is **Total Probiotics**, by NutraWest. For those of you thinking you are getting enough probiotics through eating yogurt and drinking milk, these are not good enough, nor are they replacing as many types of bacteria. Besides, milk DOESN'T do a body good!

18. Ears/Hearing: buzzing, ringing, ear pain, sound sensitivity

- **Helichrysum oil** rubbed around the ears has restored the deaf to hear, as well as taken away the ringing of the ears in some of my patients.

- The ears are controlled or affected by the kidneys, so supporting the kidneys may help with normal ear function. For this I like to use a product from K'an Herb company called **Strengthen Kidneys**, and another one called **Quiet Contemplative**. The latter is more indicated for people with a fast lifestyle or busy, stressful life.

- Lymphatic drainage treatments with the ST-8 device outlined earlier can be of primary importance in these ear problems. Seek out a doctor using this therapy.

19. Difficulty with concentration, reading

- One of the most important things to remember when you find you cannot concentrate while reading is that you must never read past a word that you do not understand. You must look it up in a dictionary, write it in at least three sentences or until you feel you have mastered the word. If you go past a word without understanding it, even a simple word, you will not be able to go on with any reading comprehension and you will find it difficult to concentrate.

- **Eyelights**™ are some of the most amazing brain treatments to come along in years. These are specially designed glasses with four small red lights that can be selected to flash with different intensities in the various fields of vision. They are easy to use and work by stimulating specific parts of the nerves of the eye, which will thereby stimulate the part of the brain responsible for various tasks. They can be used to re-educate and strengthen the muscles of the entire body, improve coordination, improve reading comprehension, improve learning time and more. I have done timed mathematics tests on my on children, before and after using the eyelights… the results are phenomenal. My children were able to cut the amount of time to do the tests in almost half! This is a must for anyone with cognitive difficulties, and should be used in rehabilitating the brain and musculo-skeletal system.

20. Twitching of the face or other muscles

- Twitching is caused by irritation and hypersensitivity of the nerves supplying the muscles. In Lyme disease this is most often the result of toxins and over-acidity of the body. Detoxification is a must. MRBT... A **4" x 6" x 1 1/2" ceramic magnet,** using the negative polarity over the region of twitching, will detoxify, alkalinize, and calm the nerve and muscle.

- **Vitamin B-complex** is also needed for normal nerve function and can be an easy solution at times.

- **Marjoram oil** and **Aconite Nerve oil** both work well rubbed into any muscle problem area as often as needed.

21. Sciatica

- **Aconite Nerve Oil** applied topically.

- Oral homeopathic **Rhus Toxicodendron Cord**

- Chiropractic adjustments and ST-8 lymphatic drainage of the entire pelvic and kidney regions.

- Recent research has demonstrated microbial infection in the sciatic nerve in most cases of sciatica, so keep in mind this may not be purely a structural problem.

22. Irritable bladder or bladder dysfunction

- Pleo-Alkala, use as directed to maintain proper pH (comes with its own urine strips for testing).

- Cypress Oil rubbed directly over the pubic bone nightly.

23. Headaches

- Headaches come from several causes: structural, chemical, stress, and bio-electrical problems. No one treatment will be a true cure all. All four of these potential causes should be addressed at the same time. It is a definite truth that you are not fixing anything by taking aspirin or Tylenol type pain-relievers.

- The trace mineral **Molybdenum** is a long time favorite of many of my patients to relieve the toxins responsible for many headaches.

- Chiropractic alignment of the entire spine.

24. Vertigo, dizziness, poor balance

- Homeopathic **Cocculus comp.** has been a "silver-bullet for many of my patients with these problems for years.

- Lymphatic drainage of the head, neck and upper thoracic region using the ST-8 is a must as these problems are often related to fluid accumulation in the inner ear and cranium.

25. Eyes/Vision: double, blurry, increased floaters, light sensitivity

- The eyes are regulated by the liver. The liver is the primary organ of detoxification, so cleansing the liver and supporting the liver nutritionally will go a long way to benefiting eye dysfunction. My favorite blend of oils for the Lyme patients with toxic livers is **Juvaflex oil** with **Ledum oil** applied on top. Then place a hot (but not scalding) wet towel folded on top of the oils over the liver. The moist heat is an age old liver treatment. The oils penetrate with marvelous effect.

- Freshly prepared carrot juice at the rate of two 8-oz. glasses per day is healing to the eyes as well as the body. I recommend a macerating juicer, such as a **Champion Juicer**, due to the fact that most of the nutrients in carrots and other veggies is inside the plant cells, which must be broken in order for you to fully benefit. For a bit of increased action add celery, parsley, and apples to the carrot juice.

26. Facial paralysis (Bell's Palsy)

- **Helichrysum Oil** applied topically over the affected area as well as the front and back of the external ear has been shown to apparently cause the nerve fibers to regenerate and restore normal function.

- **Primula Oil**, by Wala of Germany, is applied topically and is used in cases of muscle atrophy from disuse, which is the case in palsy.

- Cold Laser therapy

27. Chronic asthma worse at night

- **Silphium** capsules are historically known to break up mucus and be beneficial in cases of asthma. 1-3 capsules, 2-3 times per day.

- Ozone Air Purifiers eliminate much of the particulate and chemicals in the air that may aggravate asthma.

- **F-Complex**, by NutriWest contain many of the essential fatty acids, such as Omega 3, 6 and 9's. A key essential fatty acid needed in asthma is gamma-linolenic acid which is found in various plants, such as black current seed, borage oil, and evening primrose oil. Recommended dosage, 1-4 softgels, 3-4 times per day.

- Chiropractic care has a long history and much research documenting the necessity of proper spinal alignment in all cases of asthma.

- BRADE allergy desensitization treatments work to eliminate the hypersensitivity reactions from continuing.

- The Four-day Rotation diet will go a long way toward eliminating the food maladaptive syndrome found in every case of asthma.

28. Neck creaks and cracks, neck stiffness, neck pain

- **Valor Oil** has been called "Chiropractor in a bottle". Rub this oil from the base of the skull to the sacrum. It is very soothing and works with the electromagnetic fields of the spine and spinal muscles to align the spine.

- Obviously, proper alignment is guaranteed by seeing your Doctor of Chiropractic.

- **Borrelogen™** has been reported by many people to have cleared this problem up in just a few doses sometimes.

- The **Super Magnetic Bed** is perfect for easing neck pain while setting up an anti-microbial field throughout the entire body. Calcifications and spurs may be reduced by continued use of the high-gauss strength negative polarity. Acid accumulations that lead to spurring, calcification, and neck pain is completely blocked as the negative polarity restores the normal alkalinity inherent in healthy tissue.

29. Forgetfulness, poor short-term memory

- Nutritional support of the brain is provided by **Total Brain**, a new formulation from the healing guru, Dr. John Brimhall, D.C., and NutraWest.

- Of all of the technology and advances made by medicine, not many medicines are known to cross the blood-brain barrier. The oils in the blend called **Brain Power** contain high levels of sesquiterpenes and sesquiterpones, which have been shown to cross the blood-brain barrier! These oils are highly oxygenating and healing to the brain. Rub Brain Power into the base of the skull, behind the ears and earlobes. Some have found benefit of placing a drop on the roof of the mouth, which seems to benefit the pituitary and pineal gland. Apply 2-4 times per day, or as needed.

- **Eyelights** are outlined above (P. 85) and would be beneficial in retraining the areas of the brain responsible for memory retention.

- Reading, meditating, and just listening to slow Baroque music has been shown to enhance memory. According to Janalea Hoffman, an acclaimed expert in Rhythmic Medicine, this has to do with the body's entrainment to the frequency of the music and the way most "slow Baroque music affects body rhythms and facilitates both the relaxation process and improved intellectual functioning." To learn more about using music in your healing journey, her book "Rhythmic Medicine" is a must read.

- The **Super Magnetic Head Unit** used during sleep can enhance brain function thereby improving memory. Brain cells die rapidly whenever oxygen levels drop. Try holding your breath, how long can you go? Not long – neither can your brain. If you are already at a deficit in your brain, you need the penetrating effect of high-gauss negative polarity.

Chapter 14

Advanced Techniques for Doctors of Lyme Patients

Research indicates that many individuals having Lyme disease are misdiagnosed due to the many similarities to Multiple Sclerosis, ALS, Systemic Lupus, and other supposed autoimmune diseases. I have seen tremendous improvement in patients in all of the above illnesses using this same basic treatment protocol, many of which tested positive to Borrelia burgdorferi in blood and urine tests. In light of the recent research by Dr. Lida Mattman, Ph.D., et al. identifying a newly found strain of Borrelia spirochete in all cases of MS and ALS, we are beginning to see why we were finding "Lyme Borrelia" frequencies in patients with these illnesses.

These bacteria are unique in that they thrive in the same environment most conducive to viruses...a cold, low body temperature. The usual antagonism of bacteria and viruses is missing; they are working in a terrible synergism. This is why Lyme disease affects the nervous system and joints in a majority of cases.

Normally bacteria thrive best in a warm blooded environment, which is in direct polarity to the cold blooded environment preferred by viruses. Here we find the two microbes going at it with devastating results.

Borrelia burgdorferi are anaerobic organisms, bacteria that cannot survive in a high oxygen environment. They are, like all bacteria, viruses and fungi, predominantly positively charged electromagnetically and need the body to bring down its predominantly negative polarity before it can replicate and thrive. When a tissue is cold, as in a low body temperature person, the metabolic rate, or chemical reactions that normally create heat, are slowed down. As the metabolic rate slows, all of the body fluids cool as well. The oxygen supply to the tissues becomes depleted as the blood supply feeding the tissue with oxygen also cools down. As the blood cools it becomes more viscous, or syrupy, in consistency, which decreases its oxygen-carrying capability. The body become hypoxic, hyper-acidic, and only weakly negatively charged at the cellular level – all creating a wonderful environment for Lyme spirochetes to grow and thrive.

Any effective fight against Lyme disease would necessarily need to include therapies and lifestyle changes that would increase the core body temperature, increase the body's alkalinity and strengthen the body's normal electromagnetic negative polarity.

Immediate improvement in symptoms should follow the increase in body temperature as the body fluids begin to liquefy from their cold syrupy state and the oxygen-carrying ability returns to normal. As you increase oxygen in the tissues, you decrease acidity, increase negative polarity and kill Lyme bacteria!

Lyme disease requires a very multi-faceted treatment approach. It is a systemic infection and is poorly understood by most doctors. Chronic infections lasting years are common due to the prevalent mentality of the germ theory. As in all infectious diseases it is erroneous to think "I will be well when my doctor figures out how to kill all of these bacteria." You will be well when your body is no longer a happy home environment for the bacteria and viruses, and when the balance is restored in the tissues and entire organism that is you! You would have never manifested the disease, even if a tick injected you with a load of Borrelia burgdorferi spirochetes, unless your body as a whole was way out of balance to start with.

Most people who have recovered from chronic Lyme disease are terrified of getting bitten again and contracting the disease again. These people need never be afraid again if they and their healthcare team will take the time to understand and implement the principles presented in this book.

Treatment of Lyme Disease: This treatment recommendation is not designed to itemize every possible medicine or treatment possibility, but is designed to be used as a total program of care. Efforts should be made to use or integrate as many of the recommendations as possible for maximum healing.

1. Borrelogen™
2. Microbojen™
3. Neuro-Antitox Formulas™
4. Wobenzym™-N
5. Hyperbaric Oxygen Therapy
6. Magnetic Resonance Bio-Oxidative Therapy
7. Essential Oil Support
8. Support Structural and Bio-electrical integrity through Chiropractic care
9. BRADE (Bio-Resonance Allergy Desensitization and Elimination technique)

10. Constitutional Support
11. Support Detoxification and Elimination of the body
12. Follow all guidelines for raising a low core body temperature
13. Maintain a high normal urine pH

Treatment Rationale:

• The frequency matching to a medicine or treatment modality, as in Bio-Resonance Scanning™, is believed to work by identifying the most closely matching resonance frequencies to those frequencies the body is already generating to bring the microbes back under control. It stands to reason that the body by God's design generates specific frequencies and subtle energies to maintain balance. To recoup this point, using herbs to specifically kill microbes FOR the body is no better than taking an antibiotic to kill them.

• **Borrelogen™** is the primary and flagship nutraceutical for this Lyme protocol. It is a frequency-matched botanical formula specifically designed to match and enhance the body's own energy necessary to bring into balance the overgrowth of all of the pleomorphic stages of Borrelia burgdorferi, as well as the often seen co-infections of Babesia microti, Human monocytic and granulocytic Ehrlichia, and the elusive Human Herpes Virus-6. Borrelogen™ is a combination of botanicals specifically selected for their unique combined molecular crystalline vibrational matrix, as opposed to their specific chemical constituents as in most medicines. To my knowledge Borrelogen™ is the only formulation specifically designed to frequency-match the energy matrix of the body in order to assist the body in restoring control of these microbial possibilities. A starting dosage is generally 2 droppers, 2-3 times per day, half that for children and really sensitive or symptomatic people. It can be taken with or without food. This dosage should be maintained for two months beyond resolution of symptoms. Borrelogen™ may be rubbed in topically to affected areas, such as joints and muscles, or added to bathwater.

• **Microbojen™** is a complex frequency-matched formula containing Tragopogon herba, Isatis root, Glycerrhiza uralensis root, Lasiosphaera fungus, Scrophularia root, Oldenlandia herba,

Moutan peony bark, Phellodendron bark, Poria cocos sclerotium.

Advanced Techniques for Using Borrelogen™ or Microbojen™ For Healthcare Professionals Only

Advanced Technique #1: In that Borrelogen and Microbojen are liquid supplements, it is easy to add low potency homeopathic sarcodes (homeopathically potentized body tissues) into the bottle of Borrelogen or Microbojen to help direct or drive it specifically to the affected areas of the body. In that Borrelogen and Microbojen are primarily frequency-based formulas they will not be as restricted in where they will go in the body. Their energetic information works within the body's own communication network, and seems to not be as restricted by cell membranes and absorption issues as conventional medicines. However, in tough cases, I like to use sarcodes to further open the communication pathways specifically being affected by Lyme, as the disease process itself seems to interfere with the communication and self-regulation efforts of the body.

The lower potency sarcodes, (3x or 6x) will bring up the vitality of weak, hypo-functional tissue, while higher potencies like 30x sarcodes can help the body bring down a hyper-stimulated tissue of the body. Between these potencies, a 12x will have a more balancing effect when the tissue is not under or over active and simply needs support.

Careful monitoring of the continued need of this sarcode-imprinted Borrelogen must be maintained during the use of this technique to insure that hyper or hypo-stimulation of the body tissues does not occur. If one feels the need to balance the tissue, finish the treatment with a middle potency of a 12x sarcode given by itself for as long as is needed.

Advanced technique #2: Borrelogen and Microbojen are complex botanical formulas with resonance signatures unique to the interaction of their combined ingredients. Healthcare professionals can therefore use one of the many "homeo-bioenergetic" imprinting devices on the market to take an energetic "potentized" imprint of Borrelogen and imprint it into various essential oils which are high in sesquiterpones and sesquiterpenes. These substances in the following oils are known to cross the blood-brain barrier. Once imprinted with the energetic signature of Borrelogen, the oils appear to carry it across the blood-brain barrier, naturally oxygenating the brain tissues, and glands, and also delivering the corrective healing energy of Borrelogen to affected brain tissues. Essential oils high in sesquiterpenes and sesquiterpones are frankincense, sandalwood, helichrysum, and lavender. I often use the combination "Brain Power" by Young Living Oils for this purpose, and apply it over the brainstem, scalp, and reflex points to the brain on the foot, hand, ears, and teeth two to three times per day.

(Of interesting note: "Research has shown that sesquiterpenes play a role in dissolving petrochemicals along the receptor sites near the pituitary gland and increase the amount of oxygen in those areas." (Higley C, Higley A, Reference Guide for Essential Oils 2001 Abundant Health Publishing)

Advanced technique #3: Call any microbial specimen supply house for microscopic specimen on slides and obtain a microscope slide of each of the Lyme microbes. Using the principle of "direct resonance" testing one can hold the slide over parts of the patient's body while performing a muscle test. To do this, with the patient laying supine, use the arm extended perpendicular to the body, and the palm of the hand facing out away from the body, grasp the arm just below the wrist (not over the carpal bones) and instruct the patient to "hold strong" while you gently, but firmly pull the arm in the direction of the patient's feet. You don't have to pull hard. You are simply looking to see that the patients arm muscle "locks" immediately, demonstrating good integrity of the energy supply to that muscle. Now with the strong muscle identified, move the slide over the patient's problem areas, such as the liver, colon, joints, small intestines, spine, shoulders, or wherever, each time you move the slide over an area, test the muscle strength. If the previously strong muscle goes weak, let's say over the transverse colon, and then you have identified an area containing Lyme spirochetes, or whatever the microbe is on the slide. Basically, you are frequency matching the molecular structure of the death microbe on the slide, which is "fixed" on the slide and therefore its molecular structure as not degraded or disintegrated, to the same frequency of the molecular structure of the live microbes in that area of the body. Having identified the specific spot in the body, using a pen or marker, draw the zone on the patient so they know precisely where it is. Now using the Borrelogen, Microbojen, or combination of the two, saturate the gauss pad of a 4"x6" Band-Aid brand bandage/s and cover the area. This should be replaced two times per day, and at the very least be worn to bed at night. This type of treatment works like the medicinal transdermal patches that are so popular these days. Of course the patient should continue taking the remedies internally as well.

Advanced Understanding about the Recommended Treatments:

• **Neuro-Antitox™** may be one of the most important supplements in any effective Lyme protocol. In theory, a person could have Lyme bacteria and yet have no symptoms if the toxins alone were addressed. This product should be considered especially in patients who have severe symptoms. Although Lyme spirochete toxins are known to be neurotoxins, their effect is not limited to neurological symptoms. As research has demonstrated, virtually all of the symptoms are in fact due to these toxins, making the bacteria only the indirect cause.

While the true gem in this formula is the Silphium laciniatum, the sarcobioenergetic potencies are the components that get the Silphium and other ingredients to the affected tissues. This is a state of the science technology working in the embryonic field of biophysics. One can have the world's best antitoxin, but if it cannot reach the area of the body containing the toxins it will not work. Besides serving as a driving agent, these sarcobioenergetic potencies have a harmonizing effect of the corresponding tissues of the body.

Clinical findings demonstrate these sarcobioenergetic potencies follow closely the anticipated effect of true isopathic sarcodes. That being, a low potency of D6 myocardium tissue will increase the function of the corresponding tissue in the patient, while a D12 potency will balance and harmonize the tissue, and a D30 will bring down a hyper or overactive tissue. The effect of all three potencies added together as in this formula results in an increased overall healing and harmonizing effect of the tissues involved while eliminating much of the single potency potential for energetic injury to the tissues of the patient. In that these sarcobioenergetic potencies are not true homeopathic sarcodes (manufactured from repeated dilution and succussion of a mother substance), the designation P6, P12, and P30 are used to indicate a similar anticipated effect.

• **Wobenzym™-N** seems to help remove interference in the tissues to allow the movement of healing energy and medicines. Volumes of research over many years and millions of people bring strong confidence in this well-known systemic enzyme. Its many benefits include immune system support, anti-inflammatory activity and acceleration of the rate of healing. Wobenzym™-N in my experience also helps restore the body's warmth organization through breaking up the accumulation of antigen/antibody complexes and by freeing the metabolic processes from their cold, sclerotic, low output. It seems that in Lyme disease, as in many cold/sclerotic illnesses, the body's chemical reactions (metabolism) are being held captive, and the energy-producing mechanisms of the cellular factories have wrenches in all of their gears. Wobenzym™-N seems to remove these wrenches over time by directly and indirectly breaking up excessive protein accumulations in the intracellular spaces. Excessive protein, as we have said, promotes darkness and cold, therefore Wobenzym™-N should break up the darkness allowing the light and warmth metabolism to be restored by the other treatments specifically designed to do so. Dosage is large due to the fact that these enzymes are used up as they work their way through to the farthest reaches of the body. Generally start with 11 pills, 3 times per day, on a completely empty stomach. An empty stomach is at least 2 hours after eating and 45 minutes before eating. This is not a digestive enzyme, it is a systemic enzyme. This dosage should be maintained for 1 month, then reduced to 6-8 pills, 2-3 times per day thereafter for six months to a year, or as directed by your doctor.

- **Molybdenum** is a mineral that helps to detoxify the various toxins common in the die-off of Lyme-related organisms. Dosage: 300 micrograms 3-4 times per day, with or without food.

- **Magnetic Resonance Bio-Oxidative Therapy** (MRBT) is one of the most critical treatments in restoring the total body integrity. This is not to be confused with the multi-level companies selling mixed positive and negative polarity magnetic products. These ceramic magnets are the actual magnets researched and developed by Dr. William H. Philpott, M.D., the pioneer and genius of the use of heavy ceramic magnets of not just high-gauss strength, but deep penetration of negative polarity. Research and clinical experience reveal that sustained exposure to only negative polarity of high-gauss strength has an antibiotic effect due to the fact that it creates a hyper-oxygenation of the body, helps restore the energetic properties of the cellular crystalline matrix, breaks down and eliminates the toxins and acid that support the bacteria, viruses and fungi, and restores the body's ability to maintain the normal strongly negative polarity of the inside of cells thus restoring the strongly positive exterior of the cells, which repels the positively charged microbes and is what controls the replication of microbes. If that were not enough, then the anti-inflammatory action and increased healing rate of neurological and musculoskeletal tissues of MRBT should interest every chronic Lyme sufferer. MRBT desensitizes one to substances causing allergic hypersensitivities. It is neurologically calming and promotes the increased release of melatonin which is itself antibiotic in effect as well as the substance in the brain responsible for a deep, refreshing sleep. In chronic Lyme as in all degenerative diseases I recommend the Super ceramic Magnetic Bed. We are talking about 400 pounds of ceramic magnets creating a therapeutically high-gauss negative polarity field rising at greater than 18 inches above the bed. There are 70 one-inch-thick ceramic magnets held in two 3 ft. by 3 ft. sections of 200 pounds each! (Yes, delivery men will set this up in your bed) This offers maximum yield for maximum healing. For Central Nervous System Lyme with neurological symptoms I would add the Super Magnetic Head Unit that is made with 60 pounds of ceramic magnets that focus high-gauss all the way through the head while the body is benefiting from the bed. This is the latest in non-toxic, non-invasive, high-effect therapy. I also recommend you place a bi-temporal wrap with 1 1/2" x 1/2" ceramic magnets over the temples at the level of the top of the ears and 1" in front of the ear. This will help calm the nervous system, and improve cognitive ability while easing any cerebral allergies and relaxing the hypersensitive emotions many Lyme patients experience. This should be worn as much as possible during your waking hours. Another very beneficial therapy is to strap on a 4" x 6" x 1/2" ceramic magnet over the heart (running lengthwise to the body), and another one strapped over the stomach (running horizontal to the body). These should be worn 24 hours per day if possible. Always place the negative polarity toward the skin (These magnets are comfort covered and are marked "not this side" on the positive polarity side to eliminate any confusion). The magnet over the heart will help the heart regulate itself better, kill microbes, and electromagnetically recharge the blood flowing through up to 50,000 miles of blood vessels. This may also normalize blood pressure and eliminate arrhythmia and angina. The magnet over the stomach will help correct any food allergies, improve the health and pH of the digestive organs, and help normalize blood sugar, not to mention decrease abdominal bloating and pain. Research shows that the MRBT will soften and often eliminate scar tissue. However, it is too soon to know if plaquing in the brain can be reversed, though I anticipate this at some point. Dental infections, cavitations, sinus congestion, and even cancer patients have benefited from MRBT. Although no medical claims are made by anyone due to lack of control-study research and governmental restrictions, anecdotal and clinical evidence is overwhelming.

- **Hyperbaric Oxygen Therapy** is highly beneficial. No other therapy can saturate every nook and cranny of the body. Within the first 30 minutes of HBOT every tissue of the body (yes, even the brain and nerve tissue) is saturated with oxygen. In that a cold body does not carry oxygen efficiently, external assistance is essential. Cells begin to degenerate and die in direct proportion to oxygen deficiency. All of the chemical reactions in the body require oxygen. With the saturation of the tissues with oxygen, the cellular energy goes up and the warmth organization of the body can finally get busy with its job. There are various HBOT protocols for Lyme disease, but I recommend hitting it hard and fast to start with. One hour sessions, two times per day, should be performed in the first five days. Neurological Lyme symptoms seem to respond best at 2.5 atmospheres, while joint and muscular symptoms seem to respond better at 3 to 3.5 atmospheres. Depending upon the advancement of your condition to start with, and the response to care, HBOT sessions should continue from there, one hour, every other day, such as Monday, Wednesday and Friday, for about a total of 48 sessions, or as directed by your doctor.

Chapter 15

Example Schedule of Circuit Healing™ For Doctors and Healthcare Professionals

I am providing this information as a general guide for doctors so they can know how to implement the therapies and information in this book. Of course every patient is unique and therefore the use of sensitive testing, such as Bio-Resonance Scanning™, or kinesiology during each visit to adapt treatments is preferable. One cannot rely solely upon remedies and medicines. Health in a bottle is a myth. Medicines are just one type of tool needed to assist the body in healing itself. The following schedule is designed to fully address all four ways that the body can experience illness–structural, chemical, stress-related and bio-electrical problems. We offer training seminars for doctors to become trained in these and other treatment and therapeutic techniques.

I like to print up a two-week treatment schedule such as this tailored for every new patient. This schedule is based upon seeing a new patient three times a week. Giving the patient a copy of this book will enable them to have all of the explanations of the remedies, treatments and therapies, as well as provide all of the reading assignments. Since most people are more used to conventional doctors not seeing them so often, this allows the patient to understand what you plan to do and what is expected of them. Notice that the total amount of time spent during the day is quite a lot. You will need to help the new patient understand that your goal is to hit it hard and fast at the start so that they may heal that much faster.

Be sure to follow up on each visit as to how well they performed their home therapies and assignments, and troubleshoot any problems they are having.

A Sample 2 Week Patient Schedule (patient seen Monday, Wednesday, Friday. Some patients may need to be seen every day of the week depending on the severity of the symptoms.)

During a patient's visit with us we will be addressing many health issues with them. The following will outline the next two weeks with us, as well as some of the treatments and therapies I plan to use. No two patients are alike, therefore this outline is a general plan subject to many changes as the body responds to the treatments.

The goal of every visit is to facilitate healing in the body by removing anything interfering with optimal function, while at the same time providing the information and building blocks it needs to heal. The miasmatic predisposition and inherited tendencies to the patient's unique health history will be addressed as well to hopefully attain the desired result of eliminating the inborn cause so that a disease-free life can be realized.

Day 1 Treatments:

- Adjustment of the spine, pelvis, cranium, clear any hiatal hernia manually

- Rebalancing of electromagnetic body fields with MRBT and essential oils

- Assess the Ilio-cecal valve and Valve of Houston, other soft-tissue issues

- Address the primary chemical problems, i.e., virus, bacteria, toxins, etc…

- Insure all organ circuits are up and running at maximum efficiency

- Bio-Resonance check of all supplements

Day 1 In-office Therapies:

- ST8 Lymphatic Drainage Therapy (30 minutes) Morning

- Ion-Cleanse Detoxification (40 minutes) Morning

- Infrared Sauna Therapy (30-45 minutes) Morning and Afternoon

- Microcurrent Therapy (20 minutes) Afternoon (optional)

- Color / Music Therapy

Day 1 Home Therapies:

- Magnetic Resonance Bio-Oxidative Therapy (Negative polarity over heart 24 hrs/day.

- Wear Tesla Watch (Everyday)

- Sleep in Peat Fiber Bedding (optional)

- Dry Skin Brushing (before bath or shower)

- Solum Uliginosum Bath Essence soak –this essence contains peat and other extracts formulated to stimulate the body's warmth organization and helps with rheumatic diseases, people with weather sensitivities (symptoms worse with weather changes), spinal disorders, nerve pains and chronic pains of other origin

- Iodine Skin Stain Test

- Practice Meditation technique of choice.

- Record morning and evening body temperature

Day 1 Reading Assignments:

- Quiet Mind

- Meditation Techniques

- Diet Chapter/Eating based upon your blood type

Day 2 Treatments:

- Perform and address multiple neurological disorganization issues

- Scar Therapies, Low-level Laser, MRBT in conjunction with essential oils, balancing of the body's electromagnetic fields

Day 2 In-office Therapies:

- ST8 Lymphatic Drainage Therapy (30 minutes)

- Ion-Cleanse Detoxification (40 minutes)

- Infrared Sauna Therapy (30-45 minutes) Morning and Evening

- Microcurrent Therapy (20 minutes) optional)

- Color / Music Therapy

Day 2 Home therapies:

- Magnetic Resonance Bio-Oxidative Therapy (Negative polarity over heart 24 hours/day

- Dry Skin Brushing (before bath or shower)

- Solum Uliginosum Bath Essence soak–This essence contains peat and other extracts formulated to stimulate the body's warmth organization and helps with rheumatic diseases, people with weather sensitivities (symptoms worse with weather changes), spinal disorders, nerve pains and chronic pains of other origin

- Iodine Skin Stain Test

- Practice Meditation technique of choice from this book.

- Record morning and evening body temperature

Day 2 Reading Assignments:

- Controlling Your Thinking

Day 3 Treatments:

- BRADE #1 Organs… (Bio-Resonance Allergy Desensitization and Elimination technique) hypersensitivity treatments, using color, sound, laser, isopathic remedies, essential oils

Day 3 In-office Therapies:

- ST8 Lymphatic Drainage Therapy (30 minutes) Morning

- Ion-Cleanse Detoxification (40 minutes) Morning

- Infrared Sauna Therapy (30-45 minutes) Morning and Afternoon

- Microcurrent Therapy (20 minutes) Afternoon

- Color / Music Therapy

Day 3 Home Therapies:

- 25-hour food avoidances from BRADE treatment

- Magnetic Resonance Bio-Oxidative Therapy (Negative polarity over heart 24 hrs/day

- Dry Skin Brushing

- Detox Bath #1 (Hydrogen Peroxide/ Epsom Salts/ Ginger)

- Iodine Skin Stain Test

- Practice Meditation technique of choice from this book.

- Aerobic Walking

- Record morning and evening body temperature

Day 3 Reading Assignments:

- Who Are You on the Inside?

Day 4 Treatments:

- Cranial Fixation/fascia release in multiple postures

- Adjustment of spinal/structural problems

- Determine and address miasms

Day 4 In-office Therapies:

- ST8 Lymphatic Drainage Therapy (30 minutes) Morning

- Ion-Cleanse Detoxification (40 minutes) Morning

- Infrared Sauna Therapy (30-45 minutes) Morning and Afternoon

- Microcurrent Therapy (20 minutes) Afternoon (Optional)

Day 4 Home therapies:

- Magnetic Resonance Bio-Oxidative Therapy (Negative polarity over heart 24 hrs/day

- Detox Bath #1 (Hydrogen Peroxide/ Epsom Salts/ Ginger)

- Iodine Skin Stain Test

- Practice Meditation technique of choice from this book.

- Aerobic Walking

- Record morning and evening body temperature

Day 5 Treatments:

- BRADE #2 Glands… hypersensitivity treatments, using color, sound, laser, isopathic remedies, meridian stimulation

- Adjustment of structural problems

- Rebalancing of electromagnetic body fields with MRBT and

essential oils

- Bio-Resonance check all supplements
- Insure all organ circuits are up and running at maximum efficiency

Day 5 In-office Therapies:

- ST8 Lymphatic Drainage Therapy (30 minutes) Morning
- Ion-Cleanse Detoxification (40 minutes) Morning
- Infrared Sauna Therapy (30-45 minutes) Morning and Afternoon
- Microcurrent Therapy (20 minutes) Afternoon
- Color / Music Therapy

Day 5 Home therapies:

- 25-hour food avoidances from BRADE treatment
- Magnetic Resonance Bio-Oxidative Therapy (Negative polarity over heart 24 hours/day
- Strengthening/Nutritive Bath
- Iodine Skin Stain Test
- Practice Meditation technique of choice from this book
- Record morning and evening body temperature

Day 5 Reading Assignments:

- Redesigning Your Life to Overcome Illness

Day 6 Treatments:

- BRADE #3 Hormones… hypersensitivity treatments, using color, sound, laser, isopathic remedies, meridian stimulation
- Adjustment of structural problems
- Rebalancing of electromagnetic body fields with MRBT and essential oils
- Address Miasms

- Recheck all remedies to ensure microbes have not mutated around the remedies and that all of the body circuits are up and running at 100% efficiency

Day 6 In-office Therapies:

- ST8 Lymphatic Drainage Therapy (30 minutes) Morning

- Ion-Cleanse Detoxification (40 minutes) Morning

- Infrared Sauna Therapy (30-45 minutes) Morning and Afternoon

- Microcurrent Therapy (20 minutes) Afternoon

Day 6 Home Therapies:

- 25 hour food avoidances from BRADE treatment

- Magnetic Resonance Bio-Oxidative Therapy (Negative polarity over heart 24 hours/day

- Dry Skin Brushing

- Solum Uliginsom Bath Essence soak –This essence contains peat and other extracts formulated to stimulate the body's warmth organization and helps with rheumatic diseases, people with weather sensitivities (symptoms worse with weather changes), spinal disorders, nerve pains and chronic pains of other origin

- Iodine Skin Stain Test

- Practice Meditation technique of choice from this book.

- Mild Aerobic activity

- Record morning and evening body temperature

Day 6 Reading Assignments:

- Read "47 Thoughts to Live On"

It is recommended that a Magnetic Resonance Bio-Oxidative Therapy Bed be used continuously for six months to a year beyond the disappearance of symptoms, and then sleep on the bed periodically for preventive purposes thereafter. This creates an environment in the body that is optimal for health and healing. Although claims are made for "cure" using magnetic devices, the truth is that they simply create hyper-oxygenation, alkalinity, allow the cells to function on oxidative phosphorilation instead of fermentation, empowers the body to repel viruses, bacteria and fungi, and detoxifies the chemical and heavy metal toxins. If that were not enough, the negative polarity stimulates the immune system and increases the rate of healing in every tissue. All of these are requirements for destroying the mechanisms that lead to cancer and other degenerative illness.

Section 3

Changing Your Internal Environment So Lyme Microbes Won't Grow

Chapter 16

Lyme and Low Body Temperature

One of the very common findings I have noticed in chronic Lyme sufferers is a low body temperature or at least a very unregulated distribution of temperature in the body. I am not here promoting the hyperthermia treatments that are being used to kill Lyme spirochetes. I am not necessarily opposed to their use, but this chapter deals primarily with the importance of restoring and maintaining a normal core body temperature. This is true not just in Lyme disease but in every degenerative disease of our day.

Your core body temperature is the temperature taken under the tongue. When human physiology books refer to the "normal" core body temperature it is presented as a range sometimes listed between 97.0-99.0°F . Understand that the "Normal Range" for temperature or even the normal ranges in blood tests are based upon the average person of our day. That is why "normal" changes periodically, because as our average population continues to get sicker the Normal Ranges must be adjusted. So in this discussion I am speaking about what is an *optimal* core body temperature – 98.6-99.6°F.

Much emphasis is usually placed upon feverish conditions; however, a low body temperature is a much more sinister condition. Where a fever can be viewed as an active developmental and corrective process of the healthy body, a low body temperature can never be viewed as a normal or healthy condition, nor is it a mechanism for a learning or developmental process in the body. A low body temperature creates a happy home for viruses and chronic infections, and is a sign of degeneration and gradual cellular death.

Low body temperature is the plague of the 21st century. People with low body temperature have a weak reaction to even the most ideal medicines and therapies. As the body's core temperature becomes cold, the energetic crystalline matrix experiences a systemic collapse as tissues condense and cellular tensegrity, the infrastructure of the intra- and extracellular matrix, loses its structural conductivity and integrity. The cooperative and collective intelligence of the human organism is short-circuited as the body temperature cools. As a result, all cellular functions decrease. There is a decrease in the production of all hormones, neurotransmitters and other body chemicals necessary for normal healthy balance. As a result, there is an increased susceptibility to infectious disease. As temperature drops, the acidity of the body increases and the normally predominantly negative polarity of the cells become more positively charged. I will go into the polarity issues in more detail later.

The colder the body becomes, the more prone the person becomes to depression and other psychological abnormalities and all degenerative illnesses of the body, mind and spirit.

Until the causes of the lowered temperature are addressed and corrected, the best that can be hoped for is only temporary or mild improvement of symptoms and a gradual but steady overall decline in health.

Viruses prefer and promote a cold environment and replicate at a much more rapid rate when the body is cold. Viruses are killed and further replication is impeded by maintaining a warm body. Some bacteria such as Lyme spirochetes also prefer and promote a cold environment and can remain in a chronic state as long as their cold environment is maintained. Therefore, in the interest of the prevention and treatment of any viral, bacterial, or chronic illness, this topic must be understood.

The ultimate body coldness is seen in death. When observing a corpse many clinical gems can be gleaned and correlated to degenerative states of human suffering. In death, the blood and lymph fluid of the body solidify and the body becomes stiff and cold. In the same way, in many chronic cold illnesses such as Lyme disease, fibromyalgia, chronic fatigue, diabetes and cancer, we see that the body becomes progressively colder. As the body cools, the electrical oscillations of the fluids in the body slow down and there is a shift in the body's polarity which promotes infectious microbes and cancer.

We can see the same principle of what happens in the body by observing the same dynamics in a water molecule. When the electrical oscillations of a water molecule slow down it becomes a solid, ice. As we speed up a water molecule's electrical oscillations it liquefies and ultimately becomes a vapor.

The colder a body becomes, the slower the electrical oscillatory rate and therefore the thicker, more viscous, or syrupy the body fluids become. The more viscous the fluids become the more difficult it is for the body to push the fluids through the body. The lymph fluids that are normally supposed to bathe the outsides of all of your cells become progressively stagnant as it is too thick to move efficiently. Now, consider the fact that just like your skin is constantly dying and flaking off and being replaced, so it is that every cell in your body is in a constant state of dying and being replaced. Only now the cold, syrupy lymph fluid cannot wash the dead cellular debris away. As a result the body becomes a toxic waste dump!

Muscles normally have a high demand for energy. Due to the constant contraction and relaxation mechanism of muscle tissue, muscles assist in eliminating their own cellular waste products. In a cold body however, the liquidity of the fluids inside of the muscles is gone, and the muscles cannot move the toxins and cellular debris. The deeper you go into the belly or center of the muscle, the more difficult it is to move the toxins. All muscular contraction grinds to a halt, like an engine with no lubricating oil. The belly of the muscle develops a knot that can be felt when massaging the muscle. This is the knotted, painful, muscle condition commonly known as "trigger points" of Fibromyalgia Syndrome, which is being diagnosed in millions of people every year. If the low body temperature is allowed to persist and no therapies are applied, even in a palliative manner as in massages to move toxins manually out of the belly of the muscle, the condition follows that of the water molecule. The belly of the muscle, due to the increasing coldness and decreased muscular activity, progressively over time reaches the point of zero electrical oscillations at which time the tissue solidifies in a calcified stone in the belly of the muscle.

Interesting research that supports this concept has been performed by Dr. Carolyn McMakin, D.C., using the electrotherapy called microcurrent. The microcurrent is applied through direct contact on these trigger points via vinyl/graphite gloves connected to the microcurrent machine. The trigger points virtually vanish under the gentle touch of the glove when applying the correct electrical frequency. What may be happening here is that the stimulation of the muscle through microcurrent is externally increasing the electrical oscillatory rate of the thickened fluids in the muscle resulting in temporarily restoring the normal liquidity of the fluids, allowing the muscles to once again contract and pump out the toxic accumulation. The results are somewhat temporary due to the fact that the underlying condition that created it in our scenario, the overall low body temperature, remains unchanged. However, used in combination with various other corrective measures, this microcurrent therapy can speed healing in many cases. *Relief of Fibromyalgia Through Microcurrent Therapy* by John W. Addington, ImmuneSupport.com 7-11-2001

To continue on with the other degenerative aspects going on in the body, we can once again see that the body is set up on electrical circuits, all of which are interdependent and interconnected. One circuit in the body cannot go down without ultimately affecting the whole. Therefore, if the muscle is seizing up and becoming progressively rigid and solidified, what do you suppose the organ that is also on that same electrical circuit is doing? It is likely that to some degree it is also progressively seizing up and solidifying.

In the many miles of blood vessels, the cold, thick blood is more difficult to push through the veins and arteries. Arteriosclerosis, the progressive hardening of the arteries and the clogging of the blood vessels, is manifesting the exact same problem that is being experienced by every tissue in the too cold body. Edema in the extremities is seen as the muscular walls of the blood vessels seize up and can no longer maintain tone and the fluid leaks out of the pores of the vessels.

I look at many older patients and some not so old who are experiencing all the signs and symptoms of death in the extremities. They are dying in their extremities first, from the feet and hands up to the torso. To touch their feet is just like touching an icy, stiff, dead corpse. The foot is deathly whitish blue and etched in blue/black blood vessels from devitalized, stagnant blood.

The overcooling of peripheral blood returning from cold legs and feet causes depression of the temperature in the vital organs with slowing of metabolic processes, particularly in the brain and medullary centers. Cotran R.S., Kumar V., Robbins S.L., Robbin's Pathological Basis of Disease 4th ed. 1989 pp501. Death occurs when a vital organ reaches the point of being too cold. Your physician can name your disease, he can draw your blood and show you everything that is wrong with it, but he is simply describing the process I have just outlined. When the core temperature of the body is cold, every organ, gland and tissue is affected and becomes hypo-functional. Hypo-functional means that there are fewer hormones and less of every chemical involved with normal body and brain function. Even the psyche is affected, leading to virtually any type of psychological problem, especially depression. How many people are told that they have psychological depression from a deficiency of a certain brain chemical? Many! Can you see that of course they are deficient in "happy" brain chemicals possibly due to the overcooling of the body?

It could be said that you are dying in direct proportion to the coldness of your body. Follow this logic: Cells die in direct proportion to the depletion of oxygen. Blood that is overcooled from a cold core temperature is too thick to efficiently carry oxygen and the lung vital capacity is reduced, leading to shallow breathing. This means that the oxygen to carbon dioxide exchange rate in the lungs is minimal. Now combine the degenerative effects of the oxygen deprivation and the cold temperature and the fact that all of this and the overgrowth of microbes promote an acidic environment and you have greatly accelerated cellular degeneration and the onset of life-threatening disease.

There is an optimum body temperature which all chemical reactions in the human body need in order to maintain health... 98.6° F. I can honestly say that I have never seen a new patient come into my clinic with a normal body temperature. Just this week a 66 year old woman came in as a new patient with a temperature of 94.6! She is in dire straits for certain. She could not feel her feet and to touch her legs was like touching the legs of a corpse. The legs even looked dead and grey, streaked with blue/black veins of stagnant devitalized blood. Even in classic hypothermia as seen in people stranded in blizzards, it is well known that the circulation of blood in the arms and legs is reduced dramatically, almost to zero, in order to provide protection and warmth to the vital organs. These people will also cease to feel cold and will experience numbness, loss of coordination, mental confusion and heart rhythm problems. It sounds like I am describing many elderly people, and some Lyme sufferers doesn't it?

One way to treat weather-related hypothermia is to give the person warm sugar drinks. Sugar is a cheap, fast burning fuel for your body and therefore generates a lot of heat in the process. This may be why so many people suffering from lifestyle-induced cold core temperature are plagued with sugar cravings. Many of them consume copious amounts of sugar in the form of soda pops, chocolate, pastries and various candies. It may be a craving that is driven by the body's desire to generate fast heat to keep the body functioning. Sugar cravings should diminish as the core body temperature problems are resolved.

Keep in mind that the body has been too cold possibly since birth, due to suppressive medicines, vaccines, fever reducers, heavy metal and chemical toxins, and energetically dead foods. The retraining and resetting of the body's thermostat is just the beginning of healing the body of chronic illnesses. The normal body temperature must be held steady possibly for a year or more in some cases before the body can undo the damage of a lifetime of coldness.

Everyone can afford a simple thermometer. Track your temperature when you first awaken in the morning, before even getting out of bed. This reflects your core body temperature, when it is not being influenced by what you just ate, drank or your activity level. Many of you will likely be surprised to see just how cold you already are. This is the result of generations of suppressive therapies and an imbalanced life. You must save yourself.

Many doctors will undoubtedly say that you need to take a thyroid medication to bring up the body temperature; however, this is the same mentality of taking a Tylenol for a headache. If you don't believe me then ask anyone on the prescription thyroid medicines what happens when they go off of the medication. The body returns immediately to the previous cold condition. Definitely support the normal functioning of the thyroid, by detoxification, organic iodine and nutritional support, but see the coldness for what it really is, a sign of multi-organ system breakdown and longstanding or even generational imbalance. Besides, it is really the hypothalamus that regulates your core body temperature, along with your degree of motivation and sex drive. The hypothalamus is actually "upstream" from your thyroid. It helps the pituitary regulate the thyroid.

The healthy body has daily temperature fluctuations (diurnal) with the coolest temperature in the early morning hours, and the warmest being in the evening between 8-10 pm, after having rested for half and hour. Tracking of the difference between morning and evening temperature should reveal, in a healthy person, a difference of at least 0.9° F (0.5° C). People with a low body temperature and an overall degenerative condition will find that this temperature variation is minimal. Another unusual finding of dysregulated body temperature is that the evening is often colder than the morning reading.

The body's best chance at long-term healing increases in direct proportion to the restoration of normal body temperature and its normal diurnal fluctuation.

You and your healthcare team must address your body from every direction and with every balancing tool available. You can never truly overcome this condition with pills. Therapies must engage and reactivate and stimulate the rhythmical, metabolic and nerve/sense aspects of your body, addressing the body, mind and spirit.

In a cold body there is always a disruption of the rhythmical aspects of the organism; that part of you that establishes balance between the metabolic and nerve/sense aspects of your body. No other medicine can restore this better than Iscar®, a European, injectable, prescription homeopathic medicine. Iscar does not artificially cause the body to heat up in the way many dietary supplements do, such as ephedra (ma huang) commonly used in weight loss supplements.

Other supporting therapies designed for restoring the rhythms of the body must be applied. These therapies might include color and sound therapy, hot and cold contrast therapy, life-activity planning, breathing and voice therapy, rhythmical massage therapy, curative movement therapies, and indeed, every other treatment from your doctor will address in some way the rhythmical aspects of your body. Peat clothing and oils also have unique properties that make this natural plant fiber ideal in the restoration of the warmth organization of the body.

Low body temperature must be addressed to bring the body back to balance. The temperature must be elevated to end the dying process of the body and to help the body eliminate the cellular debris or the "sludge" in the body.

Treatment: (Even though Iscar is the primary treatment, if you cannot incorporate Iscar injections, do as many of the following therapies as possible and track your temperature)

(For your convenience, there is an order form in the back of this book.)

- Iscar® injections (Weleda) in the morning, when the body temperature should naturally be rising (see rationale below)

  Women: Iscar-Mali® (initial phase) every other day

  Men: Iscar-Quercus® (initial phase) every other day

- Temperature monitoring and graphing (upon awakening, and between 8-10 pm after a 30 minute resting period)

- Infrared Sauna Therapy – detoxifies body and restores circulation of blood and lymph

- Dry skin brushing morning and evening (entire body)

- Bath Therapies…Nutritive bath, Detox bath #1 and #2… take one bath per night before bedtime, alternating in the above sequence

- Mustard foot baths… at least once per day, preferably in the morning or early afternoon

- Teslar Watch®

- Peat/wool blend products (I recommend at least the mattress pad and comforter)

- Peat/wool socks: wear all day, especially in cold weather

- Peat/wool shoe insoles…always

- Peat/wool kidney wrap…worn during waking hours, especially in cold weather

- Peat/wool hat/cap…indoors and out due to the fact that heat escapes through the head as heat rises

- Peat/wool bedding…mattress pad and comforter

- Peat/wool apron computer shield… whenever using a computer

- Peat/wool seat cover…good for putting underneath a laptop computer when using it on your lap

- Equisetum Oil (Wala/Raphael) over kidneys… apply over kidneys 2-3 times per day

- Cuprum/Nicotiana Ointment (Wala/Raphael) apply daily to soles of feet morning (If using the mustard foot bath in the morning, apply ointment afterward)

- Solum Uliginosum Oil and Bath Essence… This oil and essence is great for restoring the warmth organization of the body. They also are beneficial for chemical sensitivities, and those suffering from weather-change related sensitivities. The oil and essence are low odor products made in Germany, both can be added to a bath for all over body application. May be applied as needed.

- Iodine Skin Test and Treatment (see instructions in therapies section)

- Daily Color Therapy… follow instructions for Color Therapy at Home in the "Beneficial Therapies" Chapter

- Hyperbaric Oxygen Therapy… Two 1-hour sessions per day for first 5 days, then two to three sessions per week thereafter

- Chiropractic spinal, pelvic and cranial alignments combined with specific homeopathic, nutritional, glandular and myofascial support using Bio-Resonance Scanning™, or other body circuit balancing technique…as dictated by your healthcare professional.

- Chi Oxygen Exerciser®… work up to 20 minutes per day (Or other movement therapies)

- Dietary Changes… see Dietary section dealing with low body temperature

- Lifestyle modification

- CRT (Computerized Regulation Thermography) tracking of progress

Iscar® Treatment Rationale:

There are many benefits to the use of Iscar in this protocol. The primary benefit is the retraining and resetting of the body's thermostat, ultimately to the norm of 98.6 or even slightly higher.

A very good sign of healing as the result of Iscar therapy is the re-establishing of the normal rhythms of daily temperature. This rhythmical pattern is expected to vary around 0.9° F or slightly more, between the early morning temperature and the evening temperature. The body temperature should assume a more regular pattern even after discontinuing the Iscar injections.

Iscar has been historically used for the treatment of people suffering from cancer. As a matter of fact it is the most prescribed cancer medicine in all of Germany. It is however, not a "chemo" type medicine as most cancer medicines go. It does not work as a chemical scalpel to force the tumor to stop growing or shrink, while destroying the immune system, as most chemo medicines. Iscar is used in cancer for all of the same reasons as listed above – to re-educate the aspects of the body that allowed the body to create cancer in the first place.

Research performed over the last 75 years shows that people with cancer who were treated with Iscar survive years beyond those treated with conventional chemo drugs. Keep in mind that Iscar is always used in combination with many other therapies, such as the therapies listed in this section.

The only reason I bring up cancer therapy using Iscar is due to the fact that almost all of the Iscar research on the internet and in books is dealing with its benefits for cancer therapy.

Concerns may be voiced of not using Iscar unless you have cancer, to ensure that it will still work if you get cancer. This argument is potentially flawed since the ultimate goal is to not get cancer in the first place.

In a reference from a European medical journal I read and subsequently lost, the author stated that a person with a core temperature of 96.5 or below is a cancer patient, whether cancer had been diagnosed yet or not. With this in mind, the rationale for using Iscar to reset the body's thermostat and all of its other benefits is warranted.

With an estimated one in three people getting cancer at some point in their life, and some authorities even saying one in two people, can we afford not to start addressing low body temperature, the one thing that ties all cancer and chronic illness together?

Other benefits normally experienced with Iscar therapy are:

- An improvement or disappearance of sleep problems

- The clearing up of constipation…decreasing overall toxicity of the body

- Increased urine output and balancing of the fluid organization of the body

- Normalizing of body weight

- Improved sense of well-being

- Improvement in states of depression

- Decrease in overall tiredness; increased energy

- Decrease in various aches and pains

- Decreased occurrence of headaches

- Increased attack by the body on any cell-replication problems

- A regression of warts that occasionally plague post-menopausal women

- Increased resistance to infectious illness

- Increased immune function

- Increased ability of the immune cells to identify and kill "foreign" cells

Expectations for post-Iscar injection:

- Optimally an increase in body temperature of between about 0.5° to 2.0° F (0.3° to 1.0° C), returning to normal within 24 to 48 hours. Reduce amount injected if body temperature goes above 100.4° F, and do not inject again until temperature returns to normal. Gradually return to the normal dosage. Without the generation of a "fever" or increased temperature after injection, the Iscar has not been effective. Your normal body temperature should increase about 1.4°F (0.8°C) to 1.8°F (1.0°C).

- A distinct reddening reaction of the skin at the sight of injection that may be accompanied by itching. This reaction area may expand and smooth out and slowly disappear about 10 hours after injection.

- Slight pain and discomfort is reported in about 16% of people and is not a basis for discontinuation.

- If laboratory testing to monitor improvement is important to you or your doctor the following items can be expected and monitored: an improvement in immunological status revealed by an increase in T-helper lymphocytes, eosinophils, granulocyte, and absolute lymphocytes, as well as a decrease in T-suppressor cells. Iscar was monitored simply by temperature and skin reactions for several decades prior to the advent of these sensitive blood tests. For the purposes presented in this book, blood testing is not considered to be necessary.

General recommendations for the use of Iscar:

- Iscar should be injected three times per week, such as Monday, Thursday, and Saturday. After every fourteen injections, a week's pause is recommended. Continue Iscar injections optimally for at least one year, or as directed by your healthcare professional. The goal is to achieve lasting changes and the continuation of normal thermo-regulation even after discontinuation of Iscar. Depending upon the severity of the illness, Iscar may be continued for life.

- It is best to inject Iscar in the early morning, preferably before 10:30 am, since the body temperature is naturally increasing gradually throughout the day. It is important to have thirty minutes of relaxation following injection. If mornings are too hectic, injection can be made at night time, followed by the important thirty minutes of relaxation. However, all efforts should be made to modify your lifestyle to allow morning injections.

- Injections of Iscar are normally made only subcutaneously (under the skin) with the needle at an angle of about 45 degrees into the fatty tissue of the abdomen.

- Inject Iscar in a circular pattern about 3 to 4 inches away from the belly button, using the belly button as the center of the circle. Avoid the waistline where pants would rub and irritate the injection site.

- If the injection site is painful, do not attempt to relieve the pain unless it is excessively painful. In this case, Arnica massage oil (Weleda) may be applied topically or as a warm compress. Remember, inflammation around the injection site is an expected and beneficial reaction indicating that the body is reacting in a normal way to the Iscar.

Chapter 17

Causes of Low Body Temperature

There are many potential causes to a lowered body temperature, each of which must be analyzed and brought into balance by you and your healthcare team. By eliminating the various causes, one can promote health and healing. Potential causes may include:

- Lifestyle

- Diet

- Heavy metal accumulation

- Vaccinations/Immunizations

- Antibiotics/Anti-fever medications

- Symptomatic treatments of all kinds, over-the-counter medicines, herbs, vitamins, prescription medicines

- Electromagnetic pollution

- Synthetic clothing and materials

- Toxic homes and environment

- Over-controlled interior climates of homes and workplaces

Your Lifestyle Influences Body Temperature

A sedentary lifestyle and the over-stimulation of the nerve/sense aspects of life lead to imbalance. Too much time and energy is being committed to what can be basically called living in your head. Balanced living requires one to live to the same degree in your body.

The techno/information age has done us no true favors in regard to maintaining a normal body temperature or in regard to longevity. It seems that everyone assumes that just because there are more centurions alive today, that our younger generations will also live longer. I doubt this will be true. While it is true that the human body should be able to live approximately 125 years, today's younger generations are aging faster and manifesting the previously considered geriatric or old-age diseases while many are still in childhood. Even with all of the advances in medicine, and increased nutritional and dietary awareness, Americans now experience some of the worst health in the world.

Obesity is a problem now in every age group in every developed country. Though obesity is a multi-faceted problem, it can be seen as the body's efforts to insulate the body from the overcooling of its core temperature. Many people have tried many different diets to lose weight, only to be disappointed. The body may be simply saying, "No way, I need that body fat to help preserve the little bit of heat in the vital organs!"

Many people commit the vast majority of their lives in front of the television, computer, reading, dreaming, sleeping, fantasizing, talking, learning, or daydreaming. People are proud of the fact that they exercise three times per week...what is that? Three hours compared to about one hundred and nine hours per week spent on the nerve/senses aspects of their bodies!

Diet Effect on Low Temperature

Eating energetically dead food is a drain on the body's energy reserves. Food serves to do more than just satisfy your appetite. Food should also do more than simply provide you with nutrients. Food should bring with it energy! Energy-rich, live food imparts to the body its energy at roughly half the speed of light, long before its nutrient content can be digested, absorbed, and distributed to the body. What most people eat is the dead skeleton of something that was relatively good for you before it was processed and poisoned to death.

Food either contributes energy to your body, or steals energy just to process the low quality nutrients. Even food cooked with love and the intent for good of the receiver has a higher vibrational quality. This brings to mind the Biblical scripture that says to do everything with a joyful heart and with thanksgiving as unto God.

I want you to understand this one point...God did not design our body to require a Ph.D. in nutrition and diet to feed it. I truly believe that God designed our bodies to function quite well on a wide range of diets. He had to know that people in various parts of the world would not have access to the same biodiversity of food. One thing I am sure of is that God did not intend for us to render our food useless before eating it.

The majority of your diet should be from organically and/or biodynamically grown fruits, vegetables and meats. Fruits and vegetables should be harvested at peak ripeness on the plant for maximizing its developmental process. God put these foods here for your benefit; let it do its job by allowing it to ripen naturally.

You will need to make the conscious decision to either buy your produce from a good health food store/grocery, or grow it yourself. I recommend that you get out and grow your own produce and learn the different healthy ways to store and preserve it. The very process of preparing the ground, composting, planting, tending, and harvesting is forcing the body to engage the metabolic heat producing aspects of your being. Gardening in its learning curve, direct contact with the earth, and its rewards through producing life, is very healing to the body, mind and spirit.

Most of the produce in the grocery store is harvested while still green, then gassed or chemically treated to achieve the correct color and texture and to extend its shelf-life. The process, however, never allows the food to reach its full energetic or nutritional potential. What little energy this produce has is destroyed by cooking. Our society is dying prematurely all around us. Chronic fatigue plagues almost everyone. Cancer, the ultimate cold disease, is now said will be diagnosed in one out of two people with an estimated one in three dying from it.

Toxic and synthetic foods are one of the most prevalent causes of lowered body temperature. This includes a wide range of food additives in the form of preservatives, dyes, pesticides, fungicides, flavorings and flavor enhancers, and sweeteners. We are being poisoned from conception onward.

Food companies think it's a great way to do business…I'm suddenly reminded of the slogan of one leading company, "No one can eat just one." Of course no one can eat just one – in fact it is difficult not to eat the entire bag in one sitting, what with all the chemical additives that are over-stimulating your taste buds and appetite centers of your brain. Synthetic foods are good business all the way to the bank, and it also just so happens to support your health insurance company, pharmaceutical company and the entire medical community in that it ensures them that there will be a steady stream of chronically dependent people to feed money into their pockets.

Wittingly or unwittingly, each of these companies are part of the problem.

Heavy Metal Toxicity and Low Body Temperature

Heavy metals are one of the primary causes of low body temperature and immune system depression. Many microbes cannot be brought back under control until the heavy metals have been removed from the body. High and low level infections can be ongoing for decades in spite of high dose antibiotics and intravenous antimicrobials when heavy metals are present. Heavy metals promote the over-acidic, low oxygen, low temperature environment which microbes love.

The term heavy metals refers to the over-accumulation of many different types of metals in the fat cells, central nervous system (brain, brainstem, spinal cord), bones, glands or hair. Heavy metals may include mercury, lead, cadmium, palladium, platinum, arsenic and nickel, just to name a few.

Of interest concerning low body temperature are the metals palladium and platinum. Researchers from the Notre Dame University and the Wichita State University, in the most detailed study of its kind, found that the catalytic converters in automobiles are spewing out palladium and platinum in the exhaust fumes. It is now understood that we are driving through an invisible cloud of these metals and are breathing them into our lungs and potentially consuming them in our foods as these clouds of metal are now known to deposit up to 150 feet on either side of the roadways. Crops, farm animals, and even your kitchen and home are constantly being poisoned by the fallout of these metals.

Interestingly, palladium is known as "The Depressive Metal", due to the fact that it is known to cause depression in people. It is also known to cause overcooling of the body. Now consider what malady is plaguing most of America...depression and low body temperature. Coincidence or good science? If we go on to consider research concerning platinum, a story was published in a recent edition of Environmental Science and Technology, reporting that platinum is an allergen that aggravates asthma sufferers and causes other respiratory difficulties. Platinum toxicity has also been associated with cancer and birth defects. (The Wichita Eagle Newspaper, Monday, November 26, 2001, front page story, Denise Neil)

Remember how this entire book has been talking about how we must change the body's internal environment so that it is not a happy home for microbes? Heavy metals play a large role in setting you up for chronic infections and repeated infections. The effects of all the various heavy metals cannot be addressed completely in this book, however, one can see that the detoxification of the body is a an ongoing chore. We live in an incredibly toxic environment. Even when we seemingly live a healthy lifestyle, toxins will remain an issue.

The problem with most efforts to detoxify the body, especially in someone with a low body temperature, is the fact that many of these heavy metal toxins are deposited deep within the body tissues. These deep tissues are cold and rigid, and many times too solidified for even the most clever detoxification medicines and therapies to reach. This is difficult for many people to comprehend, but consider how a body with poor lymphatic fluid movement and poor circulation cannot effectively deliver the detoxifying medicines to the various areas of the body.

In order to effectively detoxify the body it stands to reason that the doctor and healthcare team must address the low body temperature. Restoring the normal body temperature will then restore the normal liquid-fluid flow dynamics that would allow the detoxification medicines to reach and remove the metals and toxins.

Another primary source of heavy metal toxicity are the dental materials used for the last 100+ years, primarily mercury, which is used in many "silver amalgams". These amalgam fillings were so controversial when first introduced in the late 1800's that it split the only dental association of the time, the National Dental Association (NDA), into two groups. One group said no one should ever use mercury in the mouth due to the fact that it is so very toxic and is known to leach out over time, poisoning the body. The other group of dentists liked how easy it was to work with and how inexpensive mercury amalgams were. Remember, in the 1800's, gold was the preferred dental filling material. The two factions debated the issue until a new dental association was born, the American Dental Association – our present day leading dental association, ADA, which you see approving most grocery store brand toothpastes. Interestingly, it was the ADA who liked the mercury fillings which became the norm of our society. Of historical interest, the first use of the name "Quack" when referring to a questionable doctor was used to label these dentists using mercury, since mercury was then known as "Quacksilver". Today it is estimated that over 100 million mercury amalgams are placed in teeth every year in the U.S. alone. One can only marvel at the power and influence various associations in our country have over our standard of living, especially when considering that doctors and dentists have been persecuted and prosecuted, sometimes losing their license to practice in the U.S. for attempting to spread the word about these issues and relieve suffering through the removal of amalgams. Recent legislation has been proposed to outlaw the use of mercury in amalgams.

Some countries, such as Sweden, have already banned its use and will even pay up to 50% of the cost to have it removed from their citizens, stating that the cost of removal is cheaper than paying for the long term chronic illnesses as the result of these amalgams. (Definitive Guide to Cancer, Goldberg, B., Diamond J. Future Medicine Publishing Inc., 1997) (Of a side note, many European countries do not allow the use of fluoride in water and toothpaste due to limited benefit and excessive health complications.)

Mercury is 1000 times more toxic than lead, while the methyl-mercury vapor coming off of fillings during chewing is 100 times more toxic than elemental mercury.

These "silver amalgams" actually contain up to 50% mercury by weight, 35% silver, 13% tin, 2% copper, and a trace amount of zinc. (Let the Tooth be Known…, Are Your Teeth Making You Sick, Dawn Ewing RDH, PhD, ND, 1998, Published by Holistic Health Alternatives)

German research has shown that mercury from pregnant mother's amalgams are directly related to high levels of mercury in their fetuses. (Definitive Guide to Cancer).

I have seen many patients who no longer have any teeth, only dentures, who are incredulous that they have heavy metal toxicity still from old amalgams long removed. The teeth were likely removed due to long term degenerative changes in teeth that were likely full of amalgams, crowns, root canals, and bridges, all of which were releasing various metals into the bones and tissues of the jaws and indeed the entire body. Dr. Stephan Edelson, M.D., medical director of the Environmental and Preventative Health Center of Atlanta, Georgia, explains that "mercury vapor (methyl-mercury) is readily absorbed into the blood because of its solubility in blood lipids (fatty molecules). This process contributes to between 80 and 100% absorption through the lungs from which the mercury is then carried to virtually every tissue of the body, including the brain. (Definitive Guide to Cancer and Kudsk, F. "Uptake of Hg Vapors in Blood *In Vivo* and *In Vitro* from Hg-containing Air" Acta Pharmacologica et Toxicologica 27 (1969), 49) Therefore, the burden all of those years of metals leaching from the teeth and from other sources are not relieved by simply removing the teeth. You must understand that it is no simple matter in detoxifying the body of heavy metals.

Biological Dentistry is as different from conventional dentistry as doctors practicing Biological Medicine are from conventional doctors. These dentists strive to restore the integrity of the teeth as part of the completely integrated organ circuits. They understand that the metal in the teeth create galvanic electricity that blasts through the organ circuits causing many of today's worst illnesses. Biological dentists seek to replace potentially harmful dental materials with safe materials that are as close to the normal enamel as possible or as biocompatible as can be found.

Let's briefly touch on some of the other sources of heavy metals so that you may understand how to avoid further accumulation. Exposure to cigarettes and other tobacco products are a source of the heavy metal toxins, lead and cadmium. Lead can also come from old paint in your home, cooking utensils, ceramic glazes and solder on water pipes. Aluminum comes from many cooking pots and utensils as well as antiperspirants and deodorants, aluminum foil, and is found commonly in tap water. Cadmium can be found in some soft drinks, fungicides, various types of plastics, instant coffee and teas. The continual breakdown of metals in every machine releases an endless variety of metals into the air we breathe; consider atomic particles of titanium coming off of the turbines of the approximately 70,000 jet airliners flying over the U.S. at any given time.

The list of metals and their potential for interfering with the proper function of the human body is endless. When considering these issues, one becomes even more aware of the need to reduce the exposure to potential sources of heavy metal toxins as well as the need to detoxify the body on a long term basis. So, stay away from the mindset that you can detoxify for a period of time and be done with it.

So the question ceases to be, "where did I get all of this heavy metal?", but now moves to "How do I now get rid of it?"

General guidelines for Heavy Metal Detoxification:

- First identify the primary heavy metal toxins in your body, either through Electro-dermal screening, Bio-Resonance Scanning™, Applied or Clinical Kinesiology, CRT (Computerized Regulation Thermography) or through various laboratory tests.

- Following all of the guidelines for raising low body temperature is a prerequisite to any successful heavy metal detoxification plan.

- Various nutritional supplements, herbal formulas and metal chelation products have been tested and reported in peer-reviewed journals and found to greatly reduce the body's load of heavy metals. Always consult with your healthcare professional due to the fact that simply "stirring up" the toxins may just relocate the metals in a more sensitive area of the body causing a more severe malady, and should be therefore not attempted as a home treatment.

- Before any type of detoxification treatment is started or any silver (mercury) amalgams are removed, one must make certain that the lymphatic system is open and able to efficiently clear out the toxins that these treatments will be stirring up inside your body. The best way to address the lymphatic system is the ST8 Lymphatic drainage therapy. (Described in more detail later) It is important to continue ST8 treatments throughout any detoxification program so that the organs of elimination can function without becoming overloaded. Research has shown that chelation therapy, an intravenous method of releasing heavy metals from the body, can be damaging to the kidneys due to the overtaxing of the kidney's ability to clear out all the metal into the urine. The ST8 will help avoid this type of problem, as well as also stimulate the release of metals from every tissue in the body, as a result of a congested lymphatic system.

- Far Infrared Sauna therapy is one of the best ways to release not only heavy metals from deep within the tissues, but also to release all lipotrophic toxins (toxins stored in the fat cells). Far infrared saunas are not to be confused with regular steam saunas which many people cannot tolerate and may aggravate some illnesses. Far infrared saunas do not involve excessive temperatures and the infrared penetrates up to one and a half inches into the body to release deeply embedded toxins and bring them through the skin to be wiped off with a towel.

- Research supports the use of homeopathic metals to induce the release of metals from the body. Usually a low potency homeopathic (6x-12x) is best to cause a release of metals from the body. With this form of detoxification, if the goal is to remove mercury from the body, your healthcare professional would use homeopathic mercury in a 6-12x potency. If the desire was to remove aluminum then a 6-12x potency of homeopathic aluminum would be used, and so on.

- Ion-Cleanse Hydrotherapy (See Therapy Section)

- Drinking distilled water during a metal detoxification program can help remove metals, due to the fact that distilled water is de-mineralized water. This makes it a good chelator of metals as the distilled water can chelate (pull or attract) metals from the tissues so then the body can excrete them via the urine. (General recommendation is up to 3 quarts per day during detox program only) Distilled water should only be drunk during the heavy metal detox program due to the fact that it may ultimately pull beneficial minerals out of the body when used long term.

Chapter 18

Other Influences on Core Temperature

Sympathetic Treatments

Any kind of medicine designed to suppress the natural processes of the body can be said to be sympathetic and potentially harmful in the long run. Sympathetic treatments usually counteract whatever the body is attempting to accomplish. This is the proverbial allopathic medicine for the most part, although natural medicine is guilty of much the same.

Such medicines might include antipyretics, antibiotics, decongestants and pain-killers.

Antipyretics are fever-reducing medicines, like most of the acetaminophen type over-the-counter (OTC) drugs. By now you understand better the role that fever plays in the healthy body. To suppress or artificially bring down a fever, especially in children, really messes up the body's thermostat, causing it to be too low.

Prescription antibiotics are definitely a sympathetic and suppressive treatment that is contrary to maintaining a normal body temperature. Antibiotics, like the name suggests, are "anti" against, and "biotics" life, so "against life". Many people seem to think a swollen and hot lymph node is a sign that they need an antibiotic. The swollen lymph node is a sign that the body is working and fighting microbial overgrowth. To take an antibiotic is to send the message to the body that it is not needed anymore, and to stop attempting to control microbes. Antibiotics say "step aside body, we will do the work for you." As a result of taking antibiotics, the body is disrupted in mid-stride. The balance is lost. The rhythmical aspects of the body are no longer synchronous. Fluid regulation and transformation and transportation is disrupted, leading to dehydration of the blood and lymph, and ultimately the tissues. Antibiotics kill friendly intestinal bacteria, further creating an internal environment that is cold and dysfunctional.

Natural medicine practitioners are just as guilty many times when they use "natural" antibiotics. These botanical substances will kill microbes sometimes better than antibiotics due to their more complex molecular structures. But after everything I have presented here, is the point of optimal treatment to kill the microbes for the body? No, the body simply requires balance and support to bring microbes under control. I always wonder when some botanical medicines and colloidal silver-type medicines claim to "kill every microbe known to man" if they ever stopped to consider the over 400 species of friendly bacteria (probiotics) known to inhabit the healthy digestive system that help us digest our food correctly and produce B-vitamins for us. No doubt there will be times when a person has waited too long and the life or limb must be saved through antibiotics, natural or otherwise. Chronic Lyme is usually not one of these times.

Decongestants are used to dry up mucus, even though the mucus is the body's way of removing toxins and microbes and generally getting rid of substances clogging up the inside of the body, moving it to the outside for expulsion via the nose and mouth. Decongestants create a condition of dehydration in the tissues. I spoke to a person in a consultation who had taken a leading prescription decongestant that had caused the entire body to become dehydrated, and the skin was now leathery from an out-of-control fluid disturbance globally. Degeneration of the organs is the end result. In my opinion there is no time where these types of medicines are a good choice. Natural expectorants and bath therapies to encourage liquefying and moving mucus, combined with addressing the causes of the mucus, is infinitely better and works with the efforts of the body instead of against the body.

Even vitamins and supplements when used inappropriately can be a sympathetic treatment that in the long run can work against the body's natural tendencies. This will shock many of you, however, no one takes more vitamins and supplements than the chronically ill. I have seen it hundreds of times that people are taking fistfuls of vitamins in high doses just to feel halfway normal. Most of them have been taking them for years, since if they ever quit taking them, they are soon sick again. If you have to keep taking something, even something supposedly good for you, in order to feel good, then it is a sympathetic treatment only. If it were truly "fixing" something then eventually it would be "fixed" and you would not need to continue taking it. Whatever is at the core of the body's problem is not being addressed and may continue to worsen. Granted, most will benefit from supplementation with vitamins at some point due to the overall poor nutrient content of most of the food we consume.

Many times I have heard of miraculous "cures" from promoters of a leading supplement company, however in the final analysis, if the "cured" person ever quits taking the supplement the illness many times returns. The only time I would say this is acceptable is when the person has scarring of organs and surgically removed organs, or otherwise permanent damage; sympathetic treatment is all that is left for these people. True cures from vitamins will be seen only when they are addressing the core of the problem, and when they are thoughtfully applied to support the overall healing process.

Electromagnetic Pollution's Effect on Body Temperature

Often our patients are surprised to hear me speak so much about the electrical aspects of their body. Conventional medicine focuses so strongly on the blood, so many times it is the first time they have heard that their body is electrical. The entire body is controlled through electro-chemical interactions. These electro-chemical interactions of the body are sensitive to the influence of the much stronger electrical fields found in every home and virtually everywhere in our powerline-wrapped earth.

The body operates on direct current electricity, while the electricity in the wiring of your house works on alternating current electricity. This difference can disrupt the normal function of the body.

At no other time do these house appliance electrical fields seem to affect the normal functioning of the body more than while we are asleep. The primary purpose of sleep is to rebuild, regenerate and repair the body. If one stops to consider that most bedrooms have electricity running in all the walls, the ceiling, and the floor, whether or not the lights are on, one can begin to see how many electromagnetic fields are pulsating through our body during this all-important healing time of our day. Electric alarm clocks, electric blankets, electric heating pads all create even more disruptive fields and should be thrown away.

Computers have become a standard of life in many homes. Research shows that the emitted electromagnetic fields are definitely harmful, as demonstrated by the increased miscarriages associated with prolonged computer usage by pregnant women. I had a patient come for care suffering from chronic debilitating fatigue and profound weakness of the muscles. I found that she is a professional editor and author. When I treated her she rapidly became much stronger in her muscles. When I found out she wrote her books on a laptop computer laid on her body while in bed (due to excessive fatigue and weakness), I decided to test her newfound muscle strength with the laptop laying on her. She immediately could not lift her arms at all! Is electromagnetic pollution a potential problem? Definitely.

There are several high-tech devices designed to protect against this form of pollution. However, one my very most favorite is low-tech. Peat/ wool blend bedding and clothing create not only a shield against electromagnetic pollution, but also promote the normalization of the body's warmth organization, fighting low body temperature. Peat/wool or peat/ silk fabric has been shown to hold no static electricity. The peat/wool shoe inserts provide a barrier against static electricity so common in this synthetic carpet world we live in.

Like wool, peat has a very low flammability index, basically smoldering only instead of burning like synthetic fabrics.

There are also peat/wool aprons, vests, and pads to shield the electromagnetic pollution from computers, an absolute must for pregnant mothers using computers.

My other favorite provides protection against electromagnetic pollution as verified by independent researchers and doctors the world over – the Teslar Watch®. The Teslar watch was developed by the gifted genius, Cortland Reeves, at ELF Laboratories. Research shows that not only do the Teslar watches protect you, but they also increase the energy of every cell. You see, life is a constant fight between forces weakening the body and the forces of the body trying to restore the lost energy.

Many of the Lyme patients I see have been fighting the illness so long and antibiotics have so weakened their body, that if their body was a light bulb, it would be very dim indeed. These Teslar watches provide a way to energize the body 24 hours a day in a way that does not require nutritional supplements or prescription drugs.

Chapter 19

The Warmth Organization of the Body

Today's society suffers almost uniformly from a chronic condition of dysregulated warmth organization throughout the body. We no longer see the inflammatory diseases so common up until the mid-twentieth century. Plaguing society today are the cold, sclerotic illness, such as chronic fatigue, fibromyalgia, chronic viral and bacterial infections, multiple sclerosis, and the ultimate "cold body" disease…cancer.

Conventional medicine focuses on the microscopic analysis of the body, counting the number of this or that type of cell or microbe. Biological medicine and Circuit Healing™ on the other hand, recognizes healing of the body as a completely integrated organism. However, attention can and should be focused upon supporting specific aspects of the human being, such as supporting the restoration of the normal warmth organization throughout the body.

Doctors must become experts at recognizing and addressing the various conditions of dysregulated warmth in the body and extremities. Several possibilities exist. There could be cold hands and feet, warm hands and cold feet, warm oral temperature and cold thorax, local cold spots, or global coldness, just to name a few. Each of these cold conditions should be a clue to the doctor of the unique imbalance in the body, to the same degree as abnormal findings on blood tests.

At times a doctor may get caught up in the microscopic view of the patient and miss the truly vital information gained from simple observation. We must all become masters of reading the signs so readily available by observation on the macro-scopic scale. One hundred years of microscopic analysis has gained the U.S.A. some of the worst health in the world. The common, but flawed, theme taught in most medical schools is that if one can determine what substance that the body is low or high in, then supplementing with that nutrient or lowering the high substance will correct the illness. This "pieces and parts" mentality is one of the primary reasons our society is failing, and chronic illness of all types is the norm.

Observing and tracking the regulation of warmth throughout the body is one component of the lost "art" in the healing arts. Once one recalls that in the end the body must do the healing, not the medicines, the importance of warmth becomes obvious. Specifically, the electrical oscillatory rate of every healthy cell in the body is sustained by the correct amount of warmth. Too much warmth, either inflammation or fever, increases the electrical oscillatory rate and subsequently increases the breakdown of protein. Too much coldness causes a decrease in the cell's electrical oscillatory rate and the fluids begin to thicken and the cell degenerates and becomes increasingly dysfunctional and toxic.

It becomes clear that the best medicine in the world for a given condition may not be able to work when the body is too cold. When the body is chronically cold it becomes non-reactive, meaning the body ceases to respond appropriately to medicines and its environment.

The next question must be "What regulates the warmth organization of the body?" To answer this question one must understand that there is more to the human body than the eye can see. From an electro-energetic perspective, the body is almost not here. Electrons spinning at billions of cycles per second around a nucleus provide us with the solid feel of the body. The fact is that the body, energetically speaking, is not very dense. Many types of energy pass freely through the human body, such as quarks, neutrinos, and other energetic particles. Armed with the new realization that we are more electro-energetic than pieces and parts, we can begin to accept that there are varying fields of electro-energy, inseparable within and surrounding the body. These fields of energy have been named for scientific agreement. The etheric field, otherwise known as "ether body", is that electro-energetic level that regulates the warmth organization of the "physical" body.

The challenge of the doctor is to determine how best to recognize and treat the imbalance in the ether body. One may think that simply recognizing the coldness of the body is enough, however, the coldness of the body is a symptom of the disturbed ether body. Treatments must address the imbalances in the ether body. This is the reason that taking thyroid medicines such as Armor Thyroid or Synthroid to combat a cold core temperature is most often purely treating the symptom; they do nothing to correct the ether body.

Generally we break down the body during the day and rebuild it again at night while we sleep. The only reason we sleep is to repair and regenerate the tissues of the body. Nighttime and sleep is the time of highest etheric field energy. The etheric field governs both the warmth organization and the regeneration of tissue.

144

Illness and healing are aggravated especially at night due to interference of the etheric field by the chaotic and disruptive nature of the electrical fields emitted by the wiring running in every wall, floor, and ceiling of your bedroom. The wiring in your bedroom can definitely be disruptive to the body. While we obviously can live many years while being bathed in these disruptive electrical fields while sleeping, in the search for health and healing, one must eliminate every known issue that might interfere with the body's natural ability to regulate its warmth and its ability to regenerate healthy, vibrant tissue.

The electrical fields of your bedroom are one of the primary disruptors of the body's etheric field and therefore must be shielded.

A peat mattress pad and comforter along with wearing a Teslar Watch® can provide important support by shielding the etheric fields from the interference fields of the electricity of your house, and by the peat helping the ether body to concentrate inward.

At times the body responds to cold spots or regions within the body by producing an inflammatory reaction to warm it up. This may be seen in pain syndromes that come and go suddenly, and from no obvious traumatic cause. This body mechanism is inefficient in resolving coldness in the body, not to mention that most people have been conditioned by doctors to fight pain with pain-killers. Pain-killers promote a chronic cold condition in the body.

Contrast foot baths can be used to great benefit in that alternating cold and hot foot baths seeks to stimulate the body's restorative warmth organization and circulation. To use this therapy one should soak the feet in hot water for one minute, and then soak in cold water for 30 seconds. This should be repeated three to five times in a session, two to three times per day, for several weeks. The effect can be enhanced by adding one teaspoon of 2% copper sulfate solution to the hot water. Copper is known to be warming to the body; as the old saying goes "rubbing a copper penny warms the hand."

Another possible cause of disturbed warmth in the body is the congested and dysregulated fluid organization. The excessive accumulation of fluid overwhelms and basically puts out the fire warming the body. This condition is usually the result of a sedentary lifestyle and poor elimination of wastes through the skin. The best corrective therapy for this common ailment is the regular use of an infrared sauna, which allows for 3-6 times greater sweat production than the much hotter conventional steam and dry saunas. Greater results can be realized by taking 3-6 pillules of the homeopathic remedy Ferrum phosphoricum 6x potency, taken about 30 minutes to an hour before entering the sauna. This improves the warmth reaction of the body and increases sweat production.

Low potency (3-6x) homeopathic Apis can be applied locally to fight cold spots and will help restore balanced warmth, negating the need for the body to produce inflammation.

No medicine is better at treating disturbances in the global warmth organization of the body than subcutaneous injections of the German prescription homeopathic medicine Iscar™ when combined with corrective associated therapies, such as color and music therapy, rhythmical massage therapy, curative movement therapy, and the use of peat bedding.

A primary cause of disturbed warmth organization in the body is the global phenomenon of electro-magnetic, chemical, and heavy metal toxicity within everyone alive. There seems to be no relief in sight, and generally no time that ongoing detoxification won't be necessary. The air we breathe is full of heavy metals, such as titanium, palladium, platinum, and every other conceivable metal and metal alloy from the millions of automobiles, jets, and factories. It is absorbed into even the best biodynamically and/or organically grown foods, as these toxins are carried on the wind to the farthest reaches of the most remote locations on the planet. Until radical improvement and change in industry and society as a whole occurs, we will suffer from toxicity. Environmental toxins are very disruptive to the warmth organization of the body. Until the toxic load in your body is reduced, no success can be expected in regard to correcting the warmth organization and subsequently the restoration of your health.

Circuit Healing™ addresses and supports the restoration of all the electro-energetic fields as well as the physical needs of the body. The need for addressing all levels of the body should be obvious, since one can support the etheric body forever, but without decreasing the toxic load, restoration of the body's warmth will not be made manifest.

Chapter 20

Peat Fiber Products; Healing the Body's Warmth Regulation

You may be surprised to find a textile fabric as part of our recommended healing protocol. You will soon read how this unique plant fiber can actually be a very important promoter of health and healing.

To fully appreciate peat products, one must first understand what makes it unique in this world of high-tech fabrics. Peat is a natural fiber from the Upland Moors of Sweden. It is harvested from peat bogs at a depth of 150 feet. Unlike most plants which die and decompose, peat moss is preserved in these deep bogs. The peat harvested for fabrics are fibers that are centuries old. These fibers were around long before our planet was enshrouded in electrical powerlines and long before the advent of cell phones and microwaves. The peat fibers, because of their old age and due to their unique chemical structure, have centuries of stored forces of growth and development from an originally healthy, vital natural world, free of environmental toxins and electromagnetic pollution.

I was introduced to health promoting and protective properties of peat while studying natural medicine in Eckwalden, Germany, and was amazed to see Medical Doctors at the large German Anthroposophical Hospital, the Filder Clinic, treating all manner of disease using natural medicines and therapies, including peat products.

I advise everyone to use a peat mattress pad and comforter to put on their bed. The primary purpose of sleep is to repair and regenerate the body. What most people do not realize is that the electricity running through the wiring in the walls, ceiling, and floor of your bedroom emit electro-pollution in the form of electrical fields. The alternating current electricity in wiring is contrary to the direct current electricity of the human body. The peat in the mattress pad and comforter creates a shield around the body during this most important time of healing…sleep time.

Because of peat's unique properties it also helps restore the warmth organization of the body. The overcooling of the body's core temperature is at the source of most of today's chronic illnesses. Many people also suffer from cold hands and feet as the result of overcooling of the core of the body.

It must be understood what actually heals you of all illness – through God's design, your body does the healing. The body's subtle energy is the healing force responsible for every true cure. Peat repels electromagnetic pollution enabling the unobstructed healing of the body. If you had a cut that was not healing, you would seek to find out what is interfering with the natural design of your body to heal. If you are suffering from any illness that is not healing, peat offers you the peace in knowing that all external interference is removed while you are sleeping.

Section 4

Stress and Lyme Disease

Chapter 21

Childhood Stress and Lyme Disease

Childhood Lyme infections can be somewhat easier to address, due to the pristine nature of most children's bodies, and if it is caught early. At the same time, Lyme in children can be devastating, depending upon their health heritage and the degree of balanced life and stress in the child's life prior to becoming sick. These issues will dictate how well a child processes through the illness.

In a child's life, stress comes from all directions. In children, as in adults, prolonged stress predisposes one to illness.

Stress always affects organs. Every type of stress will target a specific organ. The liver is specifically targeted and damaged in the long run by intense and usually suppressed feelings of resentment, frustration, and irritability. Worry seems to preferentially affect the kidneys, and so forth. You see, imbalance creates illness. Restoring balance is the pure goal of biological medicine. **Stress can start the domino effect that leads to the weakening of the body's ability to control microbes.**

Even though most children have a high natural vitality, once a child is in trouble from a chronic infection, the treatment decisions become crucial. All efforts must be made to support the body using biological methods to address the child at all levels: physically, mentally, emotionally, energetically, and spiritually. High-power drugs and children do not mix well – the resulting imbalance is nearly impossible to reverse. Treatments must work with God's design of the body, and never opposite of this natural design.

Every direction a child turns they run into a barrier designed to force them to conform to a society-dictated norm. Parents should recognize that each child is unique in the world and has a unique path and strengths that should be nurtured. A child's life requires more balance than an adult, due to the fact that they are constantly evolving and developing who they will be as adults.

Did you know that at the time of birth, the nervous system is still developing? And as the child grows the number of nerve fibers will increase dramatically? Those certain neurological developmental stages must be realized, because before it is all completed, the child's nervous system will determine the best nerve pathways, and will naturally reduce the number of nerve fibers by half? This is why it is important that a child learns to crawl before it walks. If the child learned to walk first then developmental problems would occur as the nervous system would not recognize the nerve pathways used for crawling as important and would eliminate them. Truly a situation of "if you don't use it, you will lose it!" Developmental balance must be the goal of parents and teachers in every aspect of a child's life.

Parents and teachers must help children remain balanced, and recognize the seven year, cyclical nature of childhood development. A discussion of the different cycles is beyond the scope of this writing. Many aspects of the Waldorf School educational philosophy are, in my opinion, superior to the prevalent educational philosophy which seems at times to over-stimulate the intellect of a child. A good reference tool for parents and educators is the Association of Waldorf Schools of North America and their biannual publication, *"Renewal; Journal for Waldorf Education."*

Children are many times viewed by their parents as a bother to adult agendas. Parents must take an active role in creating ways to bring balance to the lives of their children. A child with chronic Lyme has the greatest potential to almost spontaneously heal with the treatment protocol outlined in this book, when all conditions are brought to balance.

Creativity, handwork crafts, focus, eye-hand coordination, intellect, morality, independent thinking, social development, imagination, intuitive thinking are but a few areas that with proper guidance can help establish the unique path each child must travel to reach a balanced adulthood. The hoops we force our children to jump through in our country's educational system do little to develop these areas. Doctors have documented for about a hundred years that children who are driven to be over-achievers and who are over-stimulated mentally by the present educational methods become pale, pasty-faced, lackluster and easily fatigued. This clearly represents imbalance, when children raised and educated in a balanced manner are noticeably more full-blooded, with rosy-cheeks and full of healthy vitality. Educational stressors that cause imbalance are part of the problem. Parents would be well advised to look into Waldorf-style educational philosophy, even if it means home schooling when no good schools are in the area.

(Association of Waldorf Schools of North America (www.awsna.org) 3911 Bannister Road, Fair Oaks, CA 95628-6805 call or write for information 916-961-0715 or for a subscription to their biannual journal: *"Renewal; Journal for Waldorf Education".*)

Parental emotional, verbal and physical abuse warps the developmental shields of a child, setting them up for physical illness such as chronic infectious diseases, as well as other aspects of human development, such as spiritual, moral, and psychological development. (Remember, just having the bacteria in your body does not mean a child or adult will come down with a disease from that bacteria. Stress can break down the child's ability to stave off disease.) Whether directed toward the child or between others in the family unit, words can wound the body, mind, and spirit causing illness at each of these levels. In the same manner, loving words spoken from the heart can heal all levels. We have all heard and experienced the principle of, "Actions speak louder than words"; keep this in mind and don't simply speak the words, be sure your actions in the future do not belie the words, for the wounds in this case strike deeper. You may be the actual cause of your child's illness.

It is definitely all right to admit to your child that you were wrong in how you handled a situation, and ask forgiveness. This sets forth a standard for your children to follow throughout their entire life.

Parents and teachers must practice and maintain balance in their own life in order to respond correctly to the children in their care.

One more note concerning the sick child. Many cultures, though not as common in the United States, keep infants and young children in almost constant physical contact with the mother. In America it seems at times that we are duty bound from a social perspective to force our children to fight their illness alone. To be tough, self-reliant, and seen but not heard. I highly recommend that especially for the young children that they be held a lot and even sleep in the same bed with the mother, or at least in the same room. This provides the ultimate healing energy of love. It also provides a sharing of body energy and warmth. A child should never have to deal with illness alone in their room. This will not spoil the child. You just being there and holding them as they need it is often enough.

Keep in mind; children may not be able to tell you what is stressing them out. They may be afraid of your response, or it may be that they put much of it on themselves, as in the case of the "perfectionist" child. It may also be that illness, household finances, school pressures, sibling rivalry, jealousy, or any number of things may be responsible. Your job as a parent is to provide a loving, nurturing home environment, as free from adult issues as is indicated for their age.

Detecting a child with stress problems:

One of the best ways of determining an overstressed person, child or adult, is to use a penlight and shine the light in one of their eyes. Observe the pupil, the black part of the eye; it should constrict, getting smaller. You see, the eye is like your 35mm camera; the aperture of the camera needs to be smaller in bright light so that the film is not over-exposed. The pupil of the eye works the same to keep too much light from entering the eye. The pupil should normally be able to hold a steady size opening. In a child or adult suffering from long-term stress, the pupil will not be able to hold a steady constriction and will begin to pulse wider and wider as the light is held to it. This test is testing the adrenal glands ability to cope with stress of any kind. The adrenal glands are your stress organs. They sit on top of each kidney. Chronic stress fatigues the adrenal glands ability to cope, resulting in an inability to deal correctly to even the light shined in the eyes. Really bad cases are seen when the pupils are almost always very large and will only constrict slightly with the penlight. These children are usually very bothered by direct sunlight or strong lights.

Another method of finding out if a child is stressed is to shine a penlight in their eye from the side, illuminating their iris, the colored portion of the eye. This takes some patience, but what you are looking for are little rings on the surface of the iris that following the circular shape of the iris. These rings may be only in certain areas of the iris or in really bad cases you may see as many as five layers of rings, between the inner and outer edges of the iris. Any rings always indicate stress in the body, and are actually formed by cramps in the four layers that make up the iris. We should never see any rings in children! Their young lives should be carefree and nurtured. Of course, we should never see these rings in an adult iris either.

Dealing with childhood stress:

The following are designed to address the body, mind, and spirit of the child:

• The above penlight tests reveal stress that has affected the adrenal glands and therefore the child's ability to deal with stress correctly. The adrenal glands can be strengthened by taking half of a tablet in the morning, of DSF-Formula™, by NutraWest, Inc. DSF was specifically designed as a De-Stress-Formula. At times it is somewhat impossible to completely remove all of the stressors in life, but this product helps in how one reacts to that stress.

• Diffusing essential oils in the house and in the child's bedroom can have not only a calming effect, but a healing effect as well. Anything you can smell is a chemical in the air that you breathe into the body. When you breathe in essential oils, they bring with them some of the world's strongest antioxidants and healing substances. You may remember how you used to feel when holiday potpourris set a festive mood in the house, or simply the smell of your favorite food being prepared. Some of our favorite oils for de-stressing are produced by Young Living Essential Oils, Inc.: Peace and Calming oil blend, Lavender oil, Harmony oil blend, Frankincense oil, Valor oil blend, Forgiveness oil blend, and Surrender oil blend. You will find your own favorites after trying a few, but let your child pick the oil for each day. These oils are usually well tolerated even by the chemically sensitive and asthmatic children.

• The homeopathic remedy "Rescue Remedy" was specifically designed to remedy all forms of stress, especially the acute stressors like a death in the family, auto or other accidents, or any stress that threatens the integrity of the body, real, perceived, or otherwise.

• Increase family and house organization. Children need some semblance of order even in the midst of their disorder. Consistency of house routines, chores, expectations should be the rule. A disorderly and trashed-out house breeds stress and chaos, while a spotless house creates its own stress for children. There must be a flexible balance maintained in the household.

• Read and teach the principles presented in this book on keeping a quiet mind, controlling your thinking, taking your authority, and practicing color therapy at home. All of these principles are wonderful to teach your children. My children are far ahead of where I was at their age. They keep me in line now, when I stray!

• Make the difficult decisions that will eliminate stress in your child's life. This may be anything, moving to a better neighborhood; deciding to home-school; getting a different job that will allow you to be around more or one that will be less stressful for you and the family; change babysitters if you have a bad one, separate siblings into their own bedrooms or bring them together; whatever it takes to eliminate stress.

• Change your priorities so that your family is the most important part of your life. Find ways to spend quality time with the child: drawing and coloring together, reading stories and books together, find art classes that you can take together, buy models and assemble them together, ride bikes together, purchase bird books or nature books and go for nature walks with them identifying birds and flowers together. You see, it really does matter that you DO it with them, consistently and often.

- If you have not started the Nintendo-type games with your children, don't even let it in the house. Children get lost in the "cool" worlds of these games and their real world can not compete, leading them to discontentment and resentment towards you and the issues of the real world. It is training your child to live in their head only.

Chapter 22

Adult Stress and Lyme Disease

Chronic Lyme infections affecting adults should be viewed as a sign of imbalance, and is usually the result of excessive or prolonged stress in life.

Infections can begin by the following possible scenario: Life is out of control, you haven't exercised in years, you work such long hours that you are too tired to eat right, the children need your attention but you can't handle it, so you yell at them, wishing you could have a vacation away from everything. You are worn down to the point that no matter how long you sleep you still are tired all day. The television news announces that a flu epidemic is sweeping the city...through suggestion and weakness you find yourself feeling a scratchy throat coming on, your neck is beginning to ache, and you think you may have a fever...and the rest is history as your body forces you to sleep, take a break, and removes your appetite as it attempts to catch up and repair.

Another such scenario might be: You have a very important meeting coming up, at which you have to give a presentation. Rumor has it that if you mess it up, then the boss is going to fire you. In your fear you feel your throat tighten up and begin to get scratchy. You then think, "A bout of strep throat is the last thing you need", but it gets worse and you can barely speak.

Many people feel somewhat subconsciously that illness has liberated them from responsibility, and others find it is "just one more thing that is screwed up" in their life. You must not be a victim of your life.

I have had many people tell me that they get sick in cycles. They suffer infections in cycles of every three weeks, or every so many months, or even a certain season of the year. If you keep making the same mistakes, you will continue to suffer the same consequences.

Make a list of all of the aspects of your life that you know are out of balance. Draw up a step-by-step plan for each to restore balance. Reduce stress. If you don't like your life, then you are way out of balance and should make a list of reasonable changes that you would like to see in your life. Then draw up a step-by-step plan to achieve each item. Stop doing what doesn't work. Many times we hold tightly to a way of life because it is easier to stay in the rut than it is to get out of the rut. Choose today to take a different path. Change yourself. If you are in torment about your life, then change the way you respond to the stressors in your life. Sometimes you cannot change the things that stress you out, but you can change the way you respond to that stress.

We all choose how we respond to stress. To some degree, the way you respond to stress is a learned process. Without realizing it you may be influenced in your response to stress by the people you socialize with. The people you surround yourself with may be lewd, crude, and generally angry people, while other people in your peer-group may be quite the opposite, suppressing their true feelings, inwardly bitter, and are basically victims of the unfairness of life. Maybe when growing up, your family members were yellers and verbally sarcastic and abusive. So, it is easy to see that stress can seem like a normal way of life to you.

Television programs of family violence, lawsuits and juvenile delinquent representations also seem to be attempting to represent "normal" life. I recommend that you turn off the television, or get rid of it all together, since it is the absolute worst teacher of your mind and morality. The adage "garbage in, garbage out" is appropriate here.

We should strive to walk in light, love and wisdom. Choose to change in spite of your environment or upbringing. Replace hate, fear and negativity with optimism, love and a positive outlook. You will be surprised at how good you will begin to feel and how your environment will change in response to your light and balance.

If your job is a stressor, then ask yourself, "What job would I like to do where I would be the most fulfilled and the happiest?" Write it down, and make a step-wise list of how you can make it come true.

If what you have been doing has created the reality of today, then if you want a new reality, you must change what you're doing to get that new reality. I'm not proposing that the grass is always greener on the other side, but I am telling you that you must change, and change for the better, in order to get a better reality tomorrow.

Admit your mistakes, seek forgiveness for your part in all conflict, and move ahead. You must get out of simply surviving your day.

Often adults with chronic disease suffer from depression. The doctor says, "Well, Mr. Doe, you are deficient in happy hormones, take this psychedelic drug and you won't feel anything anymore." Don't even go there! Read the book, "Prozac; Panacea or Pandora" by Dr. Ann Blake Tracy, Ph.D. These drugs are a trap that leads to years of declining health, as well as mental and emotional disturbances. They also lead to an average of 50-60 pounds of increased weight and diabetes, not to mention the fact that one cannot simply stop them once started due to the severe withdrawal effects. Experts say that they are "slow-fuse LSD", which was also a prescription medicine for psychosis until banned for its adverse effects.

Prescription drugs are not the way to deal with adult stress! Read the book listed above to find out why they are terrible, and how one must get off of them.

Chapter 23

Two Person Energy Balancing For Stress Resolution

Energy Clearing of Two People

Any time two people come into contact there is an intermixing of their energy. It does not matter if they are married or simply come into casual contact as with a handshake. The potential for residual and harmful effects is greatest for people who are in frequent close contact, such as married couples.

Whether you are holding hands, hugging, loving, or spending hours sleeping together, your energetic fields are repeatedly coming together. It would be good to know that you are not 'blowing" each other's electrical circuits just being near each other! Even the best of marriages would benefit from "Two Person Energy Balancing."

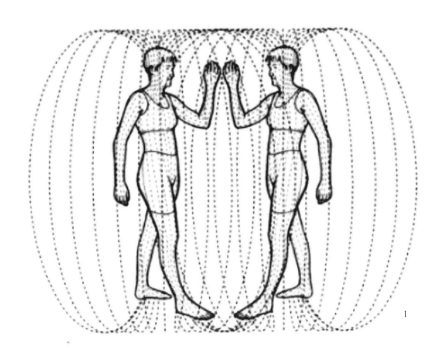

Have you ever gone to an amusement park and stood in front of one of those funny mirrors that distort your image? The mirror stretches your image or squashes it and distorts it is all kinds of ways. That is the way I see the couple's bodies when they get together as a condensed cloud of energy that gets distorted when they are near each other.

Energy distortion occurs anytime there are disruptive events inside and outside the body. In truth, the electromagnetic fields emitted by the wiring in your house, electric blankets, and even the alignment of the planets and solar flares cause distortion of the body energy fields, just as these events alter the growth of the plants and the level of the ocean tides.[2]

Together, distortion can occur even if they are madly in love with each other. The distortion of the energy fields causes imbalances physically, mentally, and emotionally. The removal of all distortion between two people is the goal of Two Person Energy Balancing.

This is the whole point of the "MIND/BODY" movement. It is not "New Age", it is a new realization that every aspect of the human being is interconnected, interdependent and inseparably interwoven. Imbalance anywhere will necessarily imbalance the whole mind, body and spirit.

Two-Person Energy Balancing was developed to specifically address imbalances that occur when two people's fields are causing energetic distortion.

The Scientific basis of Two Person Energy Balancing

"Energy Balancing" is a new concept to most people. Therefore, I hope this brief explanation will help bring it out of the 'shadows' and into the light for you.

Anytime people touch or come into each other's space there is an energy transfer. The human body is widely documented as being electrical, electronic, and otherwise electromagnetic.[2] Thanks to advances in technology these 'energy forces' of the body are no longer considered 'mystical' or as was considered in the past,'unworthy of true scientific study.'[3]

We now recognize that the boundary of a human being does not stop at the skin. It is a scientific fact that energy fields are unbounded by physical matter and indeed physical matter is at its very matrix simply energy.[4]

The body at all levels is by nature an intricate, coherent, dynamic, energy organism. The energetic fields of the body determine the shape, form and function of the body, mind and spirit.[5]

Understanding now the energetic nature of the body, one can begin to see how there can be potentially beneficial or harmful changes when one mixes energies by coming in contact with someone else. It is a scientific fact that the body's fields change from moment to moment in relation to events inside the body or outside of the body, such as when two people's fields come in contact.[6]

It is interesting that research has determined that the heart produces the strongest electromagnetic energy.[7] The heart's electrical output is distributed throughout the body via the circulatory system.[8] You might say it is the 'power generator' for the entire body. The magnetic fields of the heart reach out 15 feet from the body.[9] (So the next time you hug someone, you may want to hug them left side to left side, so that your strong heart fields can really say hello.) All of this is not to say electrical and magnetic fields are the only types of fields the body emits. There are other fields such as infrared and photonic emissions and it is likely that there are still other fields of energy yet to be discovered.[10]

Our understanding of human physiology and pathology has taken leaps forward through the development of sensitive superconductors, SQUID magnetometers, galvanometers, electrocardiograms (ECG) and many other types of electromagnetic devices.

Potential Benefits of Two Person Energy Balancing

- Improved rate of healing

- Better sleep

- Smoothing out of emotional ups and downs

- Improved energy

- Disappearance of mysterious aches and pains

- Better mental clarity

- Improved interpersonal relationships

- Improved communication

- Improvement of chronic symptoms

An energetic irritation can occur between two people which can almost be viewed as an allergic reaction. This "irritation" is a unique form of stress caused by the imbalances within the two bodies. One's resistance to the effects of stress is weakened in any chronic illness such as chronic Lyme disease. Never before has science realized the full potential that one person may exert over another by just being in the same vicinity.

The information contained herein is provided to improve your understanding the nature of this problem in this type of energy medicine. The treatments outlined herein are not stand-alone treatments, but are only part of a well-rounded wellness program of care. Two Person Energy Balancing is not intended to cure disease in the classic sense of the term, but to help remove any interference stressor hindering the body from functioning correctly.

The Treatment

How does one go about treating energy fields? Well, one treats energy with energy. And since everything is made up of the same thing, vibrational energy, potentially every type of treatment or therapy can be used.

Clinical Neurology research has determined that the more sensory input the body receives for the purpose of energy balancing, the better and deeper the effect. Therefore, the doctor will use as many vibrational tools as possible all at the same time. These tools may include low-level laser therapy, medical tuning forks, meridian stimulation, colored glasses, music/sound therapy, chiropractic adjustments, essential oils, homeopathy and nutritional supplementation.

The original treatment protocol to balance two people was developed by Dr. John W. Brimhall, D.C., and was presented in his "Health Paths" post-graduate lecture series (Kansas City-Atlanta, June 2002). Two Person Energy Balancing is not a cookbook process that treats everyone the same. Each doctor performing this treatment tests and treats as directed by Bio-Resonance Scanning™, or other sensitive testing method, therefore the actual treatments and tools utilized may vary from session to session.

It must be first determined if the two individuals are truly 'blowing' each other's electrical circuits. Each person is tested to see how well his or her body is working, without the addition of the other person's energy. Then the two are asked to hold hands and are retested to see if any electrical circuits are disrupted that previously were fine. Clinical testing has shown that almost everyone blows out in some way during this test. It has nothing to do with liking or disliking the other, it is simply how your energy fields blend.

The doctor, through Bio-Resonance Scanning™, or other sensitive testing technique, will determine the therapies needed to balance the two people using as many different therapeutic sensory inputs while they continue holding hands. At the end of the treatment, no energy circuits in either person should 'blow out' when retested. Periodical repeat treatments may be needed because so many external influences can affect a person on a daily basis.

How soon will you notice a difference? Only time will tell in regard to noticing change. The treatment itself is dealing with subtle energy, and the effect may be subtle, revealing itself only through introspection over the course of time. We have had couples report that after Two Person Energy Balancing, they were able to finally talk out and resolve their differences, thereby improving their relationships. Others just felt a greater comfort and well-being around their spouse. I know of at least one couple who came in determined to get a divorce and after this treatment came back the next day hand in hand with great smiles of renewed love and thanking me profusely. The effect for this couple seems to have been long lasting, as at last contact they were still reportedly happily married.

Some co-workers who work in close cooperation with each other have noticed greater synchronicity after receiving this treatment.

There is the possibility of improvement in some chronic symptoms, such as fatigue, depression, pain and hormonal imbalances. The actual potential for benefits is limitless. In chronic Lyme disease one needs to remove any interference to the body's ability to heal.

Chapter 24

Redesigning Your Life to Overcome Illness

Chronic Lyme affects more than just the physical structures of cells and tissues. It messes with the mind, body, and spirit.

To even hope to re-establish a state of wellness, your therapies must address the entire problem – not just attack the bacteria. One must immediately "clean house" – your internal physical, psychological, and spiritual house. A total lifestyle change is mandatory – the Lyme bacteria were allowed to grow unchecked in your body by the lifestyle and choices you have made! You must change the equation completely in every aspect of your life, constantly strengthening every area. Critical self-analysis will no doubt identify numerous weak links in your life, as well as many strong points. "You are only as strong as your weakest link". I see this in many chronic Lyme patients. Some of them have always eaten well, taken vitamins and herbs, and for all appearances lead a healthy life. What is not readily seen are the indulgences, intense chronic stress, bio-accumulative toxins from work or household sources, inherited traits, and hidden aspects that poison the body as a whole.

As long as we see the bacterial overgrowth as the cause rather than the condition of the organism's existence, chronic infections will remain a mystery. Lyme is no more a disease of bacteria than a traffic jam is a disease of cars. A lifetime study of the internal combustion engine would not help anyone to understand our traffic problems... A traffic jam is due to a failure of the normal relationship between driven cars and their environment and can occur whether they themselves are running normally or not. In the same way chronic Lyme is a disease of the human organism as a whole and not a disease of bacteria.

There are many ways to treat yourself as a "complete organism", most of which do not require that you hock your children's inheritance. Lifestyle changes should be your primary focus, combined with the efforts of your doctors.

Always remember, it is your body, the only one you have! It is your responsibility to protect it from harmful treatments. Don't trade one problem for another. <u>Be sure your doctor is treating the "human organism" as a whole, and not just attempting to simply destroy Lyme spirochetes.</u>

More times than not, with the latter treatment, since it does not treat the whole organism, Lyme infection reappears with a vengeance as soon as the antibiotics are removed.

New habits must be formed. The formation and process of developing new habits stimulates the regeneration of tissues. It is a known fact that the years of ingrained habits grind your inner being into a non-reactive sedentary mechanism. Forming new habits will re-awaken this healing force. Of course forming good habits are going to benefit you the most. This awakening force allows your body to separate good healthy cells from dysfunctional cells, and stimulates the reactive forces against the total illness. Don't blow this off as being too odd! Use your imagination to come up with a list of things you want to make a habit out of. Make a list – write it down! This list may include anything at all, i.e., change your handwriting, answer the phone with your other hand and ear than usual, hold your fork in the opposite hand to eat, not eating junk food for snacks, if you smoke - stop, find and develop new hobbies outside of your normal interests, read instead of watching TV, exercise whenever you feel like taking a nap, hang your clothes up every time, get up immediately without hitting the snooze button. You see, it doesn't really matter what you decide to make into a new habit. <u>It is the process of doing it that wakes up this incredible healing inner force.</u> If you contemplate this issue you may be able to recognize that part of you that has been asleep from being so comfortably in a rut. Too many of us work hard to achieve a comfortable life, so it will be difficult for some to even want to change – you wanted to know how to beat this diagnosis of Lyme; I'm telling you – do it to increase your chances.

Focus and capture every thought before you think it! Maintain a positive mindset, no matter what the disease looks like or feels like, or how events and people want to depress or enrage you. To do this you will be required to activate the above previously described habit mechanism, since it is not normally a habit to always think positively. An inner peace in your spirit can be achieved only by exercising/practicing with vigilance different ways to come into complete control of your spirit mind. There are several techniques geared to this end. Curative Eurhythmy is one method of expressing visual sound of your spirit through movement. A certified teacher is a must. Eurhythmy is a scientific method developed in Germany and Switzerland which is utilized in hospitals as a curative technique. As you progress in this therapy you will be more centered and more aware of your connection to all of nature. In this process you can focus more clearly and not be knocked about by events and negativity around you. It also activates strong healing within every nook and cranny of your being. If you cannot find a Eurhythmy class in your area then choose some form of movement therapy such as aqua aerobics or non-spiritualistic yoga type classes that are offered in most health clubs.

Curative artistic therapy: Profound healing forces lie hidden in art. The opening up and submission by a person into activities which are new and unfamiliar, once again, speak directly to the depths of one's being. The possibilities for artistic therapy include the entire spectrum of art – music, painting, sculpture, and dance. In general, our creative forces have been paralyzed by the advent of television, movies, and radio. Knowing how integrated every aspect of our existence is, i.e., science has documented that a person purposely thinking depressing thoughts cause alterations of depressed function reaching every cell and electrical signal in the body. So, it is easy to see (and it will become easier to see, with the more you distance yourself from these sedentary activities) that for hour upon hour we stare absent-mindedly, exerting no effort at all, imaginatively or otherwise, laying waste to and atrophying the ego and formative forces in the body. An Artistic Therapist is highly trained in carefully guiding the ill patient to the realization of formative energies to be found here, so that the unfolding of personality can occur in a non-violating fashion. Deep acting healing can be found in the arts. These therapists are not just the Joe Public person who is good with a brush or musical instrument, but one trained specifically for therapy of ill people. If you cannot find an art therapist in your area then definitely find and participate in some form of art classes usually offered by various education centers.

Sunlight, regardless as to how the information highway negatively reports, is vital to total health. Ultraviolet light stimulates the skeletal system and increases the formation of blood and bone. Up to a cumulative of one hour of sunbathing (allowing the sunlight to touch all of the body) has been demonstrated to enhance overall body function. Everyone has heard of "cabin fever". This is caused by lack of sunlight over prolonged periods such as cloudy winter days. The sunlight on the skin activates metabolic processes that produce Vitamin D. Depression and psychotic behavior, as well as a decrease in your body's metabolism, occurs from a lack of sunlight. There are varying degrees of this condition that one can see especially in people who are ill. It is vital to move even the bedridden into the sunlight as it acts as a dimmer switch on the entire human organism to crank up the power.

Fill your house with live plants. Plants clean the air as they "breathe", especially broad, large-leafed plants. They permeate the air with healthy, negatively charged electrical particles called ions, not to mention clean oxygen. The ion concentration in a house directly influences health, healing, and your sense of well-being.

We have all heard the saying, "...it is an ill wind that blows no good", this phrase refers to a phenomenon documented the world over. When the winds blow from a certain direction in specific locations in the world, the number of accidents, deaths, suicides, and hospital admissions rise. Science has finally determined that these winds are predominantly positively charged electrical ions. Positive ions promote disease. People enjoy waterfalls and feel happier and better near them because the water droplets in the air are negatively charged. Negative ions promote healing. So, plants in your home will promote healing and an overall increased sense of well-being. Do not use pesticides, herbicides, or any chemical additive as it will end up in the air you breathe as well.

One "no brainer" is to follow the treatment protocol set up for you by your doctor. It definitely won't work if you don't follow it correctly – be diligent. Believe in your doctor. If you can not believe in your doctor, then find a new one that you can believe in. There can be no room for doubt and negative energy between you and those trying to help you. Don't dabble with one doctor and another doctor. Therapies and treatments don't always mix. If you are the praying type, (and I hope you are) PRAY for your doctor! The doctor cannot heal you – he can only remove interferences and awaken the healing power within your body. The pressure is somewhat on him, but it is really on you. YOU make it happen. YOU must perform. Most of healing occurs at the changing of your mind. YOU walk your healing out into manifestation every minute of every day. The doctor only sees you for a small amount of time in a day – the healing doesn't stop when you leave the doctor's office; the responsibility simply shifts completely back to you!

Deep breathing exercises are very important. One of the primary functions of blood is to supply over 50 trillion cells with oxygen, and yet the majority of Americans would be medically classified as "shallow breathers". The lungs are one of your body's primary pathways of getting rid of toxins and waste. As you breathe out, or exhale, you are eliminating cellular debris and toxic gases. If the Lyme is to ultimately die, the body must cleanse itself of the byproducts of these bacteria. Practice anywhere, but ideally out in an area in the countryside where hopefully the air is cleaner and you're surrounded by vegetation giving off healing negative ions. Breathe deeply through your nose, then allow the lungs to naturally release the air through your mouth, without forcing out.

Keep all parts of your body warm. Many people don't realize how poorly their body is regulating the temperature in the various parts of the body. This is a component of your body's overall vitality. Try to feel it yourself, or have a spouse or friend feel and compare the temperature from every part of your body. Don't be surprised by what you find. Lyme Disease dysregulates overall body temperature and makes it cooler. There are several external ways to combat this problem. There are also internal remedies to increase and vitalize these forces. Warmth is vital to healing.

Change your terminology. I see people with Lyme disease that speak of the disease as "my Lyme this...or my Lyme that..." . They have an intense intimate connection to the Lyme. It is not a part of you! Don't accept it, even verbally. Always refer to it as "the Lyme" or "it". Don't acknowledge negativity such as saying, "It's really getting the better of me today", or " I feel like I'm fighting a losing battle". Negative thinking affects you as a total organism and drains away the healing energy every time. Measure successes in very small increments. Rejoice over them. Constantly guard your thinking and your tongue.

Visualize health and healing. Plan and keep times of quiet, uninterrupted meditative thought and visualize in your mind's eye, with great detail, what the disease looks like. Then visualize it in great detail being attacked, breaking apart, disintegrating, being carried away in dead pieces in the body fluids. See your body's immune system army hammering away at it. Then, with great attention to detail again, see yourself as totally well and physically fit, happy, and with a positive outlook on life. Do this as often as possible. Remember, your body is watching these visualizations also, and will strive to achieve it.

I tell you these last statements in an attempt or plea to your mind to understand why biological medicine and alternative medicine methods are so vital as a part of your healing regime. It is painfully obvious that antibiotics and vitamins and such are not winning in most cases.

This book outlines what may seem to be odd therapies and odd methods, but they are based upon valid science, usually established from research performed in Europe.

Chapter 25

47 Thoughts To Live On

1. In times of change, learners will inherit the earth, while the learned will find themselves beautifully prepared to deal with a world which no longer exists.

2. What you say, and what you think, is every cell's command – be sure the commands you are sending are not perpetuating the illness.

3. It's not "all in your head", but illness requires your head to be into and in line with your healing.

4. Determine and focus your mind on your body as you would have it be, and then never waver from that image. Your body will hear the command and make it so.

5. Focus on the illness and it will grow; focus on healing and it will be.

6. Doctors can help your body to heal, but only you can give your body the permission to heal totally.

7. What you need to learn is to never speak a negative. When you have a problem, never tell more people than necessary – your brain is listening.

8. This is a law of nature: Believing = Receiving, whether negative or positive.

9. Believe that you will be completely well again the way you believe that the letter you just mailed will actually reach its destination, or the way that you believe that the Statue of Liberty is in New York even though you have personally never seen it.

10. In dealing with pressure, you have to realize that all pressure begins in the mind. You allow yourself to be pressured. Consciously choose to depressurize.

11. To speed healing, you must get the hurt and dirt out of your life.

12. Change involves work.

13. You will never get the answer to a question you never asked.

14. Truth is truth, come hell or high water.

15. We fear what we do not understand. The cure for fear is understanding the truth. Understanding comes from acquiring knowledge. Wisdom is gained through applied knowledge.

16. Where knowledge fails, heart sustains.

17. Negatives are like ticks on a blood hunt. They stick to you. Eliminate the negatives and accentuate the positives.

18. All strain is drain.

19. Positive thoughts combat negative thinking.

20. Thinking patterns determine your heart, your heart determines your health.

21. Be patient with yourself.

22. Don't sacrifice your whole life because you have a wound in one area. Lyme disease is not who you are.

23. You do your best. Trust God to do the rest.

24. Action cures fear. Non-action strengthens fear.

25. Be an active participant in your own healing.

26. What you are doing today will determine your tomorrow.

27. It's really not how long we live that counts, but the quality of our lives while we are living.

28. The more healing you have to do, the more disciplined you have to be to get the desired healing done. The more sick you are, the more disciplined you must be to regain your health.

29. You are the sum total of the decisions your ancestors and you have made.

30. Wellness is not a state of being, but a state of mind.

31. The greatest part of education is learning to think for yourself.

32. I see my life far beyond today and tomorrow. I see my life from generation to generation causing them to live a stronger heritage.

33. We plant the trees so that someone else may enjoy the privilege of sitting in the shade.

34. I wish I were the man I know to be; however, I always strive to do better.

35. Minds are like parachutes: they work best when they are open.

36. Why continue to go to the world for answers when it's the world that confused you in the first place?

37. One must be as willing to unlearn as to learn.

38. All life is dependent upon decision; accomplishment is attained by carrying out that decision.

39. Be assured of this – you never have a headache due to a deficiency of aspirin.

40. Looking back gives you a stiff neck.

41. Healing never occurs by accident: it is always the result of high intention, sincere effort, intelligent direction and execution.

42. If you keep doing what you've always done, then you will keep getting the same results.

43. To change your life you must change your mind.

44. It's your body, it's your decision on how to treat it.

45. Health in a bottle is a myth.

46. Practice every moment of every day to remain unchanged and content, by any internal or external circumstance.

47. Let go of yesterday. The past is roadkill. Live completely in the moment you are in.

Chapter 26

Predispositions to Illness - Miasms

Did you ever wonder why you act the way you do, or why you suffer with certain types of illnesses? How you act and the things you suffer from may have more to do with your ancestors than with your lifestyle. The theory of miasms may explain some of what makes you tick. This is not "new age" and is not genetic aberrations, but is more of an energetic phenomenon.

A miasm, by definition, is a predisposition, or tendency, of certain psychological and physical problems that you either inherited or acquired within your own lifetime[1-2]. Miasms are not to be confused with genetic abnormalities, such as missing or mutated genes. Miasms are more of an energetic abnormality. John Davidson, a researcher and author on bioenergetics, states that, "miasms are essentially an energy disharmony, disease pattern or imbalance."

Research dating back over 200 years documents the reality of these energetic problems. Miasms are usually started by improperly treated illnesses that can go back as far as seven generations of your family tree. In other words, some of the tendencies you have, could be the result of illnesses your parents had, or medications they took before you were born, or even by your great, great…grandparents' illnesses[2].

For over two hundred years, scientists have been tracking the miasms caused by specific illnesses. Today we have immense collections of data outlining what kinds of problems future generations may experience due to different illnesses. Gonorrhea, syphilis, tuberculosis, cancer, and many more, all will generate a specific set of problems unique to the illness when suppressive therapies are used to treat them. Antibiotics are a suppressive therapy and, some agree, are the major culprit to creating miasms. The antibiotics do kill the bacteria that cause these different illnesses, but they do nothing to address the damage already done by the bacteria on a physical and bio-electrical level in the patient's body. For example, if you find that you have termites in you house, you can call an exterminator to come out and kill the termites. By killing the termites you have made it where the problem should not get worse, however, you have done nothing to correct the myriad of tunnels through the woodwork of your house. To make matters worse, you now have a very toxic chemical insecticide in your house. These tunnels and toxins, in a nutshell, are what cause miasms to occur.

How are miasms passed from generation to generation?

When a girl or boy is born, they carry the family blueprints in their eggs and sperm. These blueprints are being constantly modified. You might say it is an ongoing project that is passed on to each new generation. My sperm carry the blueprints unique to the Jernigan family. When combined with my wife's blueprints each generation put in their two cents worth on how the child should be made. Throughout both sets of blueprints there are energetic flaws, miasms, which out of the ignorance of past doctors, went uncorrected. The union of these blueprints results in a child. This child came to this world created with his or her unique set of blueprints. Let us assume for the sake of demonstration that this is a boy child whose parents got properly treated and passed on no miasms. His blueprints have no flaws. The years go by and he gets an ear infection, which due to social pressures, the parents have treated with antibiotics. Instantly, the blueprints in the little boy's sperm are modified. His sperm will now create offspring that may have tendencies to similar problems, i.e. ear infections and the psychological problems unique to the miasm. The boy will live through these minor illnesses.

The boy grows up and for example's sake, we'll say he is sexually promiscuous before he is married, and catches gonorrhea. Gonorrhea has been identified as the cause of a major type of miasm. Gonorrhea infection, and the standard treatments, causes major modifications to the blueprints in his sperm. He later settles down and marries a nice girl. This is where it really gets interesting – keep in mind that the blueprint in the sperm is being modified bio-electrically (or energetically).

Can a Miasm be sexually transmitted?

When the above couple has sexual intercourse the man's sperm is deposited within the woman. Research has verified that the sperm are viable up to three days, so for three days the woman is forced to integrate some of the miasmic energy of the sperm! In a bizarre way the woman becomes linked to that man energetically. This may be some primeval mechanism to ensure the procreation of the species, much like the way many birds and animals mate for life. It may also ensure that miasmic corruption of blueprints is kept to a minimum – possibly such as inbreeding problems seen in the breeding of purebred dogs. It is theorized that this may also be why some wives continue to stay with a husband who physically and emotionally abuses them.

Even if this couple never has children, the woman will suffer primarily on a psychological level because of the miasmic transfer from the husband's sperm. It is primarily on the psychological level since it is the most vulnerable to energetic change, however over the course of many years, the woman may experience physical symptoms as well, caused purely by the miasm.

If this couple were to have children, the father's miasm-damaged blueprint would be passed on to the child, predisposing the child to similar problems and tendencies which, if left untreated, will be passed on for another 5 generations.

What if a woman has had multiple sex partners?

In theory, each man's sperm can adversely affect the woman on a miasmic level. Besides the fact that the Holy Bible teaches against premarital or extramarital sex, this may be the scientific reason behind God's preference for monogamous marriage. Having multiple sex partners means that potentially each of the woman's partners imprinted their miasmatic garbage upon the woman and may impact her and her offspring.

Like father, like son!

The Bible even mentions that the sins of the father are passed on through the blood seven generations. So, the next time you hear someone say, "I'm just like my Mom, a worrier", or "I have my Dad's hot temper", or "Everyone in my family has diabetes" or "Everyone in my family dies of cancer,"you can recognize it for what it really is – a miasm running through the family up to seven generations.

Marriage Concerns

I know it is not romantic, but you should be concerned about your potential spouse's family health history. If nothing else you and your significant other should be tested and treated for miasms before you start a family.

How are miasms corrected?

The only recognized way to effectively eliminate existing miasms is with the proper homeopathic remedy. In the above gonorrhea scenario, the homeopathic nosode called Medorrhinum would be the appropriate remedy. Normally only one to three doses is necessary to remove the miasm from the blueprint. "Energy is never lost, only transformed or relocated and homeopathic cure attempts, therefore, to smooth out the disharmony of the miasm, as the basic cause of disease…The release of the entire miasmatic trait would result in a complete cure… If therefore, a miasm is successfully treated, the energy field is re-polarized."[2]

The best way to avoid acquiring new miasms is to combine the proper homeopathic remedies with whatever other treatments you choose. Only a doctor trained in homeopathy, or a professional homeopath trained in the treatment of miasms should address these types of issues.

Section 5

Wellness Physicians of the 21st Century

Chapter 27

Doctors of Chiropractic
"The Wellness Physicians of the 21ˢᵗ Century"

I have become aware that many people are surprised that I, a Doctor of Chiropractic can address such a wide range of illnesses. Some people seem to think Doctors of Chiropractic can only deal with "stiff necks and low back pain." This is partly due to the political stance that the chiropractic profession has had to maintain in order to exist. However, this is no truer than thinking a Medical Doctor can only prescribe drugs.

Any medical doctor, osteopath, naturopath, or doctor of chiropractic can and are receiving post-graduate training in Euro-America Biological Medicine. I have been asked innumerable times, "Why don't M.D.s do this?" To answer this, one must realize that most M.D.s work in hospitals or group practices. These doctors cannot just decide one day to do Biological or natural medicine in these settings. The hospitals and insurance companies dictate what they can and can't do, and rightly so, since the hospitals are ultimately liable for their doctors' actions. Even in small group practices, the safety of the whole keeps one doctor from doing things differently. If all this were not detriment enough, most medical doctors have a "non-compete" clause in their contract with the hospitals that forbids them to practice within a 50 mile radius from any hospital owned by that corporation. In our area, most of the small outlying hospitals have been bought out by large hospital corporations, making it nearly impossible for any of their doctors to set up a Biological Medicine practice in any but the most remote areas.

Doctors of Chiropractic are uniquely qualified to specialize in Biological Medicine due to their intensive education in working with the structure and function of body. They are trained to facilitate healing through natural means, instead of relying on drugs to force the body to perform illusions of health.

Doctors of Chiropractic believe that the body has innate intelligence. Innate intelligence is that part of each of us that knows how the heart should beat: it's the regulatory and control mechanisms behind how the body heals a cut; how the body knows how to breathe without your conscious participation. Once again, treating disease is the realm of the conventional medical doctors – Chiropractic and Biological Medicine have no desire to treat any disease, but focus upon restoring the integrity of the body, mind, and spirit, thereby leading to the disappearance of disease. Of course, there is a place for heroic medicine in the form of drugs, surgery, and such. In crisis definitely save the life first and foremost, but once the crisis has been averted, restoring the body, mind, and spirit to maximum integrity through biological and natural means, working to restore the perfection of God's design, is optimal.

From day one of training, the Doctors of Chiropractic are taught the research that proves that the body has an innate intelligence and the body is designed to heal itself. From day one of training, the Doctor of Chiropractic learns only to facilitate healing. From day one, the Doctors of Chiropractic are taught to diagnose different pathologies. From day one, the Doctor of Chiropractic learns to optimize neurology, physiology, histology, and chemistry of the body to facilitate healing. Doctors of Chiropractic do not have to unlearn invasive and toxic methods and relearn that God designed the body to heal itself, and that there are thousands of tools that are not harmful and do not need a PDR to explain the side-effects.

As you will see in the chart later, Doctors of Chiropractic are fully trained in every area of health and healing. Doctors of Chiropractic must have a Bachelor's degree before being admitted, they must complete their "Pre-Med" elbow to elbow with the other prospective M.D., D.O., D.D.S. and D.V.M. students. Once accepted into Chiropractic College, students are taught an almost identical curriculum as every medical professional for four years, up to the point where every doctor must specialize.

It is up to each graduating doctor to determine how they are going to apply the knowledge they have gained. It must be understood that all schooling is an agreed upon minimum amount of information. For a bachelor's degree, you will know at least this much; for a master's degree, this much; for a doctorate, you will know at least the agreed upon minimum also. So, even at the doctorate level, the knowledge is not the ultimate knowledge in the field. That is why doctors must have additional hours of State Healing Arts Board approved, continuing education credits every year of their career… to learn specialized knowledge in their field of interest. This continuing education in a specialized field may represent over a thousand more classroom hours. Our doctor's field of interest and "specialization" is in learning to address the degenerative and chronic diseases, using natural methods. This is called "Euro-American Biological Medicine."

Keep in mind, no doctor can go any further than they have been taught!

Biological Medicine is Post Graduate, specialized training that not every doctor receives; therefore your conventional physician may not know how to advise you regarding its use. You must seek out a doctor specializing in Biological Medicine in your area. One resource for finding these doctors is the Marion Foundation, which can be accessed on the internet or key in a word-search for "Biological Medicine."

So, if you are looking for a Doctor of Chiropractic in your area, you just need to call around and say to the receptionist, "I realize that your doctor sees many different problems, but I am curious as to which type of patients he or she sees the most?" At the Somerleyton Center for Biological Medicine we would say, we attract what we affectionately refer to as the "Humpty Dumpty Bunch" where all the Kings horses and all the Kings men could not put them back together again."

The profession has different specializations within it just as Medical Doctors. To name a few, there are Doctors of Chiropractic who specialize as internists, pediatricians, sports medicine, neurology, and obviously my favorite and what I consider the crème de la crème, those specializing in Biological Medicine. You must maintain the integrity of the nervous system and the musculoskeletal system in order for the body to heal itself.

Doctors of Chiropractic are in the top 1/2 of 1% of the most educated people in the world and are absolutely qualified to treat the body, mind, and spirit. A Doctor of Chiropractic can be your greatest ally in any illness.

The following chart compares the number of hours that Doctors of Chiropractic and Medical Doctors take in their basic training before they specialize.

Chiropractic Hours	Subject	Medical Hours
456	Anatomy/Embryology	215
243	Physiology	174
296	Pathology	507
161	Chemistry	100
145	Microbiology	145
408	Diagnosis	113
149	Neurology	171
271	X-ray	13
56	Psychology/Psychiatrics	323
66	Obstetrics & Gynecology	284
168	Orthopedics	2
2419 hours	**TOTAL HOURS**	**2047 hours**

Section 6

Important Therapies for Chronic Lyme Disease

Chapter 28

ST8 Lymphatic Drainage Therapy

"This is the medicine of the future," was the response I got when I asked one of the best doctors in the country, Dr. John Thompson, D.O., about the ST8 Lymphatic therapy machine, before I bought mine. He was not kidding, I soon found out once I started using my new ST8. I feel that the ST8 makes what I consider a really good healing system, Circuit Healing™, great!

Doctors have known for years that before effective detoxification of the body can occur, the lymphatic system must be able to flush out the toxins. Many therapies I have used for years have worked to pull, drag, or sweat out the heavy metals and chemical toxins stored inside the cells and from around the cells. But, until now stimulating the movement of lymph fluid and opening the primary lymphatic drainage ducts was next to impossible to do quickly.

One treatment with the ST8, according to some experts having 15,000+ hours of manual lymph work under their belt, is equal to 6-8 manual lymphatic massages! Because the ST8 works so quickly on the lymphatic system, I have witnessed the true role that the lymphatic system plays in healing. Near miraculous disappearance of acute and chronic pain and symptoms of all kinds greatly improved, by relieving the lymphatic congestion convinces me and every patient I have used it on that it truly is the "medicine of the future".

Now finally, when we use detoxification dietary supplements, and detoxification therapies such as the ion-cleanse, infrared sauna, and dry skin brushing, we have the confidence of knowing the cleansing lymph fluid is flowing and effectively washing out from around all of the cells and tissues of the body. It is so important because if the lymphatic system is not circulating efficiently then there is no supplement that will be able to reach the toxins locked far in the nooks and crannies of the body.

Every illness will benefit from the ST8 therapy. Every doctor involved with Lyme disease should be using an ST8 to limit Herxheimer reactions, which are the bane of every Lyme patient. Remember, these Herxheimer reactions are toxins dumping into an already toxin overloaded body from the overwhelming toxic load from simply living in this day and age.

The ST8 utilizes the latest technology of electro-medicine, non-invasive scalar waves, low current, cold gas photon therapy, ozone therapy, and resonance frequency technology, all wrapped into one painless, highly effective device.

Cells in the body that become clumped and stuck together, bond electrically leading to swelling or abnormal growths. The cells are either held together or held apart as determined by their electromagnetic charge (polarity). One can think of it as two magnets with either north pole facing north pole repelling each other, or north pole of one magnet facing the south pole of the other magnet which attracts the magnets to stick together. It is this stuck together situation that the ST8 corrects by rebalancing the polarity of the cells so that the cells separate from each other. Once apart, the energetic frequencies, photons, and ozone of the ST8 boost the immune system.

Besides being beneficial in Lyme disease, the ST8 has accumulated quite a reputation in the realm of cancer. In truth however, the list of illnesses benefitted that I or the doctors that I associate with have already experienced, that it would be futile to try to list each one.

More research and testimonials can be viewed on the ST8's company, ELF Laboratory, website, www.elflaboratory.com.

Chapter 29

Magnetic Resonance Bio-Oxidative Therapy™

Magnetic Resonance Bio-Oxidative Therapy (MRBT) is the brainchild of Dr. William H. Philpott, M.D., a board certified neurologist and psychologist, with special training and practice in environmental medicine and toxicology.

This one therapy may be my absolute favorite because of the incredible range of actions, not to mention its phenomenal track record for success where all other treatments and therapies failed. In my opinion, you will get more "bang for your buck" using this one therapy, because unlike medicines which run out or quit working, these ceramic magnets never quit working, and there is no time that the body cannot continue to benefit.

I want to list just some of the actions of the MRBT so that you can appreciate how it can turn the tide on just about any disease.

Magnetic Resonance Bio-Oxidative Therapy:
   (Negative polarity only)

1. Converts the tissues from acidic to alkaline (All bacteria, virus, parasites, fungi and mycoplasma need and promote an acidic environment wherever they are living and will die in an alkaline environment)

2. Re-establishes the normal cellular polarity back to the predominantly negative polarity needed by normal healthy cells to repel microbes. (All bacteria, virus, parasites, fungi, and mycoplasma have a predominantly positive polarity... you may be saying that opposites attract, so normal tissue attracts microbes, however in the body when the tissues become weak and diseased, the normal negative polarity drops too low, crippling the defense mechanisms of the cells. So the positive polarity microbes are in an energy fight with the weak cells. When the cell's polarity is restored and full strength, it inhibits the replication of every microbe. Viruses need your RNA in order to replicate, however they cannot penetrate and replicate when the cell polarity is high,

and they also cannot replicate in an alkaline environment. They need and try to establish an acid environment.)

3. Increases the tissue oxygen levels. MRBT hyper-oxygenates the cells. All microbes are inhibited to some degree by high oxygen levels, and some microbes are actually killed by oxygen. Through hyper-oxygenation of the body, certain enzyme systems are supported that are needed for energy production in the body in the form of adenosine triphosphate or ATP. ATP production is therefore increased to be used for energy by every cell in the body.

4. MRBT governs sleep by evoking the production and release of melatonin from the pineal gland. Melatonin is also antimicrobial and helps reset the bio-rhythms necessary for health and healing. Melatonin is a potent anti-cancer substance.

5. MRBT normalizes brain wave activity and relieves cerebral allergies that lead to all manner of psychosis and depressive states. Some cases of hospitalized neurosis and psychosis have been completely relieved within 10 minutes of using MRBT in conjunction with food allergy testing! Many of the people I have treated who had Lyme disease were also suffering from depression, anxiety, seizures and such. Lyme so disrupts the normal functioning of just about every organ system that just about no food is being digested correctly and is therefore causing what Dr. Philpott calls a Maladaptive Syndrome. (See chapter 13 on dietary recommendations for correcting Maladaptive Syndrome with Lyme disease.)

Magnetic Resonance Bio-Oxidative Therapy: (Positive polarity only for a select few situations)

Positive Polarity MRBT can be used for a select few situations:

6. Positive Polarity over the thymus, not to exceed 30 minutes, can stimulate the immune system. It can also be used to stimulate the adrenal glands (increases adrenal-cortical hormone production)

7. Can be used in 5-minute alternating practice sessions with a trained therapist in stimulating the return of neuronal function, which has been damaged or impaired by pressure, acid/chemical neuritis, infection, or degeneration.

Can you begin to see why Magnetic Resonance Bio-Oxidative Therapy is my favorite therapy? It is safe enough for me to universally recommend without hesitation even for children and the very old. There are no contra-indications but there are companies selling therapy magnets which use a mix of negative and positive polarity. Because positive polarity supports cancer and supports the excitation of the psychotic patient, and promotes the spread of microbes, and positive polarity promotes acidity and lowers the tissue oxygen levels, I do not and would not universally recommend these mixed polarity magnetic products. Just in case you are still not convinced, according to Dr. Philpott, the effects of "prolonged exposure to a positive magnetic field can produce a toxic vasculitis, neuritis, and addiction due to evoked endorphins, serotonin, microorganisms, and cancer cell replication."

Not all magnets are created equal. The latest advancement in magnets are the neodymium magnets. These magnets' specific therapeutic uses have a gauss strength of 12,000 gauss, but have only a therapeutic field penetration of about 25 gauss at 1 1/2" from the surface of the magnet, so if you are needing to saturate the body with negative polarity as is desirable in Lyme disease, this magnet would not do the job. It is great for superficial problems like muscle and joint pain.

The biggest and best penetration is from the ceramic industrial magnets, which while only rated at 3950 gauss, they provide up to 18" of therapeutic penetration at 25 gauss. The way all this works is the higher the gauss, the better, with at least 25 gauss needed to provide therapeutic effect.

Once again, MRBT in almost all applications uses only the static (non-pulsed) negative polarity.

Specific Ways MRBT Works

MRBT changes the partial-pressure of oxygen meaning that there is an increased movement of oxygen through the tissues and an increased utilization of oxygen in the cells, which increases the energy metabolism.

The entire body can be influenced bio-energetically by the physical dimension "magnetic field" at a therapeutic gauss intensity. It is known that in different diseases the electrical resting and threshold potentials of cells differ from normal values, thus impairing the cell function. With MRBT, the ions present in the cells and in the colloidal system are magnetically influenced. As they are exposed to the static negative magnetic fieldlines, the ions are pressed against the cell membrane producing a hyper-polarization, which has a corrective influence on the intracellular metabolism, particularly on the energy metabolism. If this procedure is applied over a determined period of time, it leads to a normalization of the electrical potential difference. As a result there is improved ion dynamics at the cells' interface, resulting in the increased utilization of oxygen in the cell. This increases the production of energy for healing and overall cellular function in the form of ATP (adenosine triphosphate). The resultant increase in ATP from using MRBT can be measured.

MRBT, ATP and Chronic Illness

ATP, adenosine triphosphate, is one of your body's primary energy molecules that is produced by every cell for everyday functioning and for healing. ATP is produced by the mitochondria, the energy factories in every cell. You burn up to 40% of your total body weight in ATP every day. This means that if you weigh 100 pounds, you are using up 40 pounds of ATP every day. Thankfully, you can recycle the resultant ADP (Adenosine Diphosphate), that way you don't just disappear completely in about three days! Below you will see how this 40 pounds of ATP is used in your body. Its use can be broken down into thirds, so consider as in the above 100 pound person, 13.3 pounds of ATP is being used every day for the following three general ways.

ATP use can be broken down into three major functions:

- ATP production is extremely important, especially in Lyme disease, because one-third of all of the ATP produced in your body is used to pump out the sodium from the neurons via the sodium/potassium pumps. In states of chronic illness the body's metabolism becomes compromised and the energy production in the form of ATP slows down. Without enough ATP to pump out the sodium from the nerve fibers, the nerve fibers begin to degenerate. As degeneration of the nerve occurs, you experience tingling, muscle weakness, numbness, and the ultimate progressive dysfunction of multiple organ systems. So, you can see the importance of your doctor maintaining or re-establishing the ATP production of your body.

- One third of the ATP your body produces is used to facilitate enzyme reactions. If the body's enzyme reactions do not have the ATP to function correctly, many of the chemical reactions in the body will not happen quickly enough to be of any good. This enzymatic breakdown leads to multi-system dysfunction, affecting all aspects of sense of well-being and strength. MRBT increases the metabolism (all of the chemical reactions occurring in the body) by hyperpolarizing the cells, which is beneficial in turning up the ATP production for these enzymatic/chemical reactions.

- The last third, or 13.3 pounds, of the ATP is used for energy to run all of the contractile muscles and non-contractile tissues of the body. In this area ATP shortage is noticed most remarkably in muscle fatigue and atrophy. When all is functioning correctly, the muscle fibers are "pumped up" from weight bearing exercise and the muscle fibers are filled with energy producing mitochondria, which are little organs inside of the cells that are simply ATP factories. When multiple systems become dysfunctional and multiple electrical circuits are "blown" the demand for energy is great, but the body is unable to generate the electricity it needs to keep the mitochondria working. One by one the mitochondrial energy factories shut down, ATP production falls sharply and the muscle atrophies or shrinks in size and strength. In order for MRBT research to have demonstrated an increase in ATP, it must be re-energizing the mitochondrial energy factories.

Your body's metabolism becomes sluggish during chronic illnesses, and ATP production goes down because the demand for energy wanes as the cells become *hypo*-functional. The mitochondrial energy factories gradually begin to shut down to just a "skeleton crew" and only enough mitochondrial energy factories remain to barely "keep the lights on". To say that a therapy increases the production of ATP means that the energy factories are fired up again in response to reinforcement from the cells becoming less hypofunctional and more functional again.

A healthy functioning cell needs a lot of energy and can get it when all the players are present and working. Once there is enough ATP the body can get busy repairing, replacing, and rebuilding. As the tissues become healthier, the body's natural resistance to infection is re-established and with other appropriate treatments such as antibiotics the infections can be completely eliminated.

MRBT is only now getting a foot-hold in some of the leading research hospitals in the United States, but research on the medical therapeutic use of magnetic fields has been ongoing in Europe and around the world using this particular therapy for the last 25 years.

Apart from many other diseases, Magnetic Resonance Bio-Oxidative Therapy may be applied with great therapeutic success when used in conjunction with appropriate treatments in the following ailments:

- Diseases of the support and locomotor systems, particularly rheumatic and arthritic disorders.

- Neurological, mental, emotional, psychological disorders

- Cancer

- Diabetes Type I and II

- Lyme disease and any other infectious disease– bacterial, viral, mycoplasmal, parasitic, or fungal.

- Gastrointestinal disorders, i.e., Chron's, irritable bowel syndrome, ulcerative colitis, pancreatitis, hepatitis, food allergies.

- Eye disorders, glaucoma, optic neuritis, degenerative conditions of the retina and macula.

- Sports injuries such as bruises, pulled or torn ligaments and muscles, tennis elbow.

- Delayed wound healing and non-union fractures.

- Headaches and migraines

- Heart and circulatory diseases, circulatory disturbances

- Metabolic disorders

- Neuralgia

- Bronchitis and sinusitis, acute and chronic

It stands to reason that many of the above ailments known to respond well to MRBT are now becoming known to be caused by infectious anaerobic organisms. One can see the truth in the ability of the MRBT to increase the oxygenation of the tissues thereby assisting in the killing of anaerobic microbes.

When used in conjunction with Hyperbaric Oxygen Therapy (HBOT) a synergistic effect is achieved enabling deeper penetration and utilization of the oxygen into all the cells of the body. MRBT is a strong stand-alone therapy, but it will also enable you to get more out of your HBOT treatments.

Chapter 30

Infrared Sauna Therapy

There are not many therapies that can equal the vast range of healing benefits than is documented with infrared sauna therapy. Studies from all over the world report such a wide range of illnesses that are benefited by this therapy that to include a complete list would require several pages. Some of the conditions benefited are listed below.

In the realm of benefiting chronic or frequently occuring infectious illness infrared sauna therapy is a vital part of any good treatment program. This is because of its ability to detoxify the body of heavy metals and toxins that are locked up in the fat cells.

Heavy metals and toxins are known to promote an environment in the body that is a microbe heaven. They cause overcooling of the body, hypersensitivities and allergic tendencies, and direct toxic effects on the body as a whole.

When many people hear the word "sauna", they immediately conjure up images of steamy sweat rooms that are intensely and uncomfortably hot. Infrared saunas are nothing like the old steam or dry convection heat saunas. Infrared saunas operate from between 100° F to 130°F, which is still very comfortable for most people, compared to the intense heat of traditional saunas which operate between 180° F to 235° F.

While studying Biological Medicine, I was impressed to find that some of the world's most successful Biological Medicine Hospitals and Clinics in Germany, Switzerland and the U.S. use the infrared saunas for almost all of their patients. In today's highly toxic world, there is almost no person who would not benefit tremendously from the health promoting effects of this therapy.

Infrared saunas work by emitting far infrared energy, which penetrates the body just over 4 1/2 inches! The deep penetration of heat is much more efficient than traditional saunas.

Infrared is a fascinating technology. Scientific research has now resulted in saunas that emit a finely tuned infrared energy output that closely matches the body's own radiant energy. What this means is that almost 93% of the infrared waves are absorbed into the body. With this much absorption of the infrared waves, the body heats up, but the air in the sauna remains cooler. The cooler environment of the sauna is much more pleasant to sit in, and air is not so hot to breathe.

So many of the chronically ill patients I see know that they should work out and do aerobic exercise as part of living a balanced life, however the illness they suffer usually prevents them from performing truly meaningful workouts. Many are too sick, too tired, too depressed, too overweight, in too much pain to work out, or working out would cause them to feel even worse. If you are one of these people, I've got exciting news for you! Infrared sauna therapy has been shown to burn up to 250% more calories in 30 minutes of just sitting there than spending 30 minutes of intense aerobic exercise on the best aerobic exercises, rowing machines and long-distance marathons. It not only burns more calories, but it has also been shown to have many of the same cardiovascular benefits as well!

The best aerobic exercises in the world, rowing and marathons, will burn at their peak 600 calories in 30 minutes. Sitting in an infrared sauna for 30 minutes can burn 900-2400 calories! Just one infrared session of 30 minutes could burn the equivalent amount of calories as someone running six to nine miles!

So who do you know that would benefit from detoxification, weight management, cardiovascular conditioning, and increased rate of healing? Almost everyone!

Some of you may be wondering how infrared saunas can burn so many calories. Well, according the Guyton's Medicinal Physiology textbook, the body requires 0.586 kilocalories (kcal) to produce 1 gram of sweat. An infrared sauna can cause a person to lose two to three times more sweat than a traditional sauna. The Journal of the American Medical Association (JAMA, Aug 7, 1981) reported that "A moderately conditioned person can easily sweat off 500 grams in an infrared sauna, consuming nearly 300 kcal – the equivalent of running two to three miles. A heat conditioned person can easily sweat off 600-800 kcal with no adverse effect. While the weight of water loss can be regained by rehydration, the calories consumed will not be." For those needing more convincing, NASA, after extensive research, determined in the 1980's that infrared stimulation would be the ideal way to maintain cardiovascular conditioning of astronauts in the weightless environment of space during the long space flights.

I use the infrared saunas on almost all of my patients. Most people are fine with 30-minute sessions three or more times per week for several months, or year-round. Some people who feel they are coming down with a cold may benefit from staying up to one hour.

People with heart disease are concerned that they cannot get in the sauna. Researchers in Finland report that there is abundant evidence to suggest that blood vessels of regular sauna-goers remain elastic and pliable longer due to the regular dilation and contraction of blood vessels induced by sauna use. As a matter of fact, German researchers found in type I and II essential hypertension (high blood pressure) that each person after a session in the infrared sauna had a significant decrease in arterial, venous and mean blood pressure that lasted for at least 24 hours. This finding is thought to be from the persistent dilation of peripheral blood vessels, and also due to the improvement of the viscosity (liquidity) of the blood.

Research performed in the U.S., Germany, Japan and China has shown infrared sauna therapy to benefit people suffering from the following conditions. (Benefits *people,* not diseases. Biological Medicine only treats people, since it is understood now that to treat the disease does not work as effectively.) Always seek the advice of a healthcare professional before starting any therapy.

- Acne/Blackheads
- Arthritis
- Asthma
- Backache
- Bell's Palsy
- Benign Prostatic Hypertrophy
- Brain damage (accelerated healing of)
- Bronchitis
- Bursitis
- Cancer
- Cancer pain
- Children's overtired muscles
- Chron's Disease
- Chronic Fatigue Syndrome
- Cirrhosis
- Colds/flu

- Cold hands and feet
- Cholecysitis (inflammation of the gallbladder)
- Cystitis
- Dandruff
- Diabetes
- Diarrhea
- Duodenal ulcers
- Ear diseases
- Ear infections (acute and chronic otitis media)
- Eczema with infection
- Edema
- Electromagnetic pollution (effects improved)
- Exudates
- Fibromyalgia
- Gastritis
- Gastroenteric problems
- Gout arthritis
- Headaches
- Heavy metal toxicity (i.e., mercury, cadmium, lead, aluminum)
- Hemorrhoids
- Hepatitis
- Hypertension (high blood pressure)
- Hypotension (low blood pressure)
- Inflammatory conditions and infiltrates
- Keloids
- Leg and decubital ulcers
- Low core body temperature

- Lyme Borreliosis
- Nervous tension
- Neurasthenia
- Neuritis
- Nosebleeds (reduced)
- Obesity
- Pediatric pneumonia
- Pelvic infections
- Peripheral Occulsive Disease
- Post-surgical infections
- PMS and menopausal symptoms
- Pneumonia
- Rheumatoid Arthritis
- Sciatica
- Short-term memory loss (improved)
- Skin tone (improved)
- Sore throats
- Strained muscles
- Stretch marks
- Tinea (fungal infections)
- Tinitus (ringing of the ears)
- TMJ
- Trigger points (relieved)
- Varicose veins

Chapter 31

Ion-Cleanse Detoxification

We live in the most toxic time in the history of the planet! This is not hype, but a scientifically documented fact. Research has shown that every person in America is breathing, eating and absorbing chemical toxins or poisons in micro to large amounts on a daily basis.

Toxins that find their way into the body should be excreted through the organs of elimination. These organs are the lungs, liver, kidneys, colon, and skin. The problem lies in the fact that these organs can become overwhelmed by the constant bio-accumulation of toxins. When toxins cannot be excreted through the body's normal elimination processes, the body must store the toxins somewhere in the body. Toxins enter the body through three ways... by absorption through the skin, by being breathed into the lungs, or by ingestion through the mouth.

The Ion-Cleanse device appears to pull the toxins out of the tissues where they have been stored. One of the greatest advances in chemical and heavy metal toxin removal, the Ion-Cleanse has become one of the primary detoxification methods in many of America's most elite doctor's offices.

In an Ion-Cleanse session, one will immerse the feet in a footbath of warm water with approximately 1/2 teaspoon of salt added. An array is placed in the water with the feet. This array generates electrical ions in the water. Ions are electrically charged particles, either negative (-) ions, or positive (+) ions. Because the human body is approximately 70% water, we will interact electrically with the ionic field set up by the Ion-Cleanse.

With the feet in the ionized water there will be virtually no sensation, although some people may experience mild tingling of the skin.

The Ion-Cleanse works by causing the neutralization and pulling out of toxins from all over the body and out through the pores of the feet, via electrical osmosis. Electrical osmosis is the movement of electrically charged particles (ions) across a membrane from a lower concentration of ions towards a higher concentration. In this case, the higher concentration is set up by the array in the water. The array in the water receives a small direct current that causes the metal of the array, the water, and the salt, to generate positively and negatively charged ions by separating the water into hydrogen and oxygen.

Detoxification occurs as these ions travel through the body, attaching themselves to toxins. Once attached, the toxin's own electrical charge becomes neutral, which allows the toxin to be drawn out of the tissue where it was stored. The toxin can then be excreted via the organs of elimination, however many of the toxins seem to travel great distances through the osmotic attraction of the higher ionic field within the water of the footbath.

You will see the accumulation of particles in the previously clear water of the footbath. Over the course of 20-30 minutes the Ion-Cleanse water will have quite a bit of toxic material of various colors floating around. This is desirable and represents the toxins that have been aggravating or potentially causing dysfunction in the body.

Approximately 20-40% of the toxic residues in the water represent toxins and heavy metals already present in municipal water.

The Ion-Cleanse by design causes an exhalation of sorts as heavy metals, minerals, and chemical toxins are drawn downward and out through the feet. To leave your body balanced after an Ion-Cleanse session, an inhalation of sorts is set up using various mineral or herbal essences in another footbath for another 5-10 minutes. This process is designed to leave your body energized and feeling lighter.

While the Ion-Cleanse is not expected to "cure" any disease, the detoxification of the body will remove the sludge that has been clogging the tissues and hindering the proper healing of the body. Many people have reported improvement in a wide range of symptoms.

Chapter 32

Hyperbaric Oxygen Therapy

Hyperbaric oxygen (HBOT) is a therapy which allows patients to breathe 100% oxygen through a hood or mask while in a compressed air chamber. Such exposure results in a large increase in the partial pressure of oxygen in the plasma and subsequently delivers increased oxygen to the tissues. Since we have the ST8 machine we no longer use this therapy but if one does not have access to the ST8 this is an awesome therapy.

HBOT BENEFITS

1. Hyperoxygenation of the blood

2. Fibroblast Proliferation and Enhanced Function

3. Neovascularization

4. Antimicrobial action of high oxygen

5. Enhancement of leukocyte functions

6. Vasoconstriction

7. Enhancement of some antibiotic activity

8. Compression of bubbles

There are many benefits to using HBOT, but the primary benefits to someone suffering from Lyme Disease are listed below:

1. Hyperoxygenation of the blood elevates the amount of dissolved oxygen and results in the correction of tissue hypoxia (decreased available oxygen in the tissues of the body). This results in improved or enhanced wound healing, and infection control.

2. Direct toxicity to anaerobic bacteria (bacteria that cannot live in an oxygen rich environment). The second method of infection control is through an indirect effect by the enhancement of white blood cell killing of phagocytized bacteria. Elevated oxygen

increases the oxygen-free radicals and hydrogen peroxide formation in the white cell lysosomes, improving their antimicrobial activity.

3. In inflamed and swollen or edematous tissue, HBOT leads to constriction of hypotonic blood vessels which can reverse the fluid loss into the tissues and reinstate normal lymphatic drainage. Also, HBOT appears to improve capillary integrity reducing the leakage that causes edema.

4. Selected medicines become more effective with normalization of tissue oxygen or high partial pressure of oxygen.

5. One of the most important roles of oxygen in wound healing is its contribution to the immune response to infection. It is well known that leukocytes require oxygen in order to kill efficiently. In a hypoxic wound, a wound that has little or no oxygen getting to it, HBOT increases oxygen tension in tissue, thus providing the essential substrate for the oxygen-dependent leukocyte intracellular killing mechanisms.

Chapter 33

Ilio-cecal Valve and the Valve of Houston
Correction for Colon Problems

This correction can be very beneficial when you are suffering from constipation or even diarrhea. In fact, abdominal bloating and pain can many times be relieved using this maneuver. Keep in mind that many people have heard of increasing fiber for intestinal problems, but many times what is really needed is more water. You should be consuming at least 64 ounces of purified water per day.

ICV/VOH Rebound Activation:

- Using your fingers, locate your hip bones at each side of your upper groin area. You should feel a bony point just below the waistband of your pants.

- Using the bony point as one point of reference, your ICV correction point is right between the bony point and your belly button.

- Press straight inward at the soft fleshy point between these two reference points on both sides of the groin. Quickly rebound or release off of the point so that the flesh fairly bounces. Repeat this rebound activation of the valves three times on each side. The ICV is on the right side and the VOH is on the left.

- These valves are sphincter muscles, much like the anus muscle, which partition off the colon into three general zones. This rebound activation helps re-establish the peristalsis, or in other words, helps reset the musculature that lines the colon for the wavelike movement of fecal material out of the body.

- Without proper peristalsis, the fecal material collects, putrefies, and ferments causing gas, constipation or diarrhea, and promotes the habitat for harmful bacteria and parasites to grow. It can also lead to Irritable Bowel Syndrome or Leaky Gut Syndrome which can lead to the reabsorption of toxins from the fecal material back into the bloodstream.

- Chronic constipation can lead to cancer, liver problems, and a whole host of other problems for the body, even psychosis.

- Ideally, you should have at least two bowel movements per day.

- Constipation, gas, bad breath, and diarrhea are all signs of dysfunction in your digestive tract, which may include your stomach, liver, small and large intestines, gallbladder, and pancreas. If your problems persist after performing the ICV/VOH Rebound Activation Maneuver, then something else needs to be done. Come in and get tested. Many times, chronic diseases and chronic problems originate in the intestines.

Chapter 34

Color Therapy

When one thinks of the many different tools a doctor may utilize to assist your body in healing itself, the use of color as a therapy may not seem very powerful or even valid. Color therapy however is a viable tool, the effects of which no other therapy can duplicate. Color therapy is rarely a "stand alone" treatment, but is used in conjunction with other types of treatments to facilitate and enhance the body's healing response. Your doctor may use different colors, specifically selected by resonance testing to provide an integral key to achieving a particular correction in your body. Subtle energy treatments such as color therapy are coming of age as scientific research continues to validate their superiority over conventional toxic drugs.

Effects of Color on the Body

From a historical perspective, the sun has been known to be the source of life, not as a god, but in its creation of a suitable environment on our planet and photosynthesis of sunlight into chlorophyll in plants. The medieval alchemists sought enlightenment through gazing at celestial bodies, such as the moon and sun, with an open soul and a pious heart. From their understanding the light from the moon would specifically target and influence the lungs, and the sun would affect the heart. From our discussion above, we see that in some respects they were not far off.

You can see the effects of color on physiology and the mind, when you go to a bull fight. The matador, or bullfighter, carries a red cape. The color red is converted into a specific vibration that primarily stimulates the bull's adrenal glands. We all know that the adrenal glands produce adrenaline. When the bull sees the red cape, his adrenal glands dump adrenaline into the bloodstream, consequently activating his fighting mood, and all the blood rushes to the muscles so that he can charge the bullfighter.

Color has a direct effect on the human body and the soul. When using color as a therapy, many times the patient may be wearing a pair of primary colored glasses, red glasses for example, and upon taking them off an interesting phenomenon takes place. They will then see an "after image" color, possibly turquoise or green. This after image can be likened to looking at a bright lightbulb and upon looking away one can see a glowing image of the lightbulb – actually this phenomenon is not quite the same but may help you relate to the "after image" concept.

These after images are extremely activating sources of healing to the body. Healing forces in the body respond with complementary colors to the degree of the integrity of the crystalline matrix of the individual's body. Very ill people will experience difficulty seeing the complementary color at first, but as they continue, that part of them will be restored.

You may even know people who are innocently addicted to a color…they may drive a red car, have red carpet in their house, with red curtains, and a red ballpoint pen, etc. The unwittingly are using the color red as a stimulant to keep them going at a fast pace. They may just think they simply like the color, but in truth they need the color to stimulate their "stress organs", the adrenal glands. Similarly, people with heart disease may be attracted to the color green, which corresponds to the heart and circulatory system. Conversely, some people may absolutely be repelled by a color. This may be due to agitation caused by the color in an area of the body that is already hyper-reactive and hypersensitive.

The different colors used in therapy are in reality just different vibrations on the electromagnetic spectrum. Everything in the universe is made up of different vibrations on the electromagnetic spectrum. So, all radio waves, sound, gamma rays, x-rays, microwaves…everything is made of the same "stuff". At times medicines create healing because of the medicine's unique vibratory rate. But, your doctor may not have a medicine that will provide the necessary vibratory rate unique to a color, such as red or yellow.

Each color can enhance the healing of tissue through restoring the vibratory rate of that tissue, and restoring the light metabolism unique to that tissue. All of this enhancing of vibratory rate and light metabolism translates to the normalization of the chemistry of the tissues as well.

Color, being a much higher vibration than sound, has consequently a stronger impact upon the human body. Therefore, even finer chemical changes are effected by color than sound therapy. However, the combination of sound and color therapy work synergistically to awaken healing in the body through the formative forces unique to each.

All human thought that takes place in the mind is said to be extra-low frequency waves…yes human brain waves are also found on the electromagnetic spectrum. Thought is behind all emotion, therefore emotions are energy and affect the entire body electrically. As you will read later, you will see the different organs, regions, and psychological states that each color can bring into balance.

Research into color preference, the effect of color on concentration, performance, sense of physical and mental wellbeing, etc., have been carried out over many years. Increasing evidence has been gathered concerning the therapeutic effects of certain colors in the healing environment for recovery from illness, mental health, and in stimulation of the minds of young children. Of course, it is a given that color therapy can be used by healthy individuals to maintain their good health and help them reach greater maturity in body, mind, and spirit.

Colors can be therapeutically applied in your home to assist with your overall health. Colored plastic cellophane can be taped over a window to create a color therapy session of sorts. Also, painting the walls of your house with plant based dyes and resins, as in Lazure painting, can set a more healing tone and environment.

Even the color selection of your clothing can be beneficial to healing and overall sense of wellbeing. You may want to experiment with choosing the color of your clothing based upon the "color of the day" in the chart listed later in this book. (Chapter 35).

As with all good healing techniques, progress and the ultimate benefits of doing this therapy should be measured over the course of months, as the immediate effect may not be so apparent.

Color Therapy as used in Europe and the Somerleyton Center

The following color therapy protocol was developed in Europe by Dr. Norbert Glas, M.D., and is used in some European hospitals and clinics. It is the general protocol for color therapy at the Somerleyton Center. The primary differences being that we will use various musical instruments, such as the viola, instead of the European use of the lyre, which is a harp-like instrument. We will also use various essential oils and homeopathic remedies to help align the specific crystalline matrix pathways that we are attempting to stimulate with the color and sound.

Often people are uncomfortable the first few times they do this therapy. It is so far removed from anything they have experienced from their conventional doctor. The therapist should anticipate this feeling of uneasiness and help the patient relax, reminding the patient to breathe deeply in through the nose and out through the mouth, consciously releasing tension and relaxing the body with each exhalation. The patient should be instructed to focus their attention as to how the color and sound makes them feel, and where in the body they feel it most. One can obviously just dispassionately "look" at something, but what is desired in color therapy is for one to truly experience the color and sound all the way in the core of your being.

It can be disconcerting to sit in a room with someone playing live music specifically for you. If you have ever been to a restaurant where the wait staff sang "Happy Birthday" to you, this can be the same initial sensation of being the focus of attention in a color/sound therapy session. One may feel underserving, or may feel silly, or even feel they may not be doing it correctly if no after image color is seen. Remember that this is a healing process. And like all healing, it takes time to reach the full benefit. The stronger and healthier you become, the better the after image production becomes, and the greater the sense of wellbeing produced during these sessions.

The Actual Treatment

The patient sits in a completely dark room, completely isolated from distracting sounds outside of the room. A color therapist uses a high power light box to project a certain color against a white wall for a minute to a minute and a half. There is a different color for every day of the week, except for Sunday, which is white and no color therapy is done. Ideally, the patient would do this therapy every day of the week, except for Sunday. This ideal situation is however, unrealistic in most doctor's offices since the patient may not be able to come in every day. Even doing this therapy just every now and then will still be beneficial, definitely better than nothing at all!

After the requisite time the therapist turns off the colored light. The goal is that the patient would be able to see an after image color in the darkness when the light is turned off, otherwise known as a complementary color or "after image" color. The more ill the patient, the less able they will be to generate an after image color. It is this after image color that is very healing to the body, therefore it is the goal of this color therapy to restore the body's ability to generate a strong after image. This after image may only last for a few seconds.

The color of the day is shined upon the wall three times in a color therapy session. After this the therapist plays a specific musical scale on a lyre, which is also unique to each day of the week. The therapist plays the musical scale in the keynote that relates to the color of the day, which will enhance the effect of the color therapy of the whole of your being. As with the after images of color therapy, the tones of the lyre or musical instrument, create an after tone between the notes. It is the after tones and after images that are sought for restoring balance. Each of these therapies works at the physical, psychological and soul level.

Finally, the patient has experienced the color, and the associated tones of the lyre. Now the lights are turned on and the patient is handed a quartz crystal of the same color as the color of the day. From the body's perception level, to hold and observe this colored crystal represents the consolidation, or condensed, solidified, colored light.

This completes the color therapy session. The entire process takes about thirty minutes, and is ideally performed in the morning.

The purpose of the combination of color light, color sound, and color crystal is to help reset the normal daily and weekly rhythms of the body. Each of these therapies affect a different aspect of the body's nervous system. Research in neurology as reported by Dr. Richard Amie, M.D., demonstrates that the more ways we can affect the body from a sensory perspective, the deeper and longer lasting the healing effect.

The rhythms of the body being addressed with this therapy are strongly associated with the many hormones produced by the body, as well as the rhythmical nature of every organ and tissue of the body. It is the body's rhythmical nature that is upset in any illness.

Therefore, color therapy such as this should be done every day of the week, except on Sunday, ideally for several weeks to months. Thus Monday is violet, Tuesday is red, Wednesday is yellow, Thursday is orange, Friday is green, Saturday is blue, and Sunday is white, therefore no color therapy is done on Sunday.

In a world of chaos, imbalance, and loss of the normal bio-rhythms, color therapy trains and reminds the body of the natural order of things. It is part of a well-rounded treatment protocol for any illness, and indeed to avoid illness. To lose rhythm at any level of the human organism is to lose the ability of the body to transmit coherent information, and adapt to its surroundings. The inability of the body to adapt to the ever changing internal and external environment always results in illness.

It might be said that any area of the body which experiences a breakdown in the ability to adapt will manifest as a symptom. Each color used in color therapy addresses a different part of the body, due to its unique frequency. So, one may be able to generate great after images, otherwise known as complementary color to the color green, for example, but not be able to generate a complementary color for the color violet. This would be due to a disturbance in the crystalline pathways which the color violet must travel and may be due to a problem in the organ or tissues normally stimulated by violet, i.e., the cerebral cortex.

Chapter 35

Different Colors Used In Color Therapy

VIOLET: Corresponds to the region of the brain and higher mind. Violet synchronizes body rhythms. The main areas, which the violet ray seems to influence, are the physical brain and the spiritual nature of the higher mind. It provides nourishment of a subtle energetic nature to those neurons in the cerebral cortex that contribute toward a greater understanding of our divine nature. Because violet has positive therapeutic effects upon various mental and nervous disorders, it may be effective in relieving headaches, neuroses, and even certain forms of schizophrenia and dementia. Violet can enhance the power of meditation tenfold.

INDIGO: Corresponds to the pituitary gland, left eye, sinus, nose, sight. Controls physical and higher aspects of vision as well as olfaction and physical hearing. Various types of eye diseases, like cataracts, may be treated by indigo. May also be helpful in treating disorders of hearing and loss of smell. Indigo balances inspiration, focus, concentration, insight, imagination, devotion, clear thinking, peace of mind.

BLUE: Corresponds to the throat, thyroid, parathyroid, lungs, and mouth. It is the center of communication and self-expression. Sometimes called the center of will or power. Blue softens body tissue, reducing tension, and removes obsessional ideas and behavior patterns. Diseases in the throat area such as laryngitis, sore throats and goiters respond to blue.

GREEN: Corresponds to the heart, circulatory system, arms and hands. Green balances openness, compassion, unconditional love, forgiveness, acceptance, contentment, nurturing, generosity, harmonys, assertiveness and heals loss. Green is associated with the higher mental and higher emotional energies, such as love and compassion. Many heart diseases have their root in the emotional nature. Green has soothing influences upon the sympathetic nervous system, and can therefore soothe stressed out individuals and benefit heart diseases like angina and hypertension.

YELLOW: Corresponds to the solar plexus, the digestive system, stomach, liver, gall bladder and pancreas. Reduces introverted personality. Balances logic, humor, efficiency, organization, warmth, radiance, flexibility, self-awareness and self-control. Yellow can stimulate rational thinking and one's intellectual nature. Yellow can benefit ulcers, various stomach problems and indigestion.

ORANGE: Corresponds to the lungs, reproductive organs, genitals, gonads, prostate and spleen. Diseases influenced by orange may be asthma, emphysema and bronchitis. Distributes life-giving oxygen throughout the pulmonary system. Balances sensuality, passions, procreation, vitality, optimism, enthusiasm, family-orientation and tolerance.

RED: Stimulating and energizing, speeds up the rhythms of the body. Corresponds to the base of the spine, adrenals, kidneys, bladder, colon, spinal column, legs and the blood. Balances the physical self, self-preservation and survival instincts, sensory, and courage. Red helps balance the vitality of the physical body. Diseases such as anemia and severe fatigue may benefit.

AQUA: Corresponds to the thymus and is a helper in working through grief. Aqua balance is a merging of heart and words to produce loving expression.

MAGENTA: Corresponds to the vitality of the system offering healing support and emotional balance.

**Relationships of Musical Instruments, Sound, Color,
  Body and Daily Rhythms**

Instrument	Color	Keynote	Body*	Day
Wind	Violet	B	Brain	Monday
Reed	White	A	Pituitary	**
Fine String	Blue	G	Throat	Saturday
Piano	Green	F	Heart	Friday
Harp	Yellow	E	Liver	Wednesday
Thick Strings	Orange	D	Lungs	Thursday
Bass Tones	Red	C	Adrenals	Tuesday

*For a more complete explanation of areas of the body influenced by color and sound see section on "Different Colors Used in Color Therapy."
**There is no color (White) for Sunday

Using Color Therapy at Home

The easiest way to practice color therapy at home is to purchase a set of color therapy glasses. A good set of the six most commonly used colors will cost about $95.

If you have just completed our two-week program of care at Somerleyton Center, then you have experienced color and sound therapy six days per week. By now you are well on your way to seeing the complimentary colors that are so healing to your whole being. We did this therapy with you to restore the light metabolism of the body and to reset the glandular/hormonal/rhythmical aspects of your body as part of your healing process.

Since you came to us desiring a new and better reality, and hopefully we have helped you realize this goal, you will need to continue doing color therapy Monday through Saturday at home to attain even higher gains.

Start each day by wearing the colored glasses of the day. Refer to the chart on the following page for determining the color of the day. Wear the glasses in good lighting, preferably in sunlight. Allow about three minutes before removing them. You should see the complimentary color briefly, as an after-image. It may help to look at something, like a white wall immediately after taking off the glasses in order to see the complimentary color.

After the complimentary color fades, put the glasses back on and repeat the process two more times for a total of three times. The entire treatment should only take 15 to 20 minutes and you can do it while brushing your teeth or getting ready for the day.

It is not necessary, and may in fact be detrimental, to wear the colored glasses for longer periods of time, unless directed to do so by your doctor or color therapist. Be careful walking about, climbing stairs or driving when wearing the colored glasses because shadows and distances may appear differently through the glasses.

Not only will performing color therapy at home help to maintain healthy balance and rhythm in the body, but it will also be a beneficial tool to help start your day peacefully and in tune with the world around you.

You may even get more out of your morning meditation and prayer time by combining or doing your color therapy just prior to these activities.

For the person desiring the ultimate benefit at home, a lyre can be purchased on which the scale of notes that correspond to the color of the day can be played directly after you are finished with the third and last color and complimentary color for the day.

Colors of the Week:

Day	Glasses	Complementary Color
Monday	Violet	Yellow
Tuesday	Red	Green
Wednesday	Yellow	Violet
Thursday	Orange	Blue
Friday	Green	Red
Saturday	Blue	Orange
Sunday	No color therapy on this day	

The colors of the week as listed above are used in this way to primarily address the rhythmical aspects of the body and to this purpose should be used in this sequence. A color therapist or doctor may use other colors on these days in conjunction with other therapies to achieve specific therapeutic goals.

Essential oils that can enhance your color therapy

These oils are definitely not the only oils that can be effectively used to enhance your color therapy and are not presented in any preferential order. The oils recommended here can be diffused into the air during the color therapy session or a drop or two can be placed on a cotton ball and inhaled. Each type of oil has its own vibrational rate, which affects a specific region of the body. Experiment with the oils listed and you will find which ones work best for you. You may be able to select the oil for the day as dictated by intuition on that day.

(I like to use an ozone air purifier in the house so that the smell of Monday's oil does not combine with Tuesday's and so forth…this also keeps your house and clothing from smelling overwhelmingly like an herb shop.)

Monday Oils – frankincense, rose, white angelica, cypress, lemongrass, birch (oil blends- Joy, Awaken and 3 Wise Men – YLO = Young Living Essential Oils, Inc.)

Tuesday Oils – myrrh, nutmeg, rosemary, sage, geranium, basil, (oil blends – Endoflex (YLO)

Wednesday Oils – German Chamomile, helichrysum, ledum, grapefruit, lemongrass, (oil blends – JuvaFlex, Peace and Calming – YLO)

Thursday Oils – Fir, eucalyptus, ravensara, hyssop, (Oil blends – Raven, Aroma Life – YLO)

Friday Oils – Lavender, ylang ylang, thyme, sandalwood, cinnamon, marjoram (Oil blends – Valor, Citrus Fresh, Christmas Spirit – (YLO)

Saturday Oils – Myrtle, oregano, peppermint, lemon, clary sage (Oil blends, Sacred Mountain, Present Time, RC, YLO)

Chapter 36

The Biophysics of Color Therapy
**(You may want to skip this section if you are
not interested in the nitty-gritty scientific
details of the effect of color on the body)**

There are two primary functions of the eye. One is to translate the electromagnetic vibrations of light into patterns of nerve impulses that are transmitted to the brain. The other function is to provide an entry point to access the "fiber optic" network that provides light/photons as nutrients to every tissue of the body.

If you recall our discussion of the body's crystalline matrix network in the earlier chapter, "A Theory of Intermicrobial Communication", you will remember the potentially science-shaking implications. Crystalline matrix pathways connect every aspect of the human being to its internal and external environment. These pathways therefore enable the body to adapt at virtually the speed of light to changes in and around the body. In this color therapy chapter we will see further supporting evidence leading us closer towards moving the theory of bio-crystalline-fiber optics from scientific theory to scientific fact.

Alfred Kastler, Ph.D., (1902-1984), a French physicist, was awarded the 1966 Nobel Prize in physics for his work in developing methods that used light of specific photon frequencies (colors) to manipulate the energy levels of electrons in atoms. His work to my knowledge has never before been applied in biophysics the way I am postulating here.

One of the primary goals in color therapy in humans is to restore the bio-crystalline photon pathways. The pathways are known to be open and working when the patient is able to see an "after image" of a different color than they were being treated with. For example, if one is treated with the red color, the after image one should see is green. What Dr. Kastler called "Double Resonance" may be why this after image is created.

His theory of, "Double Resonance", which he developed in the late 1940s, states that when you apply a specific frequency of a beam of light, which is carefully selected to excite atoms to a particular energy level, that when the atoms return to their unexcited state, they emit energy in the form of LIGHT! In other words, when we use specific colors (frequencies) in color therapy, the frequency excites the atomic and molecular structure of the specific organ and tissues targeted by that color, which when the color therapy light is turned off the atomic and molecular structure returns to its less excited or new excitation state. When the tissue comes down from its excited state it emits its corresponding light frequency (color) unique to the tissue's molecular characteristics and specific to their energy level.

Disease is the result of a disturbance in or collapsing of the bio-crystalline pathways of the body. I theorize that all of the best natural healing methods work by influencing and manipulating these pathways in the body. It is the opening up of and maintaining the integrity of these bio-crystalline-fiber optic pathways that restores and ensures the long-term health of the human body.

Each tissue of the body if you will recall is made up liquid crystals which will reflect different wavelengths of light (color) depending on the orientation of its molecules. The organ or tissue depends on the temperature of the organ or tissue to maintain its crystalline orientation. Therefore, each organ or tissue one desires to influence will require a specific color. This is why the heart is specifically stimulated by the color green, the adrenals red, and so on.

One can begin to see the tremendous potential for facilitating healing using this knowledge. Dr. Dietrick Klinghardt, M.D., Ph.D., has developed a new type of color therapy device that incorporates this technology. His device enables the doctor to embed homeopathic or bioenergetic frequencies within wavelength of specific colors. When a patient gazes into the color being projected, the transmitted energy may work to destroy the molecular structure of viruses, bacteria, parasites and toxins hiding deep within specific tissues of the body. (Dietrick Klinghardt, M.D., Ph.D., 1ˢᵗ Annual Conference on Lyme Disease, Belleview, Washington 2003)

The optical properties of any liquid crystal can be manipulated by subjecting the liquid crystal to a magnetic or electric field. Doing so changes the orientation of the liquid crystal's molecular structure. We saw an example of this phenomenon demonstrated in the story of the lady from Alaska earlier in the chapter "Healing at Home." Recall that by using the Magnetic Resonance Bio-oxidative therapy, she was able to regain full use of a previously paralyzed leg, foot and toes. The magnetic therapy resulted in a restoration of the ideal orientation of the bio-liquid crystalline matrix, which led to the reorientation of the optimal tissue molecular structure, and the realignment of the lines of tensegrity. Once this occurred, the effect instantly restored normal function throughout the bones, nerves, meridians, muscles, tendons, ligaments, and connective tissues. This is made possible because every tissue of the body is made of bio-liquid crystals. So now we see that not only can light photons (color) and sound manipulate the liquid crystalline matrix of the body, but also magnetic and electrical fields as well... sounds like alternative medicine is firmly supported by mainstream science!

So when you receive a Chiropractic adjustment, take a homeopathic remedy, eat high energy organic foods, use Magnetic Resonance therapy, acupuncture, or simply sleep with a peat mattress pad and comforter it will have direct and potentially lasting effects on the liquid crystalline matrix of your body. Every treatment or medicine is going to either enhance or harm this matrix. So do you still want surgery, and toxic pharmaceuticals? Choose your medicine well!

Through the years doctors and scientist have focused upon the easily measured electrical and chemical aspects of the human body. However, what was not realized until now is that the electrical and chemical aspects of the body are dependent upon and preempted by the light/photon mechanisms of the body's crystalline matrix, something not so easily measured by conventional methods.

One of the problems with the liquid crystals as a whole and those found in the body is that they are only crystals when they are at the correct temperature. Too cold or too hot of a body temperature and the crystals loses their coherence. This is what happens in all chronic degenerative diseases. We see this especially in the ultimate "cold disease" cancer. The body's core temperature is too cold, or a part of the body is too cold, which leads to a breakdown of coherence in the area's crystalline matrix. This breakdown in coherence means that there is a breakdown in the normal regulation and communication in that area of the body. Without communication with the rest of the body, the tissues of this region become chaotic, and begin to produce cells in an unregulated and often rapid manner, independent from the rest of the body. We call this a tumor or cancer. This tissue is cut off from the normal control mechanisms of the body and has no direct pathways to the external environment. Any successful treatment for cancer would therefore require one to reestablish lines of communication between the normal crystalline matrix of the body and the autonomous tissues of the cancer.

"Liquid crystals reflect different wavelengths of light depending on the orientation of its molecules." (Microsoft Encarta Encyclopedia, 2003) Combine a bunch of molecules and you get tissue and organs. So based upon this science we see that any molecular structure, be it the liver, heart, or lungs, will emit and reflect back through the body's crystalline pathways the color frequency unique to its molecular structure. The orientation of the molecules depends on the temperature, so once more we see the importance of maintaining the optimum core body temperature. From this we can also see why someone who is very sick has lost the ability to see any "after image" color. The reason for this lack of no "after image" color is the excitation of the end-organ's molecular structure by the incoming colored light is blocked by a breakdown in the crystalline-fiber optic pathways. Therefore, the end-organ's molecular structure will not emit photons back through the pathway for an after image, since there was not any molecular excitation.

Laser sources have atoms whose electrons radiate all in step, or synchronously. As a result, the electrons produce light (photons) that is polarized, monochromatic, and coherent, which means that its waves remain in step, with their peaks and troughs coinciding, over long distances.

Laser light is said to be "coherent light photons." Interestingly, the crystalline matrix of the body is said to be transmitting "coherent light." The really awesome realization of this is that we know lasers, or "coherent light", can carry a great deal of information and travel long distances without losing signal strength.

For years maverick physiologists have stated that the ion-transfer mechanism of the nerve impulses in the human body are way too slow to account for the huge amount of information transfer that is going on in the body. Our desktop computers operate much faster than nerve impulses, yet these computers still cannot compute as fast as humans. It sounds like the Human Physiology and Neurology textbooks need to be revised. What we used to think was running the body, the central and peripheral nervous system is just another cog in the wheel, with the crystalline-fiber optics network carrying the bulk of the information and maintaining the integrity of the human organism.

Light as a Nutrient

Photons can turn into electrons when excited. From this tidbit of information we can see how color or light can be used and is necessary as a nutrient! In a color therapy session, the color used is a specific frequency, which can through a photoelectric interaction with the end-organ, can cause the production of hormones or other chemicals as needed, through nuclear transmutation. Nuclear transmutation is like what scientists have tried to do for years – turn lead into gold. If lead could be forced to take on one more electron it would turn into gold. Although possible to some degree in a laboratory setting, the human body, bacteria, and various microbes do this at will.

The photoelectric effect is a process in which an atom absorbs a photon that has so much energy that the photon sets one of the atom's electrons free to move outside the atom. Part of the photon's energy goes toward releasing the electron from the atom. This energy is called the activation energy of the electron. The rest of the photon's energy is transferred to the released electron in the form of motion, or kinetic energy. Since the photon energy is proportional to frequency, the released electron, or photoelectron, moves faster when it has absorbed high-frequency light (such as the color, violet). So where does this newly freed electron go? It is snatched up by the nearby metabolic process to build whatever chemical is needed at the time. What about the atom that lost the electron? It experienced a nuclear transmutation and is now a new type of atom, possibly a mineral that the body needs. You see, we are not talking about losing electrons from molecules, but from atoms!

I have seen several people whose doctor found on blood tests that they are deficient in Magnesium. However, these people would tell me, "How can that be Dr. Jernigan, I have been taking "Mega-Magnesium" for three years," holding up the bottle to prove it. The answer is that there is a disturbance in the light metabolism somewhere in the body, hindering the uptake and utilization of the Magnesium. It also goes to show that the body is not just pieces and parts. Just because you are low in something does not necessarily mean that providing your body with that substance will correct the situation. You see, the body is smart. It is usually doing or not doing something for a reason. That is the goal of treatment to provide the body with the information it needs to get back to normal functioning. Of course there could arguably be a breakdown of this or that enzyme system impairing the utilization of Magnesium, but what came first the enzyme or the photons stimulating the production of the enzyme?

In summary, when colored light enters the eye, an electro-fiber optic-like network goes into motion. The photo-receptors in the eye convert the specific colors of the light into electricity. Colored light passes as photons through the body's liquid-crystaline matrix. These photons serve a twofold mission. One, to be converted into nerve impulses needed by the brain to create vision as we know it. Second, the photons travel at about half the speed of light, as a photo-nutrient, to the organ and associated tissues on that specific fiber optic, crystalline circuit. The photon is converted into electricity that has an affinity and influence on specific organs and tissues in the body. Each color effects a unique set of organs and tissues as well as mental and emotional states depending upon its wavelength.

The eyes have much to do with the light metabolism of the body, which has a direct effect upon the warmth organization of the entire body. I theorize that the eyes transform and transmit external light/color of specific frequencies in an organized manner, almost as a nutrient to the farthest reaches of the body through a fiber-optic-like network.

People with low core body temperature, chronic fatigue, cancer, or other chronic cold/sclerotic illness can especially benefit from color therapy, since these conditions are either caused or aggravated by disturbances in light metabolism.

Light metabolism, is necessary for the conduction of the orchestratic, rhythmical, creative and formative aspects of the entire human organism. The crystalline optical pathways of the body enables part of this coordinated orchestration through its properties of photoconduction. Photoconduction is where electrons in crystalline matter absorb energy from photons are then brought to the range of energy levels at which they can move freely to conduct electricity. (Microsoft® Encarta® Encyclopedia 2003) No wonder the medieval alchemists associated the light of the sun with the function of the human heart – the sun being the primary source of celestial photons and the heart being the primary generator of electricity in the body!

It is well understood that the ability to see images takes place in the direct nerve pathways of the optic nerves progressing along the optic tracts to the optic geniculus where the image is made manifest to the rest of the brain. What is less clearly understood is the close relationship of eyes to the rest of the body. In the womb, the brain is the first organ formed after which the brain stem, spinal cord, and spinal nerves are formed in that order, with the organs growing off the ends of the spinal nerves as directed by the brain. During all of this formative sequence, the eyes have not been formed and are still basically part of the brain tissue. It is only later in development that the eyes begin to emerge as an off-shoot of the brain. This early and close connection to the brain is why the eyes contain light pathways, or fiber optic connections to every tissue in the body.

The absolute absence of light metabolism in the body is certain death. The disruption of light in a specific region of the body leads to dysfunction and compaction of the tissues and fluids of the region. This is what we call disease.

One must realize that we are not dealing with inert matter when we are working on the human body. The human body is extremely dynamic, meaning it is constantly morphing or changing its shape, function, viscosity, chemistry, tensegrity, and energetics to adapt to the everchanging external environment. Because we are not dealing with inert matter, such as rocks or dirt, but the dynamic human body, all vibrations experienced by the body will have immediate and potentially lasting effects. So the vibrational nature of color and sound can cause fluids in the body to change viscosity (how syrupy or liquid a fluid is). They can alter lines of tensegrity in the muscles, bones, and connective tissues, often relieving various pain syndromes. Brain waves will change in direct and specific ways to the various colors and sounds.

Research in advanced neurology has shown that emotional trauma causes actual grooves to appear on the surface of the brain, emotional scars if you will. Color and sound therapy have been demonstrated to enable this emotional groove to be erased! If one remembers that emotions are thoughts, and thoughts are extra-low frequency wavelengths, it becomes easier to understand that using other wavelengths, such as color and sound to "erase" the wavelength effects of emotional trauma that scars the brain, is not so mystical.

There are various methods of using colors therapeutically. One can use non-prescription colored glasses, lazure wall painting, color therapy rooms, even the color choices of clothing can be applied for therapeutic purposes. Color therapy is not a random use of colors, it is used in such a manner as to create a specific electro-chemical physiological response in the organism. Sound, or music therapy as well as essential oils can enhance the overall therapeutic experience during color therapy.

Section 7

Detoxification

Chapter 37

Why Detoxify if I've got Lyme Disease?

Remember earlier I mentioned how that research indicates that the majority of symptoms in Lyme disease are caused by the release of toxins by the spirochetes? And that a Herxheimer reaction is a worsening of your symptoms due to the die-off of bacteria which break open, spilling their guts into your tissues? Well, if that were not bad enough, your daily accumulation of toxins just from living, eating and breathing is staggering! These toxins are jamming up the machinery of the cells, interfering with the regulation of the body. Toxins are a universal problem. There is virtually no one on the planet who does not need to detoxify the body on a continual basis. There is no one who should not be working to eliminate the sources of toxins in our house and life.

I hear all the time how doctors are telling their patients that it's great if they feel like crap while on antibiotics for Lyme disease! They think that indicates good treatment. I think it's poor treatment. You suffer terribly because the doctor didn't bother to make sure your body was able to efficiently eliminate the die-off toxins. Detoxification of the body must be a part of any effective Lyme protocol or one risks permanent damage to nerve and joint tissue from the toxic irritation.

Today more than 77,000 chemicals are in active production in this country. Our exposure to these chemicals is greater than at any time since the beginning of the Industrial Revolution. More than 3,000 chemicals are added to our food supply, and more than 10,000 chemicals in the form of solvents, emulsifiers and preservatives are used in food processing and storage. Ethyl alcohol, isopropanol, wood rosin, shellac, propylene glycol, silicone, ammonium hydroxide... You're eating it for breakfast if you're eating grapefruit, melon and fresh oranges from the supermarket... Thiabendazole, mineral oil, methylparabin, dimethyl polysiloxane, benzimadazole... You're eating these for lunch if you had supermarket tomatoes, avocado, apples... Fungicides botran, 2-6 dichloro-4-nitroaniline, orthophenylphenol... Sound like a good balanced dinner? You're eating these yummy ingredients in sweet potatoes, onions and limes from your local supermarket. Fungicides are put into wax to provide a longer shelf life; even peeling won't get rid of them, you eat them. They cause cancers, birth defects, damage to the immune system and other diseases.

When ingested, these chemicals can remain in the body for years, altering our metabolism, causing enzyme dysfunction and nutritional deficiencies, creating hormonal imbalances and lowering our threshold of resistance to chronic disease.

Besides food borne chemicals, we are continually subjected to poor air quality, chemically contaminated water, household cleaners, paint fumes, pharmaceutical drugs, pesticides, heavy metals (including mercury) and the list goes on and on. Today, studies show that most of us have between 400 and 800 foreign chemical residues stored in the fat cells of our bodies. This occurs gradually over the course of our lives. These chemicals enter into the body either through the skin, lungs, or they are eaten. Most of the time, these chemicals are bio-accumulative, meaning minuscule amounts accumulating over the course of years. These chemicals and heavy metals make up the "total toxic burden." When the amount of toxins exceed the body's ability to excrete them, our body will begin to store these toxins. This bio-accumulation seriously compromises our physiological and psychological health and leads to chronic disease.

Environmental Protection Agency (EPA)

Since 1976 the EPA has been conducting studies to determine the presence of toxins in the fat cells of the body. This study is called the National Adipose Tissue Survey (NHATS). The results of this study are staggering. Across the United States, the EPA took samples of people's fat cells (adipose) and analyzed the samples for the presence of various toxins. In 98% of the samples they found many toxins, including benzene, PCBs, DDE (a metabolite of DDT pesticide), dioxins, toluene and chlorobenzene, all of which are highly damaging to the immune system and compromise every tissue in the body. The EPA only looks for 100 out of the potential thousands of different toxins that could be present in the fatty tissue samples. Twenty different toxins were identified in over 75% of all the samples.

So, from this and other studies you can see that it is not so much a matter of "if" you have toxins in your body, rather how much! Remember that our goal is not to just get rid of Lyme spirochetes or your symptoms, but to remove anything that may be blocking your body's healing mechanisms. True health is not the absence of pain or symptoms, otherwise aspirin would be the ultimate longevity medicine.

Toxicity Symptoms

The following is a partial list of known symptoms often related to toxicity: allergies, acne, anxiety, burning skin, brain fog, chronic fatigue, chemical sensitivities, depression, eczema, frequent colds or flu, feeling "sick all over," insomnia, loss of dexterity, low body temperature, memory loss, mood swings, muscle and joint pains and poor concentration. The list of potential toxicity symptoms for Lyme sufferers is the entire list of possible Lyme disease symptoms since the symptoms are the result of the bacterial toxins.

As a result of this widespread environmental contamination, doctors are faced with increased rates of toxin-related cancers, neurological diseases, reduced immune function, allergies, and the newer diagnoses of multiple chemical sensitivities, chronic fatigue syndrome and fibromyalgia. Doctors are finding their usual treatments are not as effective as in the past due to the presence of these many toxins in people.

Did you know that few people actually die of cancer? Authorities say that they actually die of toxemia, produced by an excessive buildup of toxins.

Did you know that you cannot simply take supplements and laxatives to eliminate all of the toxins? You must be guided through a total body protocol to truly achieve detoxification. Consider the skin for a moment. Did you know that your skin is one of your largest organs of elimination? Your skin should be releasing two pounds of waste acids every day! Most people have spent their entire life blocking this process through lotions and powder and toxic antibacterial, deodorant soaps. So as you can see, two pounds of waste per day that is not being eliminated through the skin is going to add up and tax the body severely.

Toxins, Lymphatic Drainage, Elimination Organs and the CRT Test

The CRT (Computerized Regulation Thermography) test is one of the most reliable methods of determining the degree of toxic load on the body. If your doctor conducted this test, he probably showed you areas of your body indicating toxins effecting proper organ thermal regulation on your CRT test. He most likely also found that your lymphatic system was blocked or otherwise demonstrating dysregulation of some form on the CRT. Problems in the lymph system are common when the body is toxic.

Everyone has experienced a swollen lymph node at some time in his or her life. A lymph node is part of a chain of nodes all over the body, which is an integral part of your immune system. Lymph channels conduct lymph fluid and connect lymph nodes. Every lymph node has special immune cells, like little "pac-men" that swallow up and help the body break down toxins and microbes. Lymph fluid flows through the channels and gathers toxins from the tissue spaces between cells and in the tiny blood vessels called capillaries. The lymphatic system can be likened to an efficient plumbing system. When plumbing is clogged, then the bathroom gets a backlog of hazardous waste. As long as the lymphatic system is flowing freely through the body, it can filter out toxins. Once the lymphatic system is clogged, the liver, kidneys, skin and lungs have to work much harder to keep the body clean. Eventually, these organs of elimination become fatigued and can no longer deal with the toxins.

As people age or become less physically active, the flow of lymph is impaired. Sometimes the lymph nodes are blocked due to permanent scarring from repeated infections. Proteins begin to concentrate in the lymph vessels and nodes, which become clogged (blocked), stagnant (hyper-regulating) and inflamed. From here the organs of the body begin to show toxin strain and eventual overload which leads to illness from accumulated toxins.

Women: The lymph channels and nodes of the armpit become congested, as do the breasts, when underwire bras are worn. Studies by several researchers found that the majority of women who wore their bras over 12 hours daily were 21 times more likely to develop breast cancer compared to those wearing them less than 12 hours a day. Women who also wear their bras to bed had 125 times greater breast cancer risk. The underwire bras create a dam, causing a blockage of the flow of lymph through the armpit and breasts, which leads to the accumulation of toxins.

Dry Skin Brushing for Enhancing Skin Elimination

Healthy skin should eliminate two pounds of waste acids every day. Skin brushing before dressing, and before every bath, will remove the top layer of dead skin that would otherwise block the effective elimination of toxins through the skin.

You can look closely at the iris (colored part of the eye) in the mirror and tell how well your skin is eliminating. If you can see a darker ring around the very most outer edge of the iris then you have what is called a scurf ring. Seeing a scurf ring always means that your skin is not eliminating toxins well, and it is being reflected on the iris of the eye. It is not a disease of the eye, but simply a reflex sign of an overload of toxins at the level of the skin. You can observe your eye and watch it improve as you progress with your detox protocol.

You will need:
– Natural Fiber Skin Brush w/a long handle
(NEVER USE A SYNTHETIC BRISTLE BRUSH due to the fact that these can cause an adverse electrical charge on the body)

Instructions:
Use this brush dry, without any soaps or water, prior to bathing or dressing. It should take you about 5 minutes or so, brushing your entire body, except the face. Brush in all directions, but generally moving towards the heart. Imagine you are brushing the lymph fluid up from your feet, up the legs toward your heart. Do the same, starting at the hands moving lymph fluid up the arm towards the shoulder and on to the heart. Using the long handle of the skin brush, reach to the lower back area and brush the lymph up the spine and sides, moving it up and over the shoulders to the heart. Your skin may at first be very sensitive and you may think that you are scratching and hurting the skin. Make sure you are not damaging the skin, but after a week or so of doing this you will usually find that it feels good.

You may use a special face brush to use on your face.

Detox Bath #1 (Pain Reliever Bath)

This is one of my absolute favorite bath therapies. It is the first thing we do for our own family whenever we feel we are coming down with something. Not only does it detoxify the body and relieve pain, it seems to stop many infections in their tracks and help the body regain balance.

You will need:

4 cups Epsom Salt (Magnesium Sulfate)

32 to 64 fluid Ounces of Hydrogen Peroxide (3%, as found in grocery stores)

2 Tablespoons of Ginger (fresh grated preferably, wrapped in a thin piece of cloth or in a tea ball)

Instructions: This and all bath therapies work best by first dry skin brushing the entire body (see section on "Dry Skin Brushing"). This removes the layer of dead skin that may otherwise block the absorption of energy and nutrients from this bath and stimulates the blood and lymph fluids to rise to the skin to accept the bath.

Fill tub with warm water. Add the above ingredients. Soak for at least 20 minutes. The beneficial effects of this bath are cumulative and increase in effectiveness the more you use them.

Through medical studies, this therapy has been shown to relieve pain that did not even respond to narcotic medicines. Recommended taken for at least seven consecutive days, or as recommended by your doctor. Continued use daily, or as needed is fine.

Do not use if you are pregnant.

Detox Bath #2

You will need:
·   1 liter of Cold-pressed Olive Oil
·   1 liter of Cold-pressed Castor Oil

Instructions: This and all bath therapies work best by first dry skin brushing the entire body (see section on "Dry Skin Brushing"). This removes the layer of dead skin that may otherwise block the absorption of energy and nutrients from this bath and stimulates the blood and lymph fluids to rise to the skin to accept the bath. Be sure to drink plenty of water throughout the day prior to doing this bath, but do the bath even if you have not drunk much water throughout the day. Just drink at least 8 oz. of water before getting into the tub.

Be very careful getting in and out of the bathtub as you and everything else will be very slippery. Generally not recommended for senior citizens, those with poor balance or impaired walking, or anyone at an increased risk of falling. Use anti-slip mats in your tub and get out only after wiping the oils from your hands and feet. Step out of the tub onto a bath mat if you have a tiled or linoleum floor!

Instructions:

1.   Rub your skin from head to foot with a mixture of equal parts of the olive and castor oils.

2.   Then, with the oil still coating the skin, immerse yourself in a hot bath for 20 minutes. The bath allows the oil to penetrate to the deepest levels of the skin, but take care entering and exiting the tub as the oil will make everything slippery.

3.   Immediately after the bath, go to bed under heavy cover for 1 hour to sweat out poisons; then shower. Follow this routine every day for three days, then three times weekly for 3 months, or as indicated by your doctor.

During any detoxification program, breakdown products of toxins and other metabolic debris tend to accumulate under the skin. The skin is one of your body's largest detoxification organs, therefore it is important to keep the toxins moving through the skin and out of the body.

(Good as a stand alone therapy, but best in combination with the Lemon Juice Cleanse)

Detox Bath #3

This bath is especially beneficial if you have a history of toxic habits, such as smoking, eating excessive amounts of meat, or excessive alcohol consumption. However, even if you have not met the above description, you will still benefit from this bath as a generalized detoxifying bath. It is also very beneficial for those undergoing radiation therapy, or after x-rays.

You will need:
- Baking Soda (Sodium Bicarbonate)
- Epsom Salts (Magnesium Sulfate) or Sea Salt

Instructions: This and all bath therapies work best by first dry skin brushing the entire body (see section on "Dry Skin Brushing"). This removes the layer of dead skin that may otherwise block the absorption of energy and nutrients from this bath and stimulates the blood and lymph fluids to rise to the skin to accept the bath.

Add 1 cup of Baking Soda and 1 pound of Epsom Salts, or 1 cup of Sea Salt, to a warm tub of water filled enough to cover you. Soak for 20-30 minutes up to 3 times per week to help eliminate toxins through the skin.

Liver and Gallbladder Flush

(Best results are achieved after first doing a Lemon Juice Cleanse to ensure that the colon is healthy enough to deal with the increased work load and doing coffee enemas throughout this flush and beyond, but are not required.)

This Liver/Gallbladder Flush is a time-tested favorite of doctors around the world and is one of the best methods of cleansing the tissues of the liver and gallbladder.

Detoxification is essential to any chronic illness program. If you do not relieve the body of toxins, the chances of recovery from many illnesses are greatly reduced. This protocol can be a mildly difficult and uncomfortable process, however, a well-rounded plan of treatment such as this should minimize any discomfort.

The Liver/Gallbladder flush can be repeated monthly, but at the minimum one should do it every six months. The liver refers more pain to more different parts of the body than just about any other organ. It will be well worth the effort as many people feel greatly improved after doing one of these flushes.

You will need:

1. One gallon of Apple Juice – Organic, unfiltered, and unsweetened

2. One box of Baking Soda

3. One pint of Epsom Salts (Magnesium Sulfate)

4. One bottle of Calc-Acid (by Nutri-West™) or Calcium Phosphate

5. One bottle of Phos-Drops (by Nutri-West™)

6. One bottle of Molybdenum (by Jernigan Nutraceuticals)

7. Cold-pressed, Extra Virgin Olive Oil

8. Bentonite Clay (purified for human consumption)

9. Whipping Cream (1 pint)

10. Fresh Fruit (Preferably miscellaneous berries)

11. Two bottles of Total Liver Detox (by Nutri-West™)

12. Optional: Two 4" x 6" x 1/2" ceramic MRBT magnets

Follow these instructions completely:

1. Add 1 ounce of Phos-Drops to 1 gallon of Apple juice and mix well.

    Over the next 4 days, drink all the juice between meals at the rate of 3-4 glasses per day. Keep the apple juice chilled to avoid fermentation, but let it come to room temperature first before drinking it. Always rinse your mouth out using 1 teaspoon of Baking Soda in 1 glass of water, or brush your teeth with Baking Soda after drinking the juice to prevent the acid from damaging your teeth. Otherwise eat normally and take your coffee enemas as usual. Take 2 Total Liver Detox tablets 3 times every day until the two bottles are empty and 1 Molybdenum capsule 3 times every day until empty.

2. On the fourth day, while still taking the Apple juice/Phos-Drop combination, take 2 Calc-Acid immediately before breakfast, and 2 immediately before lunch. Drink about 2 pints of pure water that morning.

3. 2 hours after lunch, take 1 tablespoon of Epsom Salts dissolved in warm water; add juice if desired.

4. 5 hours after lunch, take 1 tablespoon of Epsom Salts dissolved in warm water; add juice if desired.

5. 6 hours after lunch, eat a dinner of Whipping Cream and fruit; the whipping cream contracts the gallbladder; any fruit is acceptable, but berries are best, either fresh or frozen. Take 1 Calc-Acid with your meal.

6. Half an hour before bedtime, put 1 tablespoon of the Bentonite in 1 glass of water, mix well (Start by adding water slowly), and drink.

7. At bedtime, drink 1/2 cup of Olive Oil; a small amount of orange, grapefruit, or lemon juice may be added, if desired. Immediately go to bed and lie on your right side with your knees drawn up; hold this position for 30 minutes. For maximum detox with the minimum discomfort you may opt for the Magnetic Resonance Bio-Oxidative Therapy ceramic magnets. Place one of the 4" x 6"

x 1/2" ceramic magnets over the liver (over right lower ribcage and overhanging the abdomen a bit), place the other ceramic magnet over the navel running lengthwise across the abdomen. Strap these magnets in place with the negative polarity side facing the body and sleep with these on for at least 3-7 days. You may feel nauseated during the night due to the release of stored toxins from the gallbladder and liver; this is normal and will pass.

8. Observe your first few bowel movements which should be rather loose, so that you can describe them to your doctor. You may see floating pellets which many doctors believe to be gallstones which were softened and passed painlessly during the night.

9. On the following day, eat normally. Take 2 Calc-Acid with breakfast, 2 with lunch, and 1 with your evening meal.

10. Continue taking all of the Total Liver Detox and Molybdenum until gone.

Coffee Enema

You will need:

1. Enema bag with hose

2. K-Y Jelly (A lubricant available in any pharmacy)

3. 1 pound Organic Coffee (Never use instant, decaffeinated, or flavored coffee)

4. 1 Bottle of Molybdenum (by Jernigan Nutraceuticals or other reputable company)

5. Cold-pressed Sunflower Oil (keep refrigerated)

6. Cold-pressed Flaxseed Oil (keep refrigerated)

Coffee Enema Protocol: generally recommended 3-4 times per week.

1. Start the Coffee Enema just prior to going to bed. Add 3 tablespoons of ground Organic coffee (not instant or decaffeinated) to 2 pints of distilled water. Boil for 5 minutes uncovered to drive off oils, then cover, lower heat and simmer for an additional 15 minutes.

2. Strain and allow liquid to cool to body temperature. (Test temperature on forearm to be sure) Pour into enema bag. Lubricate rectal enema tube with K-Y Jelly. Hang enema bag above you, but not more than 2 feet from your body. The best level is approximately 6 inches above the intestines. Lying on your right side, draw both legs close to the abdomen.

3. Insert tube no more than 3 inches into rectum (adult). Open the stopcock and allow fluid to run in very slowly to avoid cramping. Relax and breathe deeply, to let coffee flow in. Retain the solution for 12-15 minutes. If you have trouble retaining or taking the full amount, lower the bag to the floor to relieve the pressure. After about 20 seconds, slowly start raising the bag toward the original level. You can also pinch the tube to control the flow.

4. Release into the toilet. And immediately take 2 capsules, 300 mcg (micrograms) of Molybdenum with a glass of water to help chelate

out any liberated toxins. Take this dosage of Molybdenum 3 times per day for one week following.

5. After each enema, swallow 1 tablespoon each of the Flaxseed and Sunflower oils.

6. Upon waking the next morning, if you experience headache and drowsiness, an additional enema is recommended that night.

7. Depending upon the severity of the detoxification symptoms, one may increase the frequency of enemas to 2-3 times per day.

Keep all equipment perfectly clean between sessions.

Facts concerning Coffee Enemas:

Coffee enemas help to purge the colon and liver of accumulated toxins, dead cells, and waste products.

The coffee enema may seem strange at first, but research by Max Gerson, M.D., reveals that the coffee enema is effective in stimulating a complex enzyme system involved with liver detoxification (called the glutathione-S-transferase enzyme system). During the coffee enema there is a 600% increase in the activity of this enzyme system which ensures that free-radical activity is greatly reduced and that the activity of any carcinogens is blocked.

Coffee is known to contain choleretics, which are substances that increase the flow of toxin-rich bile from the gallbladder. The coffee enema is thought to be among the only pharmaceutically effective choleretics noted in the medical literature that can be safely used many times daily without toxic effects.

The Master Longevity Body Cleanse

There are few, if any, other total body cleanses that will do more good for you than this cleanse. I developed this cleanse protocol after years of using a modified version of the classic "Master Cleanse", a lemon-juice, cayenne pepper, and grade-B Maple syrup recipe. This new cleanse still ultilizes lemon juice, cayenne pepper and grade-B Maple syrup but it now incorporates Chinese wolfberry juice concentrate as well.

My longevity body cleanse program is light years better than the old "Master Cleanse." If you are going to spend the time and effort to do a cleanse of this type you might as well benefit from more than simply cleansing the tissues. The potential for detoxifying *and* healing is so much greater now that I just get excited knowing my patients are starting this cleanse. My new cleanse still provides the beneficial limonine from the lemons of the old Master Cleanse but it also provides the therapeutic grade lemon oil added in the Wolfberry Berry Young Juice®.

Every nutrient, mineral, vitamin, carbohydrate, amino-acid needed by the body is provided by the Chinese wolfberry juice. Those with blood-sugar concerns can adjust the cleanse by adding more or less of the Wolfberry Berry Young Juice.

It is a good idea to do this cleanse for 7-21 days with a maximum of 40 days, during which no other food should be consumed. I prefer 14-21 days after which foods from the "highly beneficial foods" group for your specific bloodtype (O, A, B, AB), listed in the book by Dr. D'Adamo, "Eat Right for Your Type". None of these foods should be consumed more than one time in a four day period. Basically, you should be rotating your foods in order to avoid maladaptive syndromes and food allergies in the future.

Don't be afraid to do this cleanse. The first three to five days are the hardest for most people, simply due to the lifelong habit and emotional ties to eating. This cleanse will help you in innumerable ways. The Holy Bible speaks of fasts, which this cleanse is a "fast", avoiding foods throughout. In the Bible it says, "When you fast, do not put on the sack cloth, and rend your clothes, as your reward is already determined." What this means is that if you put on a sad face and act miserable during your fast so that you get sympathy from all the people around you, then your reward will only be the sympathy of those around you. A cleanse or fast is a prime time for you to practice meditation and prayer. If you desire more than people's sympathy, you will be rewarded with a cleansing of the body, mind and spirit.

You will need per day:

1 gallon distilled Water

6 ounces of Wolfberry "Berry Young Juice"

1/8 to 1/4 Teaspoon Cayenne Pepper (red pepper), whichever amount you can tolerate

12 Tablespoons of fresh-squeezed Lemon or Lime juice (about 6 Lemons)

2-4 Tablespoons of genuine grade-B Maple syrup (not grade A maple flavored syrup). You may also increase the amount if you are experiencing low blood sugar.

1 bottle of Digestive Enzymes (These should last you about 1 month)

1 bottle Probiotics (These should last you about 1 month)

1 bottle Herbal Laxative

Instructions:

- Combine all of the ingredients listed. Always use fresh squeezed Lemons or Limes. It is preferable to use organic Lemons when possible. Drink at least 1/2 gallon to a maximum of 1 gallon of the Master Longevity Combination, spread throughout the waking period of your day. If you get hungry just drink another glass. <u>Absolutely no other food should be eaten throughout the duration of your program</u>.

- Take one capsule of the Herbal Laxative at night to loosen accumulated mucus and fecal matter in the intestines.

- Take one capsule of the probiotics (Total Probiotics – NutriWest) in the morning and one at night.

- Take one - two capsules of digestive enzyme (Detoxzyme- YLO or Allerzyme is a 100% vegetarian formula which will work fine) morning, noon and night.

*** Best if Cleanse is used at the same time as the Epsom Salt Purge and/or Coffee Enema, since it is very important to have 3-5 bowel movements per day to expel all of the now liberated toxins from the body. (Without good bowel movements, toxins can be stirred up and lodge in new areas of the body.) You are constipated if all you are having is one bowel movement per day. If you ever get the urge to have bowel movement, go immediately to the stool instead of waiting as many people are prone to do when they are busy. Do not strain excessively on the stool. Most people are surprised at how much still comes out in the bowel movements even though they are not eating anything. Much of the BM's are the 20-40 pounds of fecal matter that has gotten lodged throughout the intestines. In research performed by the world-renowned Sir Bernard Jenson, D.C., who was knighted for his work in natural healing, it was found in a study of 600 elderly people, who reported they were having at least one bowel movement every day, that later upon autopsy all had at least 20 pounds of accumulated matter lodged in the intestines.

*** Observe your bowel movements so that you can report what it looks like to your doctor, such as color, diameter, firmness, size, quantity, parasites, recognizable food that went undigested.

*** Upon successful completion of the Master Longevity Body Cleanse, you now have a clean body. It will respond differently than before the cleanse. You should absorb more nutrients from your food and gain more vitality from the food you eat. However, your clean body will also let you know immediately with various symptoms when you have eaten something full of food additives, toxins and otherwise low-vitality foods.

Expectations of the Master Longevity Body Cleanse:

To eliminate and break up toxins lodged in any tissue of the body.

To relieve strain and stress on the organs and glands of the body.

Re-establish proper fluid balance.

Cleanses all body tissues and purge poisons out of the body.

Breaks up mucus.

Strengthens and builds the blood.

Stimulates and builds the immune system.

Reverses the aging process, increases longevity.

Eliminate food allergies, and allergies of all types.

Normalizes the metabolism, including blood sugar and cholesterol.

Relieves the burden off the body of having to deal with digesting food while you heal.

Inhibits tumor growth.

Facts about the Master Longevity Cleanse:
This cleanse has all of the nutrition needed during this time. There is no need to take vitamins during this cleanse; in fact, vitamin supplements can frequently hinder getting the best results from the cleanse.

Rest and take it easy if you have to – although most people can go on about their regular business without difficulty.

It can be used three to four times per year and will do wonders for keeping the body functioning at a maximum health. You may also drink distilled water throughout the cleanse. No other drinks or foods are allowed.

Wolfberry, Berry Young Juice® This juice is the closest to the "fountain of youth" found to date. Not only does it contain high amounts of Chinese wolfberries, but it also contains five of the richest sources of the free radical fighting antioxidants from wolfberry, blueberry, pomegranate, apricot, and raspberry. If this were not enough, the juice is enhanced with therapeutic grade essential oils of lemon and orange, both of which contain the phyto-chemical, d-limonene and its derivative perillyl alcohol, is thought to block both tumor promotion and progression. The Lemon and Orange oil in the Berry Young Juice are antiviral, antiseptic, invigorating, a body tonic, antiparasitic, increases white blood cell formation, antidepressant, antispasmodic, digestive aid, and sedative. It contains high levels of Limonene

This source of wolfberries comes from the Yellow River in the Ningxia Province of central China, where it has been used for 5000 years and is listed in the world's oldest medical books. Science has documented that wolfberries are the only known substance proven to increase human longevity. Wolfberries are consumed daily by one of the longest lived societies on the planet, with people living in excess of 120 years. It is the most nutrient dense food ever found, containing 13% protein (no other fruit contains more than 5-6% protein), 21 amino acids (six times higher in proportion than bee pollen). It also contains over 80 minerals and trace minerals, carbohydrates, and more different enzymes than can be counted.

This juice contains substances which stimulate the 2 primary phases of liver detoxification. It stimulates a 48% increase in the powerful antioxidant superoxide dismutase (SOD) in the blood as well as a 12% increase in hemoglobin, not to mention that lipid peroxide levels drop 65%

The blueberry concentrate in Berry Young Juice, is high in the powerful flavonoid antioxidant, proanthocyanadin, which recent research has shown improves brain function.

Pomegranate juice in the Berry Young Juice, are high in potassium and vitamin C, and research shows pomegranate reduces the LDL or bad cholesterol.

Apricots contain a powerhouse of nutrients, containing three times more potassium than bananas, twice as much magnesium as broccoli, and four times as much niacin as spinach, as well as a having high concentrations of carotenoids.

The raspberry juice in the Berry Young Juice contain ellagic acid, a plant chemical that protects cells from genetic mutation that can lead to abnormal cell growth, like cancer. Of interest, raspberries contain over four times more antioxidant capacity than vitamin C and beta-carotene.

Berry Young Juice is crucial to the success of this cleanse. To substitute anything else is incomprehensible because of its lifegiving benefits. Even after the cleanse I recommend you drink about one fluid ounce a day, which is the equivalent of eating 1/4 to 1/2 cup of fresh wolfberries, the ultimate longevity food.

Lemons and Limes are acidic fruits, but are actually alkalinizing in the body once eaten. The more acidic the tissues and fluids of the body are, the more dysfunctional and ill you will become. Alkalinity is conducive to health and the rebuilding of tissues. These citrus fruits contain substances which stimulate the 2 primary phases of liver detoxification. An essential oil contained in these fruits called limonene and its derivative perillyl alchohol, is thought to block both tumor promotion and progression. Lemon juice is said to be one of nature's most powerful antiseptics, used internally and externally. (If you find you are extremely acidic, take the following bath to reduce the acid levels in your body: The Vinegar Bath: Put 1 cup to 2 quarts of 100% apple cider vinegar into a bathtub of warm water and soak for at least 20 minutes.)

Grade B Maple Syrup is the second run with more vitamins and minerals plus more maple flavor. Grade B is preferable for this cleanse and less expensive as well. It contains Vitamins A, B1, B2, B6, C, Nicotinic Acid, and Pantothenic Acid. The minerals include Sodium, Potassium, Calcium, Magnesium, Manganese, Iron, Copper, Phosphorus, Sulphur, Chlorine, and Silicon. This type of maple syrup is a balanced form of positive and negative sugar, and should always be used instead of any substitute.

Cayenne Pepper is necessary for stimulating proper circulation. Interestingly, cayenne is also a hemostatic substance, meaning it arrests bleeding. It is vital in this cleanse in its ability to break up mucus and increase the warmth of the body tissues which has a softening effect on hardened toxic tissues. It helps to build blood and also adds many B-vitamins and vitamin C.

Digestive Enzymes (Detoxyme™) are necessary to neutralize any gas, and toxins. There are special enzymes for digesting proteins (protease), carbohydrates (amylase), fats (lipase), and fiber (cellulase). Lactase is used to break down lactose, the component in dairy products that are indigestible in many people. Detoxyme contains other enzymes but also includes synergistic therapeutic grade essential oils of cumin, fennel, and anise. These essential oils relax the lining of the stomach and small intestines, making the detoxification process smoother. They are also beneficial in their anti-parasitic actions.

When used during this cleanse these enzymes and oils will assist in removing much of the undigested matter that can get caked on the walls of the intestines.

Probiotics – (Total Probiotics™, by NutriWest) As the sludge of years of fermented, putrid matter and mucus begin to be dislodged from the intestines, the underlying intestinal walls, which normally harbor our friendly bowel bacteria, will need to be re-inoculated with a variety of acidophilus-type bacteria. Among their many health promoting functions, they help:

(1) Reduce the level of cholesterol

(2) Curb or destroy potentially pathogenic or harmful bacteria and yeasts such as Candida albicans

(3) Through their production of lactic acid, they preserve and enhance the digestibility of foods

(4) Help produce important B-vitamins

(5) Prevent cancer and other chronic illnesses by detoxifying or preventing the formation of carcinogenic chemicals.

Mustard Foot Bath

This foot soak is used as relief from general aches and pains, toxic headaches, and overall toxic conditions. It also seems to increase blood and lymph circulation, as well as increase overall sense of wellbeing.

You will need:

- Mustard Powder

- Cayenne Pepper

Instructions:

In a basin of warm water, add 1 tablespoon of the Mustard powder and 1 teaspoon of ground cayenne pepper. Sit in a comfortable chair and soak your feet for 20-30 minutes in this mixture. You may do this 2-3 times per day if desired, for weeks to months, and definitely in periods of intense toxicity and pain.

Contrast Foot Bath

The Mustard Foot Bath can be used to help stimulate the warmth organization of the body, resulting in the improvement of the body's core temperature. To use this therapy one should soak the feet in the hot water of the Mustard Foot bath for one minute, and then soak in cold water for 30 seconds. This should be repeated three to five times in a session, two to three times per day, for several weeks. Note: To continue the warming effects of the contrast foot bath or the regular Mustard foot bath wear Peat/Silk or Peat/Wool socks and/or rub Cuprum/Quartz Ointment on the soles of the feet then wear socks.

THERAPIES SECTION

Neurological Disorganization

X's and O's Test

This tests for neurological disorganization between the left and right cerebral hemispheres. The brain processes visual information through a coordination of the right and left brain.

Symptoms of visual neurological disorganization may include disorientation, brain fog, undue confusion, getting lost going to places you should know, lack of concentration, irritability, difficulty reading schematics and maps, and problems of locomotion while visually seeing many lines that cross each other.

One woman with Lyme disease figured this out to some degree on her own. She found that she could walk up the stairs of her house, only if she would close her eyes. Apparently the balustrades of her spiral staircase were causing a visual processing disturbance, due to the criss-cross appearance as she looked up the stairs. She also found out on her own that she could walk stronger and farther if she would place the palm of her hand over her belly button. Her husband lovingly teased her saying that, "You look like you are trying to hold yourself together." However we know from clinical science, that placing the hand over the belly button acts like a jumper cable putting energy in from a different circuit (the hand) into the small intestine circuit. From knowledge of Circuit Healing, we know that the small intestine circuit is shared by all of the muscles of the abdomen and the quadriceps muscles of the thighs, the strongest muscles in the body that lift your legs while walking. This woman, at her worst, was in a wheelchair due to chronic Lyme disease! She now is a vibrant member of society, a devoted energetic mother, and a corporate executive of a multi-million dollar corporation. After years of fighting to regain her health, she has no more symptoms, and has remained symptom free for many years now. Once, when I called to check on her condition, only a few months after beginning to treat her, her husband relayed my question to her, and told me in a choked-up voice, "Oh my God! She just did a cartwheel in the middle of the living room to show me how good she is doing!" He also said, "I can't thank you enough for giving us our mom and wife back!"

It took much more than this treatment to get her back to normal, however every treatment and therapy is needed, because if the neurological disorganization goes unaddressed it is not a given that it will simply correct itself.

The X's and O's test is a simple yet effective way to enhance and facilitate the normal functioning of your body.

To Test:

• First on two pieces of paper draw on one a large circle, on the other paper draw a large X (each about 2 inches tall)

• You will need someone to help you test your muscle strength. Hold out your strongest arm straight in front of and perpendicular to your body with the hand open and your palm facing away from your body, the thumb will be pointing down towards the floor. Have whomever is going to test your strength, grasp your arm just above the wrist. Instruct them to tell you to "hold real strong" as they apply gentle pressure downwards towards the floor. In doing this you are just trying to feel what a good strong muscle test should feel like...they are not to force your arm down, but to feel the muscle "lock" firmly with gentle pressure.

• Once you know what a strong muscle test feels like, have your partner hold up the paper with the circle on it, in front of your face so you can look at the circle. While still looking at it, have your partner retest the same arm. It should stay strong.

• Now have your partner hold the paper with the X on it, in front of your face. While you are still looking at the X, have your partner retest the same arm. If the previously strong muscle goes weak, then you may have some neurological disorganization going on. This is nothing that needs an emergency room or hospitalization. In fact it can be very easily corrected.

To Correct the Neurological Disorganization:

• Place your right palm on your navel.

• Take your left middle finger across to the point where the RIGHT collar bone meets the sternum (breast bone). Now slide the finger tip down off the collar bone into the soft fleshy area just below the collar bone and just right of the sternum. You will know when you've located the correct point when you hit a spot that is very tender. Massage the tender point in a circular motion for ten seconds only.

• Now reverse the above hands, placing the LEFT palm over the navel. and using your right middle finger to massage the same point on the LEFT side of the body.

• Having completed the above, have your partner hold up the paper with the X on it, and while you are still looking at the X re-test the same muscle. The muscle should now stay strong indicating that you are no longer disorganized.

• Repeat this morning and evening. If the points do not feel tender, then you either have not found the correct point to massage, or this is not your problem. After you have been massaging them for a few days, these points may not be tender anymore, indicating that you do not need to keep doing it. If the points progressively hurt worse then you are over-massaging them, and should back off for awhile.

Iodine Stain Test

This simple test is almost too simple, it cost next to nothing and will help you to know when your body is in need of Iodine. I really like how this test demonstrates that just because you give the body a nutrient, it doesn't mean the body will utilize it. In this test, if the iodine stain that you paint on your skin remains on the skin for 24 hours then your body apparently doesn't need it and therefore leaves it on the skin. If your body does need the iodine, often it will be slurped up almost immediately, and the iodine stain will disappear within a few hours. So in this one simple test you can determine if you need more iodine, and you can provide iodine all at the same time.

Instructions:

• Get a 1 ounce bottle of tincture of 2% Iodine.

• Paint a spot using the tincture about the size of a silver dollar. Paint the spot in an inconspicuous place such as your belly, thigh, or the inside of the arm. Be sure it is dry before putting on clothes to prevent staining the clothing. Do this when you know you will not be taking a shower or bath, since it may wash off.

• If you body level of Iodine is normal, then the spot will remain on the skin for 24 hours.

• If the spot disappears in less than 24 hours, this means your body needed Iodine and took it in. (I find it awesome that our body will take in what it needs and leave on the skin what it doesn't need!) This works transdermally much like the now popular Nicoderm and Estrogen Patches, by soaking into the blood stream via the skin.

*** Important...if you are presently on thyroid medicine you may need to cut back on your dose, or ultimately stop it all together, now that your body has the iodine to manufacture the thyroid hormones it needs.

Keep applying the Tincture of Iodine every 24 hours, at different places on your body, until the spot stays there for the full 24 hours.

Purpose:

Iodine is needed by the thyroid to produce thyroxin. This test will let you know if you need more iodine, and it will also supply the iodine your body needs. Once iodine levels are normal in your body (meaning the spot lasts 24 hours) then you can stop applying it for a while and re-check periodically.

Iodine is one of America's most common deficiencies, even though the salt most of us consume has been iodized, this form of iodine seems to not function efficiently in the body. According to a study by the CDC (Center for Disease Control) the number of Americans with low iodine has quadrupled in the last 25 years. Dr. Bernard Jenson, D.C., Ph.D., found that the iodized table salt, which is superheated so that it can pour more easily, is a poor form of iodine for the body. I recommend sun-evaporated sea salt with supplemental iodine. Sun-evaporated sea salt is loaded with trace minerals and does not come with the health risks of regular iodized salt. Sea salt will actually help normalize the fluid regulating abilities of the body and has been known to normalize edema and high blood pressure.

Once again, just giving your body iodine does not ensure your body can use it. Chlorinated water, which most Americans drink inhibits the absorption of iodine, as well as a metabolic form of chlorine, perchlorate, inhibits transportation of iodine in the body. This is one more reason to get a whole house water purification system. The body will absorb two cups of the water in a 20 minute bath! I know my local municipal water is blue as any swimming pool and smells just like a pool from all of the chlorine. If our goal is to eliminate anything that is interfering with your body functioning normally, eliminating your consumption of chlorine and supplementing with organic iodine will go a long way towards healing.

Iodine deficiencies may show up as weight gain, lethargy, fatigue, enlarged thyroid, hair loss, fibrous cysts, and mental retardation. In fact, experts say that iodine deficiencies are the world's leading cause of preventable mental retardation.

In conclusion, replacing the missing iodine in you body may restore normal thyroid function, however if you find that your spot never seems to last 24 hours you need to alert your doctor and he can determine what you need to do from there. Many times when this happens, the hypothalamus and adrenal glands are fatigued and need support before the iodine will be efficiently used. Also, a special form of liquid potassium iodide can be taken sublinqually, while using this skin stain test to determine when you have adequate iodine.

Dietary Sources of Iodine: Dulse, Kelp.

Section 8

Diet and Nutrition

Chapter 38

Diet and Nutrition

The media is full of advertisements promoting this or that nutritional advancement or diet. Eating has become "rocket science" to hear many of the leading experts talk. Testimonials are one of the favorite ways to promote and market and ultimately sell you books, tapes, supplements, and diet programs. The claims are often real; however the results gained by one possibly enormous success overcoming some chronic illness are conspicuously absent when others attempt to do the same.

While eliminating poor dietary choices will always promote health, there is much to be said for the healing effects of proper diet and nutrition. It cannot be argued that eating nutritious foods is well within God's design of health and healing. Even the "process" of changing your dietary habits promotes healing in that we are creatures of habit, and the habits are what have created the reality you are now suffering. Forming new and better habits will necessarily create a new and better reality.

Nourishment from natural foods raised and prepared in such a way as to preserve the inherent vitality will always provide more value to the human organism than any modern synthetically derived or processed "super-food". Only nature can provide food with the qualities of transformative energy. Only foods started from vital heritage seed, grown with respect for the timing of planting and harvesting, and maximized through the natural treatment of the soil have the ability to impact every level of the entire human physically, emotionally, energetically, and spiritually.

The quality of a food rests upon its content of formative forces. Formative forces are the inherent energy made possible only through the proper growing, harvesting, and preparing of the food. These formative forces are released from the food as it is chewed. Did you ever wonder why we must chew our foods? Birds don't chew at all. We chew the food because the teeth are an entry point into the electro-energetic organ circuits. If one had to wait for the digestion and absorption of nutrients it could take up to six hours! Once released through chewing, the formative energy of food travels through specific teeth as dictated by the type of food, at approximately half the speed of light…roughly four times around the planet in one second. This enables the organ circuits to get the energy they need without having to wait for complete digestion. The formative energy of well-grown foods is enlivening and coherent energy. The nutrient content, enzyme activity, and bioavailability (how easily the nutrients are absorbed into the body) is greatly enhanced as well in these well-grown foods. High quality natural foods ensure that the energy and the building blocks needed to heal are present.

What brings about the maximum benefit to the body from foods is the process of selection, preparation, intentionality, and transformation of that food chosen by yourself. The very process of changing your diet has its own healing consequences. Denying yourself of habit foods, those comfort foods we all have emotional bonds to, and even the process of choosing and preparing your new foods, demands an exceptional amount of inner activity. This inner activity is very restorative to the part of the body which regulates warmth organization. This concept can be seen in another way; the habits and ruts we have been living with for years have created the reality of today. Every process of changing and getting out of the ruts of your life will necessarily cause a whole new reality. Selecting more balanced and healthy food and lifestyle choices will breed only the improvement in life quality.

While advancements in our knowledge of optimal diet and nutrition cannot be ignored, it must be said that God, our Creator, did not make the task of eating to be "rocket science." When He created this universe, He had to have known that the Eskimos would not have a wide diversity of foods, nor would the nomads of the desert. God designed the body to function perfectly under a wide range of diets...not to include dead junk foods, but the foods He provided, properly grown, harvested, and prepared.

At the Somerleyton Center for Biological Medicine, a blend of modern dietary science and natural foods is used to maximize healing. Foods are recommended based upon the phenomenal research of Dr. D'Adamo, N.D., and author of the Best Selling book "Eat Right for Your Type" which revolutionized the world's understanding of food selection. This research is combined with the 4-day rotation diet of Dr. William Philpott, M.D. It was Dr. D'Adamo who determined that the good or bad reaction of eating a specific food can be anticipated based upon changes in your blood, and based upon your blood type, i.e., blood types A, B, AB, or O.

Through his research we now know what foods are basically "Medicinal", "Neutral" or "Poisonous" to you based upon your blood type. Finally, one diet doesn't have to fit all. If you eat foods only in the Medicinal category (Highly Beneficial) it will promote and accelerate healing. Neutral foods are basically just fillers, while Poisonous foods (foods to avoid) hinder the healing process.

Dr. Philpott's 4-day rotation diet helps break any food addictions that are always present in just about everyone's diet. He recommends that one should avoid eating the same food substance twice in the same 4-day period. Food addictions are also known to cause what he calls a "maladaptive syndrome". By breaking these food addictions every illness becomes much easier to overcome. Indeed, many symptoms and their causes can be eliminated by using the 4-day rotation diet. I have found that combining the individualized D'Adamo diet of highly-beneficial foods with never eating any of these foods more than once in a four day period provides the best of all worlds.

In providing this new diet program it is understood now that it will normally force you to change your dietary habits as discussed earlier. It may involve having to eat foods that you must learn to prepare and find new recipes. This and the elimination of toxic processed foods and habit foods will go a long way to speeding you towards healing.

Approach this dietary change with an open mind and a happy heart. Life is a journey, and we are not trying to mess up your journey, but make your way easier and more enjoyable.

Does all this mean that you absolutely cannot partake of your favorite foods forever? Definitely not! This simply enables you to make better food choices. I will say those who have told me that they followed the highly beneficial foods "religiously" saw the greatest benefit.

Be patient with yourself. It has taken my wife and I fifteen years to get to the place where we are at in regards to our diet. We now grind our own organic grains, get our milk from our own Nubian dairy goat, our eggs from our chickens, our vegetables and herbs from our own land. The process of change has been an interesting journey that has no end.

A. Foods to Avoid
(Also a great idea to <u>always</u> avoid these foods, or in very limited amounts)

1. Foods high in saturated fats (pork, cream, lard, etc.)

2. Dairy products (Unless goat, and natural, unprocessed cheeses)

3. Canned food and carbonated drinks

4. Iodized or regular table salt (Use only sun-evaporated sea salt)

5. Stimulants (coffee, black tea, alcohol, etc.)

6. Fried or roasted foods

7. All food preservatives, food colorings, flavor enhancers (read food labels: MSG, NutraSweet, etc.)

8. Microwaved foods (Some L-form amino acids are converted over to the D-forms, which promote free-radical damage)

9. Refined sugar, cakes, jams, chocolate, and ice cream

10. Refined oils (non-cold pressed oils…even olive oils) Use only cold-pressed.

11. Foods cooked in aluminum cookware, or aluminum utensils

12. Tapwater, or unpurified water. Use distilled water only under the advisement of your physician, since it can leach out helpful minerals from your body.

B. Supportive Dietary Measures

1. Maintain regular and consistent mealtimes.

2. Before eating relax momentarily for 10 seconds, then begin eating. (Blessing your food in prayer – science has shown that this cleans the food, makes it more bio-available, more digestible, and consequently tastes better)

3. Pay attention to what you are eating. Chew until each bite is smooth and easily swallowed. Seek to feel the energy and taste the subtle flavors of the food.

4. Force yourself to slow down, this will aid digestion and appetite satisfaction. Eating should not be a chore. Many times food is eaten without much awareness to what is eaten, much like driving a car for miles and suddenly realizing you don't recall anything about the journey.

5. Eating by candlelight and calming music can assist in setting a relaxing tone to the evening meal.

6. Avoid alternating between hot and cold foods on a frequent basis.

7. Eat most of your daily protein in the morning or at lunch time (Stomach acid is highest early in the day which allows for better digestion of proteins…the bi-product of incomplete protein digestion is called nitrosamines and are very carcinogenic).

8. Drink room temperature, purified water (a minimum of 8, eight-ounce glasses per day). Cold water requires more work by your body to bring it up to body temperature. This can be a problem when so many people now-a-days are suffering from low body temperature. Don't drink tap water as it often contains herbicides, pesticides, chlorine, fluoride, and other chemicals. Do not drink much during the meal as this dilutes the stomach digestive juices. Do not drink over a gallon per day.

Give Thanks for Your Food
And Your Medicines

As a doctor, I am always reading God's Word to see what He says about sickness, medicine, healing, and diet. It should be no surprise to anyone, that whatever He saw fit to put in His book, then it must have been important for providing His children with a more abundant life.

We are instructed to give thanks and bless our food before eating. Why? First of all to acknowledge Him as the provider of all good things, and obviously to show that we are genuinely thankful for the food.

What does thanking Him for the food do for us? Number one, is that we are blessed by following His directive. What most don't realize is that the food is made more palatable. You are ensured that you will only take in the good of the food and nothing bad. It also ensures that you receive maximum benefit and assimilation of the nutrients.

It seems like if this is true then everyone should also be blessing and giving thanks to God in Heaven for the medicines and remedies you take. Somewhere along the way, medicines, even though we swallow them just like food, became something else that did not need to given thanks for. They are food and should be blessed in the same manner.

Now, due to the fact that scientific technique allows us now to determine the precise dosage that is needed by each individual patient, it has been confirmed that the dosage required is greatly reduced when the medicine has been blessed.

A patient of mine from Brazil communicated a disturbing story. She was told by an acquaintance that he had worked his way up in a certain overseas company. Because of his level of achievement the company awarded him with a trip to a convention in the company's country. The convention was held in the same hotel in which he was staying. Upon arrival the day before the convention, he wandered into the convention room, just killing time. All around him people that worked for the company were bringing in loads of fruit and flowers, arranging them in a circle. He stopped one of the workers asking what was going on. The reply "shook him to his toes." The worker proceeded to tell him that the formula for the company's product came from the "god of something or other" and they paid homage and "blessed" their product in the name of their "god" and that this was the secret to the incredible increases in sales worldwide."

When I heard this it made me think of the Scripture verses that states that we wrestle not against flesh and blood, but against principalities and powers of darkness. (Eph.6) The closer to the genuine, the greater the counterfeit. And the thief cometh not but to steal, kill, and destroy. (John 10:10)

If there are companies out there that are "blessing" their products (i.e., medicines) in the name of their little "g" gods, then the rationale for us to give thanks and bless our medicines in the name of Jesus Christ prior to consumption becomes more pronounced.

Do we need to worry about all this? No, we need to just be wise to the methods and strategies of the adversary; after all our Father God in Heaven is bigger. However, you must be wise to the situation and do what the Word says and 'give thanks to God in Heaven for your food' and your medicine.

Chapter 39

"No Brainer" Things To Do

1. Ladies, if you are using the birth control pill, you need to seriously think about finding an alternative contraceptive because of the intense strain birth control pills place on your body. Consider Natural Progesterone cream if you are having PMS, menstrual irregularities, menopausal symptoms, or energy and sleep problems. Proper hormone balance can make all the difference in your healing. Read *What Your Doctor May Not Tell You About Menopause* by John R. Lee, M.D. Even if you are a woman in your early twenties you may benefit more than you could imagine from this book. Dr. Lee has recently written another book entitled W*hat Your Doctor May Not Tell You About Pre-menopause*. We recommend the Arbonne Prolief™, natural progesterone cream. It is in a pump dispenser that meters out the exact 20 mg dose that is generally recommended.

    Compared to other progesterone creams in jars and tubes that are on the market, the pump is better since I find that women will begin to ration the cream as they begin to run low, not getting the physiological dose that is generally needed. Also in jars, the cream is exposed to the air every time it is opened, often leading to increased oxidation, destroying the progesterone. Beware of some herbal wild yam creams, which according to Dr. Lee, have little or no actual natural progesterone. A pregnant woman produces about 800mg of progesterone cream every day, so this 20mg dose is consider very safe. The general recommendation is to rub one pump, two times per day (am and pm). Split the amount that comes out in one pump and rub half of it on one side of the body and the other half on the other side of the body. Rub it into thin skin areas, such as the sides of the breast, but not over the nipples, the inner arms, inner thighs, or groin.

2. Avoid MSG (monosodium glutamate). This is a flavor enhancer type food-additive. Read labels on foods and spice packs. This substance is known as a central nervous system excitotoxin. Glutamate crosses the blood-brain barrier irritating brain function

and peripheral nerve tissues. Read *Excitotoxins*, by Russell L. Blaylock.

3. Avoid NutraSweet®, another excitotoxin to the brain and nervous system. A bi-product of NutraSweet® is wood alcohol, which is widely known to be very toxic to the human body. (NutraSweet® company is now in court fighting lawsuits due to the epidemic of problems being blamed on this substance) Read *Excitotoxins*, by Russell L. Blaylock.

4. Increase your water intake. Purified water is a must, because of the documented impurities, parasites, and viruses known to permeate municipal water. Although drinking three quarts of water per day will not flush out the Lyme bacteria, it will flush out many of the toxic byproducts that cause pain in the body. Keep in mind that water is required for every single chemical reaction in the body. Drinking coffee, teas, or juices cannot substitute for water, because it requires all of the water in the coffee, tea, or juice to process those substances out of the body. Drinking these will actually create a water deficit, or dehydration, since many of these drinks have diuretic (stimulates urination) actions.

5. Absolutely no soda, pop, colas or whatever you want to call them. Most of these drinks have as much as 11 tablespoons of sugar in a 12 oz. can. The sugar literally burns up the islets of Langerhan in the pancreas, the cells responsible for producing insulin. Eventually enough of these cells are lost and hypoglycemia turns into diabetes. Many of you have chronic fatigue as a component of the LD. Get off of the sugar roller coaster. Stevia is an herbal sweetener that can be found in many health food stores that is a much safer sugar substitute than the other artificial sweeteners. It is totally safe for diabetic people.

6. Eliminate all milk and dairy products. This may be too drastic for many of you, but you should be told anyway. "A sip of milk contains hundreds of different substances, each one having the potential to exert a powerful biological effect when taken independently of the others. Pus, blood, feces, allergenic proteins, naturally occurring powerful growth hormones, fat, cholesterol, pesticides with vitamin D added, viruses, bacteria (including bovine leukemia, bovine tuberculosis and bovine immuno-deficiency

virus) all combine to produce a vast array of ailments in our society", according to researcher Robert Cohen. Lyme disease is a war…dairy products act as glue in your body's war machine. Dr. Julian Whitaker, M.D., is the founder and editor of the largest read health newsletter in the world. Dr. Whitaker agrees that you should "knock off drinking milk altogether", and to "use all dairy products sparingly, and be sure to avoid products from hormone-treated cows." If you want to learn more concerning this matter read the book, *Milk, The Deadly Poison*, by Robert Cohen.

7. If you are doing something obviously bad…STOP! These are things like smoking, chewing tobacco, drinking alcohol, taking recreational drugs, eating junk and chemically dead foods, and the like.

Chapter 40

The Dangers of Cow's Milk

It turns out that the cow's milk that we all grew up believing "does a body good", actually is potentially very harmful. We are talking about the various types of milk in your grocery stores; Vitamin D milk, 2%, and skim milk, all are harmful.

I do not make this statement lightly. It is supported by a plethora of research.

The bulk of this research can be found in a recently published book, written by Robert Cohen. The book is *MILK - The Deadly Poison.*

One of America's leading alternative medicine advocates, Dr. Julian Whittaker, MD agrees with the fact that we have all been sold a lie from the dairy advertisers. The research is overwhelmingly consistent in verifying the harmful effects of the milk we are being sold.

Some of the facts brought out in research are:

- Milk is actually a poor source of calcium

- It is a milk protein that contributes to Type-1 diabetes

- A hormone in milk is a key factor in every human cancer

- The effectiveness of antibiotics is hindered by milk

- Asthma is linked strongly to milk consumption

- Milk is a contributing factor to heart disease

- Pasteurization does not work as completely as thought

- IGF-1 genetically engineered hormone in milk is the key factor in the increased occurrence of childhood cancers

- The FDA admits today's milk is chemically different (published in the August 24, 1990 issue of Science magazine.)

- Due to the high protein content of milk, it actually promotes calcium loss

- Milk allergies cause sinus problems, diarrhea, constipation, behavioral problems.

- Milk is the leading cause of chronic ear infections.

- Milk contributes to elevated cholesterol, and is linked to osteoporosis, obesity, and high blood pressure.

- Milk in recent studies causes a seven-fold increase in breast cancers, and a four-fold increase in prostate cancers.

- Traces of active medicines such as antibiotics, as well as pus and bacteria are found in the same milk you buy at the store.

- A protein from cows milk actually destroys the beta-cells of the pancreas that are responsible for producing insulin.

- It is estimated that 60% of America's dairy cows have either leukemia, tuberculosis, or the bovine AIDS virus.

What to do instead of cows milk:

Avoid drinking cow's milk all together, or at least sparingly from dairies that are beginning to offer hormone-free, organic milk and milk products. Also, a better alternative is to switch to fresh raw goats milk (read in the book...On the High Road with Goat Milk), or switch to Soy, or Rice milk which is generally available in your grocery store's dairy section.

The fact that Lyme spirochetes have been cultured from virtually every body fluid, including cow colostrum and fresh milk, with no conferred immunity makes one question the safety of such products. There is practically no better immune-boosting dietary supplement on the market than the fractionated colostrums. However, screening needs to be performed on each batch of whole colostrums to ensure there are not any Lyme spirochetes present. Keep in mind that a cow only produces a limited quantity of colostrum, and after freeze drying it there is not that much powdered colostrum. So, many cows are needed to produce the hundreds of thousands of capsules needed to supply the demand. The more cows the greater the risk of one being infected. While there is not any evidence of Lyme infection from taking an infected colostrum product, I don't recommend risking it. My favorite colostrum products are the immune-stimulating *fractionated* colostrum and not whole colostrums.

Chapter 41

On the High Road with Goat Milk

Several years ago, the world's largest, and most respected medical journal, The Journal of the American Medical Association, published an article titled "Dietetics and Hygiene," which reported:

"The goat is the healthiest domestic animal known. Goat milk is superior in every respect to cow's milk. Goat milk is the ideal food for babies, convalescents and invalids, especially those with weakened digestive powers. Goat milk is the purest, most healthful and most complete food known."

Raw-vs-Pasteurized Goat Milk:

Pasteurization of milk not only kills germ life, but destroys enzymes and changes the chemical and energetic balance of the milk. Research overwhelmingly demonstrates that pasteurization creates higher rates of degenerative illnesses in both humans and in animal research.

Although cow's milk and dairy products are popular in the U.S.A. and Western Europe, a recent survey reveals that in the rest of the world goat milk and goat products are used 65% of the time. Goat milk is usually well tolerated by those sensitive to cow's milk.

When fresh, good quality goat milk is indistinguishable from cow milk in taste. Goat milk is naturally homogenized, therefore there is no separation of cream in the raw milk.

It is usually well tolerated by those sensitive to cow's milk.

Fresh goat milk is alkaline and has a tendency to neutralize acids in the body. The cholesterol found in goat milk is more highly evolved than that of cow's milk due to the fact that the goat's thyroid is also more highly evolved which controls the fat content of the milk much better. The fat globules are 1/5th the size of the fat globule found in cows milk. Our brain uses cholesterol to form and maintain the myelin sheaths of the nerves in the "white matter" part of the brain, and in many other normal cellular functions.

In regards to cholesterol...the benefits of raw goat milk far outweigh any risks. Not to mention that we now know that high cholesterol in humans is directly caused by high homocystiene levels. And, two-thirds of all the cholesterol in your body is manufactured by your liver in response to high homocystiene...only one-third comes from your diet.

Those suffering or recovering from chronic illness, and devastating diseases will not find a better diet to follow than fresh raw goat milk. Raw goat milk from a good source is the best tonic to restore health. Malnutrition, lung and bronchial troubles, weak digestion, rickets, joint troubles, chronic fatigue, and other incurables will all respond and improve when goat milk is used.

Some people have restored their health via a total raw goat milk fast. Everything needed for life is provided in this milk. Some have lived on goat milk alone for years, simply due to how good they feel while on it. Milk less than 3 hours old is even more vital. Goat colostrum is incredible compared to cow's colostrum as an immune system booster.

Goat milk for Infants and Children

There is no better substitute for mother's milk for an infant than fortified raw goat milk. Non-pasteurized goat milk is the closest to mother's milk in nature. Mother's milk is always the absolute best food for the infant. High IQ has been correlated with how long an infant was breast fed. If at all possible, every attempt should be made to breast feed your infant. If you are having problems with breast feeding consult your local LaLeche League listed in the phone book, or your doctor.

The brain of your new born is not fully formed at birth and requires live food from the perfect source...the mother, to complete the brain's development. Not only this, but mother's milk contains many immune system components that confer protection upon your baby, until your baby's immune system can take over at about 1 year old. These important immune system factors are missing from infant formulas. Fresh raw goat milk does have many of these immune system components.

Infant formulas are devoid of living energy, or live flora, and other essential nutrients which cannot remain stable in a powder or canned form. Many children develop colic and are irritable while on synthetic milk formulas.

The bowel movements of an infant fed mother's milk or raw goat's milk are not stinky and foul, like formula fed infants bowel movements. Similarly, the bowel movements of infants fed raw fortified goat milk do not stink. The stink of formula fed bowel movements demonstrate poor digestion, fermentation, and produces gas, and many times abdominal discomfort.

Fresh goat milk is living energy, not a processed, basically dead food. There is almost nothing worse though for infants and children than the cow's milk found in most stores today. Not only are the fat globules found in cow's milk five times larger than those of human milk, but the pasteurization and homogenization, not to mention the growth hormones used to get the cows to produce more milk, and the drugs, mucus, and such render cows milk devoid of much benefit, and may lead to many problems for your child.

It has been reported that in each gallon of cow's milk from your grocery store, that there are about 30,000 cows' milk mixed in each gallon. (Did you ever see the big milk tanker trucks on the highway, with thousands of gallons of milk? How may cows do you think it takes to fill just one of these?) This is important to know, because every cow has its own unique antigen (allergic factor). With the unique antigens of 30,000 different cows in every gallon of milk, the chances of allergic reactions are practically unavoidable.

Every human mother has her own unique antigen factor also. This is why an infant fed by wet-nurse may be allergic to the breast milk of another woman.

Fortified Goat Milk

Every milk, other than Mother's breast milk, including goat milk is lacking two vitamins and a mineral important to the development of infants and children. These are Folic Acid, Vitamin E, and Iron.

The following chart outlines the daily fortification requirements for infants and children:

Daily Fortification

	0-6 months	1-3 years	4-6 years
Iron	10 mg	15 mg	10 mg
Folic Acid	0.5 mg	0.1 mg	0.2 mg
Vitamin E	4 IU	7 IU	9 IU

Raw fortified goat milk, generously supplies calcium, magnesium, phosphorus and all other necessary minerals, to build strong bones and teeth.

It is wonderful in its ability to help with children who are sickly and weak, developmentally slow, and will cure many intestinal ailments.

Weaning Formula

- 6 ounces raw fortified goat milk

- 3 ounces purified water

- 1/2 tsp of Grade B Maple syrup (or Black-strap Molasses for iron)

When the time comes to wean your baby from breast milk, it is a good idea to use this formula. Goat milk is an ideal food, since it is closest to mother's milk in composition and properties.

The milk is diluted for the first 6-12 weeks after weaning to match the liquid needs of the baby, and prevent constipation. Purified water may be used for the infant first and gradually reduced. Vary as weaning advances. After a few weeks, depending on the child and the reactions, use straight goat milk.

Moving to Solid Foods

Anatomically, when the infant begins to get his first teeth is also when the digestive tract is developmentally ready to handle something other than milk.

Always start with single pureed vegetables. By starting with one vegetable per day, you are allowing the child's brain to identify and learn how to digest that one food.

Many allergies are created when infant's first foods are pureed mixed vegetables or mixed fruits. An allergy of misidentification can be created. For example, if the first food you give your infant is mixed peas and carrots, the brain of your child will identify and learn to digest these foods in this form. Later in life, when the child eats just peas or just carrots, the brain may identify them in the way that it learned it...mixed peas and carrots. This misidentification causes the body to digest the single vegetable thereby creating metabolic antigens. Through the improper digestion of foods, allergies are caused.

If you will only begin introducing vegetables, many times you can avoid your child developing a sweet tooth. Introducing fruits first may lead to life long sweet tooth. Many children started on vegetables only, will prefer vegetables over sweets, which will only help your child manifest their maximum life potential.

Section 9

While Addressing the Body and the Soul, Don't forget the Spirit!

God-Designed Living

FOREWORD TO THIS SECTION
ON GOD-DESIGNED LIVING

by: Dr. Sara Jernigan, D.C., B.S., Wife

As Dr. David Jernigan's wife, I feel I need to give you insight to what my husband deals with every day, so that you can understand why Dr. David has been inspired to write on spiritual topics. Plus, he is so humble that the majority of the people that know him never hear or know how God works with him. So imagine this, every single day every 15 or 30 minutes, someone is asking Dr. David to heal them.

I feel that to walk into his treatment room is like walking in to see one of the great men of God in the Bible. God instructed these great believers to do many different things to heal God's people. He had them teach the people, lay hands on the sick therapeutically, anoint people with oils, He inspired Jesus to spit in mud and put it in the eyes to heal the blind, He inspired others to heal leprosy by having them go dip themselves the river, he inspired another to lay on top of a dead child seven times to bring the child back to life, he touched them, etc... If Dr. David was a "straight chiropractor," one who only adjusts the spine, the patient would just lay on the table and he would adjust them and he would say, "next!" If he was a medical doctor he would order a lab test, send them to a specialist, or give them a drug and say, "next!" But instead, God has fun working with him.

Since God has blessed Dr. David with an incredible brain to hold an incredible amount of knowledge, and the ability to separate truth from error, thereby enabling him to be free to explore different tools for healing, God will take that information and give Dr. David the inspiration of what to do for that patient. It may be something that God is usually not able to tell people because they have not trained themselves to know many different ways on how to heal people. Therefore, with some patients God is able to tell him to just pray for that person and that person is immediately healed. Other times people just need to be reminded of God's word and then they are healed. Some people for whatever reason seem to need to struggle and work hard to walk out their healing, so he will have them on all kind of remedies and home therapies.

Some people have been afflicted with devil spirits, so that when they are on the treatment table they are writhing around like the man in the Bible that was writhing on the ground and Jesus cast the devil spirits out into the swine. Dr. David has put his hands on some people and seen an evil entity come roaring out of the person and then go back inside the person. Sometimes when he is treating someone, he can feel a huge evil force menacing him. Sometimes the person changes their voice and acts like those people in horror films. As a doctor walking with God, he sees it all.

Every 15-30 minutes Dr. David is with another patient. He is actively practicing the spiritual competition that is explained in Ephesians 6. Of course, not every patient is this way, but it happens.

Like I said, if you ever spend time with Dr. David you would never realize this is going on all day long because when you walk into his treatment room he is totally concentrating on you. So you may never know that two minutes before you walked into the room that he just helped someone who was deaf in their ear for 40 years and God gave him the inspiration to apply a specific oil to that patient and for the first time in 40 years that person could hear in that ear. He may tell you what had just happened, just to help with your healing and believing, but most times he just thanks God for the deliverance and just moves on to the next person. Now with this in mind, when you read the following passage you may receive it better and may understand why he felt lead to teach on this subject.

Sincerely,

Dr. Sara Jernigan, wife

Chapter 42

Get the Hurt and the Dirt Out of Your Life

A common misconception is for one to say "I was fine before this bug bit me". It may be so, but feeling good does not guarantee that you were healthy when the bug bit you. It is my experience that most people have much unresolved hurt and dirt contributing to their state of health. Everyone at any given moment may have as many as two hundred potentially harmful organisms in their body. Why aren't we all sick? Could it be that what we call the human organism has the ability to control every pathological microbe? A totally healthy human does this very thing without you even thinking about it!

I have often wondered at the wide diversity of symptoms that I see in some Lyme patients. Lyme does not affect any two people in the exact same way. I have seen people with only one prevailing symptom though positive for LD. There are common symptoms, but there are always many symptoms that fall outside of the norm. As a doctor I have to wonder why the Borrelia burgdorferi spirochete affected the patient in this unique way. From my clinical experience I have come to the conclusion that not only can *chronic* Lyme Disease bring about new problems to your body, but it is unique in that it also brings the dirt of your life to light.

From birth to present time your body is constantly being challenged. These challenges may arise from emotional traumas such as the death of a loved one, physical, sexual and emotional abuse, physical injuries such as auto accidents, chemical challenges from medicines or pollution, not to mention stress from inherited tendencies. Any unresolved issues will be made or manifested physically or psychologically as your body becomes more dysfunctional by the chronic infection of LD.

Most people can recall a time when they injured their body. We'll say you injured the back for this example. You may have not ever gone to get it treated, and eventually the pain went away. The body adapted to the problem. The problem is still there, only now the pain and the problem are "put on the back burner" by your brain. This adaptation mechanism of the body occurs on every level, whether the level is of a physical, chemical, or psychological nature. Unfortunately, many times these insults cannot be effectively adapted to and they manifest in an ever worsening cascade of symptoms to get your attention so you can deal with the true cause.

Chronic illness breaks down the body's ability to keep these problems on the "back burner". These back burner problems are areas of weakened tissues, which may have never manifested as an obvious problem if life had gone on without a major challenge such as Lyme disease. The fact is that the Bb and any other invading organism or parasite will always go to the weakest areas of the body first. This phenomenon is seen throughout nature. One example of this is seen in the plant kingdom. Plants that come from a strong genetic heritage and have been nurtured in ideal conditions for generations have an increased natural resistance to bugs and plant illnesses. Weak plants from poor soil and poor genetic heritage are extremely susceptible to infections.

The point of all of this is that you are sum total of all of the challenges and lifestyle decisions you've made. In chronic Lyme disease, all of this will be brought to the fore-front and all of it will need to be finally addressed by you and your healthcare team.

Everyone has heard the saying, "you are what you eat". Well, you really are much more than that. You are, more accurately, the sum total of all that you have experienced. You integrate all of the good in your life, and hopefully resolve all of the bad. Anything bad that goes unresolved will affect the entire human organism.

The Bible deals with much of this topic. It says to control your thinking…by taking every thought "captive". We know now from science that whenever you *allow* yourself to become depressed, that every cell in your body becomes hypo-functional, or depressed.

We also know that when the Bible says, "not to let the sun set on our wrath" (Eph 4:26), that perpetuating that negative emotion overnight causes an energetic "computer virus" affecting the body in its entirety, in a way unique to the type of negative emotion. So you can see how important it is to exert your free will choice to control your thinking. We don't use the word "wrath" very much in today's society, but it means anger and negative emotions. Thought is the only thing God gave you complete control over in the five senses world. This line of thought may shock many of you, but it must be dealt with, because I continually hear patients carrying around a lot of unresolved anger, resentment, fear, unforgiveness, and the like. God said it, but also medical science has verified it – these issues affect the entire body. God also placed a specific time factor in the verse in Ephesians – overnight. It is this time factor that sets the "computer virus" in motion. Other verses also address the need to resolve all conflict quickly.

My good friend, Mary Lynch, M.D. is fond of saying "Drama!" to her patients who are stuck in the drama of their life and illness. It is true; many people do get caught up in the drama of their situation and will tell their tale of woe to all who will listen – perpetuating the negative emotions not only overnight, but for weeks, months and years; carrying and accumulating them like a sack over their shoulder throughout their lifetime. This perpetuates the sickness reality. Many feel that they can just "forget about it" or feel that "time will heal all wounds." Amnesia is no cure for these negative computer viruses of your body.

The ability of the immune system to function, and the ability for the body to heal itself, is directly reflected by the number of unresolved issues. The problem for you and your healthcare team is that many times you had issues that went unresolved that even you have forgotten. Out of sight is not out of mind. Many of these unresolved issues cannot be dealt with using a pill, but they very definitely must be brought to resolution.

• Your greatest avenue and **"First-Aid"** for correcting these unresolved issues, healing, and staying healthy is your one on one direct communication with God as His child, your properly maintained heart of love, and your ability to exercise your God given spiritual authority over every form of adversity, through the power God in Christ in you, working in and through you as you to will and do of His good pleasure, understanding His good pleasure is that you prosper and be in good health at all times.

You must resolve any known issues with Him. Having done so, do not look back. Let the issues be permanently non-issues. This requires one to completely clean out the "rooms in your mind" where these issues reside. Forgive and forget it. Get rid of the emotion attached to the issue, so that if the issue is brought up again in the future you don't have to go down the emotional path you used to associate with that event.

Phillipians 3:10

"Brethren, I count not myself to have apprehended; but this one thing I do, forgetting those things which are behind, and reaching forth unto those things which are before."

The fact of the matter is that the past does not define who you are today nor does it determine your tomorrow. If you do not know God as your heavenly Father, then seek Him out. (Romans 10: 9&10) Having done so, change your habit patterns of thinking. Stop watching your soap operas or your fishing shows and put your energy into reading God's Word and into reading self-improvement books. Listen to motivational or educational tapes instead of the news. Do volunteer work for worthy causes.

Eventually you will maintain an attitude of a conqueror instead of that of a victim.

If you already have a great relationship with your heavenly Father, wonderful. I'll just share with you a few verses, which I find as a doctor interesting. I am always interested in what God says about sickness. In I Corinthians 11:28-30, God mentions why some are sick as He talks about the partaking of communion unworthily...

I Corinthians 11:28-30
But let a man examine himself, and so let him eat of that bread, and drink of that cup. For he that eateth and drinketh unworthily, eateth and drinketh damnation (condemnation) to himself, not discerning the Lord's body. For this cause many are weak and sickly among you, and many sleep (die).

For this cause many are weak and sickly among you, and many are dying prematurely. Now as a doctor reading this I really take notice, especially when God our Creator Himself says that this is a cause of much illness!

The Lord's Supper, and now communion, is a memorial to remind us that Jesus Christ was the sacrificial lamb. The crucifixion and resurrection of Christ Jesus restored our ability to have direct communication with God, something that was lost to mankind in the Garden of Eden. It also gave us, who believe, the ability to no longer be servants of the Lord, but be sons and daughters of God – joint heirs with Christ. To "not discern the Lord's body" means that one has forgotten what Jesus did for all of us, and who we are in Christ Jesus. Paul is talking here about religious bigots, people who were forming different sects... those following Apollo, those following Peter, even those thinking they were superior because they were circumcised. Paul was addressing a problem that started way back in the early church, the development of sects within what was supposed to be one body of believers – these sects are what we now call denominations.

As a child, growing up in the Christian churches, I thought communion was all so cool, those cute little pieces of bread, and how neat it was to get grape juice in those cool little glasses held in round silver trays and do what the adults were doing. As I got older I recall being scared to take communion "unworthily", all of the adults were always so somber and serious about it all, but I still did not really understand what it meant to partake unworthily or how to make sure I was doing it right. I knew I had received Christ Jesus as my Lord and Savior, but I always thought communion was about whether I was DOING and BEING a good boy all the time... and I knew I wasn't acting right, or getting good grades in school, or enjoying reading the Bible, so could I or should I take part in the communion? This question got more and more serious the older I got, because even though I knew it was done in remembrance of what Jesus did for me, I thought the "unworthily" part was talking about my performance since the last time I took communion, kind of like sitting on Santa's lap and having him ask if I had been a good boy this year..."No, I haven't", I'd think, "but I tried to be good." Now, after years of suffering this way, I learned through studying the original texts, what communion is all about, and why God relates it to getting sick and dying prematurely.

Jesus was asked what the most important law of God was, he responded, "You should love the Lord your God with all of our heart, soul, and mind, and the second was to love our neighbor as our self." He did not say to love our "Christian neighbor", or the neighbor that is a part of the same sect or denomination as you, He simply said "your neighbor!" There should be no scorn and haughtiness, frowning in disapproval of those who do not believe exactly the way you do. There should not be any religious bigotry. In order to honor the Lord's Supper in communion, one must know how to manifest the Christ within them.

It is okay to be completely convinced of the correctness of the beliefs of the denomination you have chosen, but also recognize that God made it very simple as to the bare minimum for salvation and thereby inclusion in His "one" body of His children. John 3:16 demonstrates how simple God intended it to be, it is like God knew man's nature would be to complicate things, so he spelled it out very plainly, "For God so loved the world, that He gave His only begotten Son, that he that believeth on Him should not perish but have everlasting life." God also showed the simplicity of His plan in Romans 10: 9-10, "If you will confess with your mouth the Lord Jesus, and will believe in your heart that God raised him from the dead, you will be saved." This is the minimum requirement to be part of God's "one" body. Everything else that can be found as differing opinions, doctrines, theologies, and beliefs within denominations and Christian churches are things that we all can ask God to clarify for us when we are with Him in heaven. In the meantime, we must do what He said, love God and love your neighbor as you love yourself, without the sense of separateness because we are truly one body. This is what God calls "walking in the light, as He is in the light."

So, take this to heart, God's book says that many of you are sick, and dying prematurely, because you have something ugly in you, something other than love for those outside of your sect, and because of that you are desecrating what Jesus, God's Son, did for you and everyone that believes Romans 10: 9 and 10. Don't have a hard heart about this, don't fall into the belief that going to church every Sunday is enough, or that volunteering for mission trips and church activities is enough. God didn't say many of you are sick and dying prematurely because you haven't said any "Hail Mary's" or worked hard enough at being a good Christian.

How do we remedy this problem? Examine your heart for any of this feeling of separateness from every Christian denomination. Examine your heart for anything other than pure love for your neighbor. Examine your heart and despite any of what you may think of as shortcomings, love yourself. Especially examine your heart that you truly in your heart of hearts believe in and love God your heavenly Father.

So, when God's Word says examine yourself, you need to ask yourself the following questions. Could you take communion with a Methodist, Baptist, Pentecostal, Roman Catholic, Greek Orthodox, Non-Denominational, Jehovah Witness, or a believer of the Way International? Would you feel you are all part of the one Body? Or would you feel your beliefs and doctrine were the only correct beliefs and feel like you have to "pray for those lost souls of the other denominations?" Since God says, "For this cause many of you are weak and sickly among you and many sleep," I would strongly suggest as a **First Aid,** you read Galatians. In Galatians, every time it says, Jew, Greek, bond or free, you need to put the words, any denomination besides mine, any culture besides mine and have God heal you of any selfish spirit that is causing you to judge Christians and non-Christians. God put one responsibility on us in this administration of Grace and that is to love and to walk in love and we are to leave the judging up to God. (Matt 22:36-40)

Your "First Aid" is your one on one direct communication with God as His child, your properly maintained heart of love, and your ability to exercise your God given spiritual authority over every form of adversity, through the power God in Christ in you, working in and through you as you to will and do of His good pleasure, and His good pleasure is that you prosper and be in good health!

• "**Second Aid**" is your pastor, or minister. Many times someone with a deeper knowledge of spiritual matters is required. They can give crucial guidance and have insight into the knowledge of God's Word concerning your issues. Healing and true cures are available. Remember the examples in the Bible. When Jesus Christ and the disciples were able to perform great signs, miracles and healings, it was when they accessed God's Holy Power. The times the disciples could not heal the people is when they or the people had no faith. You still have to believe for healing. Believing is an action word. It is just like the man with the crippled hand. Jesus said, "Stretch forth thy hand." When the man acted on the command and stretched forth his hand, his hand then was healed, not before that time. You can't go to your minister or pastor and put the responsibility on them for your healing. You must be actively involved. If you have to keep reminding yourself to believe, you're not believing. When you are really believing, it is not an issue. (Doctors reading this need to recognize the need to speak to patients like Jesus did here "Stretch forth thy hand". He didn't say "Try to stretch forth thy hand". The word "Try" provides the opportunity or permission to not complete the task. Try, is an incomplete action from the very beginning and gives the person a trapdoor to not achieve the task.)

•   "**Third Aid**" is where you have used first and second aid and still need to find help from a knowledgeable healthcare practitioner. This is the correct order of things. If you have a deep splinter in you, you could by faith have it disappear. However, a doctor can easily remove it thereby allowing it to heal. Many people are afraid of the alternative therapies due to lack of understanding, and their desire not to do anything contrary to God's Word. I do encourage you to find a Christian healthcare provider. Keep in mind that a hammer is a great tool if you want to build a house, but if you use it to hit someone in the head and kill them, is it less of a tool? People corrupt what God has made. Most healing remedies and techniques are tools which when used correctly can aid in facilitating correction by your body. It is always your body that does the healing. No one tool can correct all of the problems in the body. If you have a worm in your liver, I cannot give you a chiropractic adjustment and correct that problem. However, if you dislocate your finger there is no pill that I could give you to put the finger back. The more tools your doctor has to facilitate the healing of your body the more likely your recovery. Homeopathy can be a wonderful tool to facilitate the correction of long forgotten issues. Professional Christian Counselors are another good avenue available. Myofascial therapies, addressing the connective tissue membranes that sheathe all of the muscles and indeed the entire body, can many times bring out in the open stored emotional issues that can be like a poison to the body, slowing the healing process. Keep in mind that when your body sees that someone is helping things, your body will naturally begin to bring things off the back burner to be finally dealt with. You may see many odd and unexplainable problems suddenly show up out of the blue. Your body really desires to be rid of all of the garbage.

Doctors are your third aid, but in an ideal situation you should find a doctor who practices using God-designed natural methods and whose philosophy of healing is to restore the integrity of your body; one who actively seeks inspiration to let God work in and through them to will and do of His good pleasure – knowing that His pleasure is that you be healthy in mind, body and spirit. By this I mean that I often hear people saying my doctor goes to my church and is so nice and he thinks I need Prozac or such. Going to church and being nice, is not enough and you should not submit to poisons and treatments that harm God's perfect design of your body.

Chapter 43

Spiritual Aspects of Infectious Disease

Doctor, Be a Healer

The spiritual realm can be a causative agent in creating imbalance in any type of illness. Lyme disease is no different. Your ability to heal and recover from Lyme disease completely is or can be impaired through spiritual imbalances.

As doctors we are called to teach balance to our patients. Many times I see people who seem to live the most balanced lives and yet are still suffering tremendously from a chronic illness. They eat right, live right, think positive thoughts, always seek out natural medicines, but for all of this they remain sick. What then is the cause? What balance issue is there to address as a doctor? Many times it is the spiritual issues that must be addressed.

I see people every day in my clinic who are starving for spiritual guidance, and are in a spiritual wasteland wanting to be fed, going to church hoping to find the answers they need only to find a message perfect for the congregation, but devoid of pertinent information to deal with the specific needs of that person as an individual. It is not really the fault of the organized church, because church is not the physical walls of the building anyway – the church is the people, the body of believers. Everyone serves a purpose in the body of Christ.

No one is in a better position to help people on an individual basis than a doctor. A doctor is the only one many people will open up to and tell the truth of how they are suffering. Many times ministers/pastors are the last to know when someone is sick, and are only called upon when one is expected to die. Doctors are continually in the trenches. It is our profession, our calling in life, to help the needy in any way we can. Doctors should be masters of God-designed healing and God-designed living.

God-designed living is the way of life that promotes optimal spiritual and physical health. God-designed living turns mere existence on this planet into an art of balanced living. I will go into God-designed living in greater detail in later chapters.

The following information cannot begin to address all of the information needed to prepare a person for every contingency. However, my desire is to arm you with enough information that healing can be reached, and to open up for you an area possibly missing in your life – a real and vital walk of power with your heavenly Father God and through Christ Jesus.

This is an area however, that most doctors fear to tread. We are taught that since we, as doctors, are in a position of influence and power, we cannot imply or even attempt to imprint or teach patients on spiritual matters. I find this unacceptable in that we are all called to teach the message to everyone for the healing of all nations. I have found that it is of primary importance in correcting the illnesses that are plaguing almost every patient. To not address it at times is to subject a patient to a life of misery spiraling towards death, unless someone, somewhere steps forward to help. If not you, then who? If not now, then when? Doctors must walk wisely as to what and when to teach, helping people as lead by their Heavenly Father.

In my "New Patient Information" packet I make a point to let people know that my clinic is a Christian/Bible based clinic, so right from the start everyone knows that this is an important aspect of our care. Those offended can then choose a different clinic.

Thankfully, we live in a predominantly Christian country, therefore many times we can remind people of what they should already know. This does not mean that you have to speak in "King James" terms, such as "thou shalt" and "verily I say unto you". Biblical principles of truth are often understood better when put into everyday language –parables were often the preferred teaching method of Jesus for a reason. Parables many times can communicate across religious denominations and belief systems.

It is important then to understand why a doctor should integrate spiritual aspects of healing. It is important because there is no way to separate body, soul, and spirit. All are interconnected. One cannot be out of balance without affecting the others. Spiritual matters cannot be out of balance without causing imbalance in your body, which in the end allows microbes, or disease to grow unchecked. It is no great mystery how this happens. This chapter will undoubtedly challenge your belief system, but in a world full of darkness, this will help you find light through the truth from God's Word concerning everything pertinent to life more than abundantly – without illness of any kind. (John 10:10, 2 Cor 9:8, Eph 3:20, 3 John.)

As I mentioned earlier concerning infectious diseases being sometimes referred to as a "contracted disease", so also are spirits of darkness under "contract". Under this "contract" agreement, the spirits of darkness have been given the right to be there screwing up your life and health. Who gave them the right? You did, usually either through spiritual ignorance or by choice or both. There is also the possibility that they gained the right or access through your generational line.

When we follow Jesus' example, as instructed in the Holy Bible, we see that his ministry and instruction included healing <u>and</u> deliverance. Deliverance from what? The powers of darkness working to kill, steal, and destroy you. Was this only something unique in biblical times? I mean come on, we are in the techno-age now! No, the Bible is very clear that powers of darkness will remain a fact of life until the return of Christ in the last days.

Doctors and the Church cannot ignore these spiritual issues if they are to be effective in bringing hope to the hopeless, healing to the broken, restoration to the sick in body, mind, and spirit, and freedom to all who are oppressed or held captive by the dark side.

Should doctors do everything for a patient? Or is it better to teach them how they can heal through a more balanced life? Obvious the latter. In the same way people need to be taught spiritual maturity, instead of simply being delivered through no effort of their own. The parable comes to mind that is paraphrased here, "You can feed an man a fish and he will be fed for a day, or you can teach him to fish and he will be fed for life".

How spiritual knowledge can be integrated into many doctor's offices poses a real challenge. Direct communication during an office visit, books, seminars, brochures, cassette tapes, and educational videos are all viable ways to increase your patient's knowledge. God did not make this spiritual topic to be rocket science or hidden from everyone except the few "high priests".

When the Holy Bible says things like, "…for this reason are many of you sick and dying prematurely…" every doctor should sit up and take notice! Much of conventional medicine is simply changing the nature of the disease, pushing the symptoms around, never truly restoring health. Doctors must become trained to be spiritual leaders in their community. They must lead by example.

At this point I want to clarify the term "Doctor." I consider the ideal "Doctor" to be a teacher, coach, confidant, healer, counselor. This type of doctor works with God's design of the human body and works diligently through natural, nontoxic means to bring the body, mind and spirit back into health and balance. It is a more perfect philosophy of care than cutting, burning, and poisoning the body into the illusion of health, through drugs, radiation, and surgery. Of course, it is a 'no-brainer' that as long as people continue to live like there will be no consequences to their imbalanced lifestyles, high-powered drugs and 'heroic medicine' will be their only hope. Doctors must become masters themselves at the art of balanced living and sell, teach, and promote the same.

There is a story I once heard that really brings this point to reality. A top student at a prestigious medical school and his favorite professor were walking along a jogging path beside a river outside of the university. The student was very pleased to have this individual time with his professor outside of the classroom environment. Suddenly they heard cries for help! They looked and saw a man drowning in the river. The student kicked off his shoes and jumped into the river. With much strain and effort the student fought the river current and dragged the now unconscious man onto the riverbank and began CPR. An ambulance had been called, which by the time it arrived the drowned man was breathing again through the heroic efforts of the student. As the ambulance drove off with the man, the student felt pretty puffed-up, proud to have been able to show off his abilities to his favorite professor. The student glanced at his professor as they continued their walk along the river, but the professor didn't seem impressed. A short while later they happened upon another drowning man, and again the student saved him at great effort. Still no great reaction from the professor, who simply acknowledged the job as well performed. As they continued their walk, the student through great heroic effort had to save two more people from drowning. As he dragged the last victim from the river, he looked up at his professor and exclaimed, "I don't know how long I can keep doing this – I'm getting exhausted!" The wise professor said, "Then you might want to run up ahead and stop the guy who is pushing these poor people off the bridge."

This is the way I used to feel in my clinic. I could save many people from certain death through great personal effort, but it was never ending. I was tired and frustrated at trying to save people who were being thrown into the "river" by the ignorance and by the misguidance of politically and economically motivated dictocrats of physical and spiritual health. I mean, does anyone really believe that they are having pain due to a deficiency of aspirin? Or that margarine, which is only missing a couple of ingredients from being axle grease really promotes better health?

There truly is no shortage of sick people. A doctor reading this may think that there are no people interested in true balanced living. That everyone is just interested in the quick-fix. I predict that if doctors become masters of balanced living, and reorganized their clinics to practice natural

Biological Medicine, that people would come out of the woodwork to be a part and learn for themselves the art of living a higher quality of existence.

For those who feel that only church ministers and pastors should teach on spiritual matters, Ephesians 4:11-12 says, "And he gave some, apostles; and some, prophets; and some, evangelists; and some, pastors and **teachers;** for the perfecting of the saints, for the work of the ministry, for the edifying of the body of Christ." Doctors are called to be teachers of balanced living in all areas of life – even spiritually.

The Bible says in the book of Hosea 4:6, "we are destroyed from a lack of knowledge." Just last week I had a minister who I have been treating as a patient tell me that he couldn't promote natural medicine to his congregation! I was dumbfounded! I wanted to say, 'you mean to tell me that it is okay for you to go to the hospital and pray for them, but you won't tell them there is a better way of living and healing that can only benefit them, that will definitely follow God's natural design of the human body?' You mean you are spiritually led to let your congregation use pharmaceutical drugs which comes from the Greek word *pharmakeia*, which is translated as witch-craft? (Gal. 5:20) You mean God tells you that you should promote drug companies that only think about how to get more and more people to take a drug? You mean God says to steward the "temple", meaning your body that God created, that you as the "shepherd" should, through silence, promote drinking pop and processed foods and allow your flock to destroy their temples that God created because it is politically incorrect. 'Don't you know, I said, that up to 300,000 children of God, members of your flock, are dying every year and will never be able to love God, teach people, or take care of their family members, and this number is just those people in hospitals, from the appropriately prescribed medicines that were so toxic and harmful that it killed them? (That is 3 million people in 10 years!) This does not sound like the work of God but the work of the adversary who only wants to steal, kill and destroy. This is your flock, you are to steward, guide, and shepherd your flock – your congregation! And you're telling me it is politically inappropriate for you to promote God's design? He replied, "We can't promote one way or the other," meaning conventional or natural medicine.

If this is the true state of things in every church, then doctors are the only hope of teaching the truths about living, working, and healing through and in line with God's perfect design. The Bible has much to say about how we are to live and heal. Real people are dying at an alarming rate from what has been promoted as our ultimate authority on health and healing, conventional medicine. One might argue that many more are "saved" through these high-powered drugs, but overwhelming irrefutable research shows that Americans suffer the worst health in the world and yet we take the most amount of prescription drugs, we have the most high-tech hospitals, and we have more doctors per capita than any other country. The fourth leading cause of death in the United States is from prescription medicines! Estimates are that 5 million people just in the United States suffer serious life-threatening prescription drug reactions, every single year.

People, it is high time that change be made toward a more natural approach to living and healing – one that follows God's design.

Ministers/Pastors need to quit being so politically correct, and so afraid of offending the people and conventional medical doctors in their congregation and step forward and save their flock and teach their flock and support doctors who will teach along side of them the truths of God's design for balanced living.

Doctors, you must step up to the plate and change your ways – learn Biological Medicine, which is a way of practicing medicine that recognizes all aspects of life must be addressed, and no treatment should be used that may harm another part of the body. And you must become a Master of Light™ to teach and lead those who are in your care. Keep in mind that God designed the temporal and seen world we live in, and the eternal and unseen spirit world. (2 Cor 4:18) The two worlds are inseparable; therefore, both realms must be addressed.

No matter how spiritually mature we become we must all still follow the physical laws God laid out. I mean, no matter how spiritually enlightened one becomes, I would not recommend standing in front of a speeding bus. I say all of this because some people will undoubtedly attempt to achieve healing from a completely spiritual method, ie., divine intervention, which while available, does not negate the need to live and practice healthy living in the physical world.

Patients, God can work through your doctor to 'will and do of His good pleasure', (Phil 2:13) but you and your doctor must seek for that relationship based upon God's way. It cannot be off limits in a doctor's office to speak of spiritual matters when appropriate.

It is not an easy topic, since not many churches are teaching the meat of the spiritual aspects of healing. Doctors and patients need to be taught the foundational truths necessary to converse on an established and agreed upon basis. Otherwise, the doctor will keep running into contrary belief systems. The following chapters will present the truth based upon God's

Word without any denominational theology.

I pray that all who read this will have the eyes of their understanding enlightened (Eph 1:18 & 19) and that your personal commitment to Christ will be deepened to the end that you will be able to understand and spread the good Word, be healed personally, and heal the sick and cast out all forms of darkness. (1 Cor 2:8, 2 Cor 4:4, Eph 4:14, Heb 2:14, I Pe 5:8, Eph 6:12)

Chapter 44

A Handbook for Optimal Life

Imagine, if you will, that I have commissioned you to write a book. And in that book I wanted you to include every issue that would be pertinent to achieving a more abundant life now and eternal life later. And it would need to be pertinent to anyone of any race, gender and age for the next two thousand years and beyond. However, the book cannot be more than an inch and a half thick.

If this were the case, you would not include things like "How to make minute rice" in your book. You would assume your readers would figure these types of non-life changing things out for themselves.

However, you would definitely be including only those things which are really important. And you would not want to be real wordy, because you are trying to fit everything into one book.

To write such a book would be a monumental task, don't you think? This is what God has already performed in the Holy Bible. Inspired will of God...through men. (2 Tim 3:17, 2 Peter 1:20 & 21) Realize as you read the Bible that if God put it in his "Book" that it must have been very important.

When you read the Word of God, the Holy Bible, you need to realize that it is either all true, or all a lie. I believe it is all true, and accurate with a mathematical precision. I feel the need to clarify this last statement. The Bible is accurate in its original form. The true accuracy of the Bible can only be found by going back to the original Hebrew and Greek text. One must realize that there have been many fundamental changes, additions, and forgeries away from the original texts. The many revisions of the Bible have watered down or outright changed the original meaning sometimes, but definitely not all the time. The Holy Bible has been revised many times, such as the King James version, New English version, New International version, etc. Changes were made in each of these versions in an effort to simplify the information or to support the popular political opinion of the time. For example, the English language will often use one word for something the original text had several different meanings, each with its own unique spelling, to enable the reader to know which meaning it was referring to. Like the English word "Receive", which when referred to in the Greek text were the words *"Dechomai"* and *"Lambano"*, each with two distinct meanings. Dechomai is receiving from God spiritually within oneself. This is a subjective reception. (Example Acts 8:12) Lambano is receiving the gift into manifestation after having received it spiritually. This is an objective reception, it means one did not just receive their life time membership to eternal life but it means they actually manifested their new holy spirit. (Example, Acts 8:15) Also, most Christians and critics of the Bible do not realize that the Bible has 7 different administrations and each administration has different rules. Gen.1:1 to Gen 3:24 is the Paradise Administration, The Patriarchal Administration comes next but ends when Moses receives the written commandments. The 3rd Administration was the Law which was the Mosaic Law that was eradicated when Jesus died. The 4th was called the Jesus Administration which ended with His death. We are in the 5th or Grace Administration which began with Jesus' death. The 6th will be the Reappearing Administration which will start with the "gathering together" (I Thess 4:17, 2 Thess 2:1) – it will end with Satan destroyed. The Last but not least is the Paradise Administration which is number 7, Revelation 21 until forever. So, if there appears to be contradictions in the Bible, one has not gone to the original Greek or Hebrew or one is trying to apply the wrong Administration during this period of Grace. (Romans 15:4). The accuracy of the Bible can be discussed at great length but the above information is just a sampling of why I believe the Word of God to be accurate.

Often times a doctor will be accused of being biased in his opinions, or research. I will tell you right now that I am most certainly biased...to the truth of God's Word, the Holy Bible.

The volumes of scientific research that I have studied boils down to validating the truths laid forth in God's Word.

There are many times that everything has been already done that doctors know to do for a patient, all to no avail. When it comes right down to it, there is nothing left to do but address the one area that is least discussed in a doctor's office – spiritual matters.

The Bible tells us that we wrestle not against flesh and blood, but against principalities and powers of darkness. (Eph 6: 12) Powers of darkness, demons, entities, forms, beings, energies, no matter what the name, the verbiage oftentimes that deals with the unseen realm of the universe is generally not adequate. Yet, this very topic is what God tells us is most important. As a matter of fact, becoming "saved" or "born again" is all about leaving the temporal and seen world of the five senses and accessing the unseen and eternal world of spiritual perception that God in Heaven says matters the most. (2 Cor 4:18)

So, consider for a moment that everything in your life is going wonderfully. The birds are singing, you are financially sound, and your personal life is awesome...doesn't sound like too much of a wrestling match, does it? However, it is not too difficult to imagine sickness, failing finances, and ruin in your personal life as a wrestling match with the "powers of darkness". It kind of sounds like the movie "Star Wars" with Darth Vader saying, "Do not underestimate the power of the Dark Side"

I have had many people as patients who were very obviously wrestling with the Dark Side. One such patient, on coming in for treatment the first time, was very weak and soft spoken; seemingly, she barely had enough energy to walk across the room. Before beginning my treatment, I prayed silently as I put my hands on her to begin treatment, committing what I was about to do unto God in Heaven, and began to silently speak the Cleaning Prayer outlined later in this book. Suddenly, and quite surprisingly, she began to thrash about the table unlike anything I had ever seen. It seemed impossible that anyone so very weak in character and energy could achieve even a small burst of such energy. I really felt like I was in a bad B-rated horror flick. As I watched somewhat shocked, it seemed that she was being shaken and thrown about from something that had a hold of the core of her body. As suddenly as it began, it ceased. Now in the same weak and soft voice she said, "I know that may seem odd to you, but that just sort of happens to me sometimes..." Okay, all of you doctors reading this, what medicine are you going to grab for? You could reach for anti-psychotics and sedatives to mask the problem, or you could recognize it for what it truly is, a wrestling match with the "darkside." I didn't have the time or backup people to address this primary issue on this first visit. However, on subsequent visits, I was able to help this woman clean her spiritual house and teach her how to maintain her newly found health. Her recovery is remarkable to see as new found strength and stability is returning to her life.

This is but one example of many really bizarre cases. Not all people coming in for treatment are this dramatic, but all are wrestling with powers of darkness. 1st John 1:5 says that God is light and in Him is no darkness at all. In the Epistles, which is the part of the Bible and in the Grace Administration which pertains to our present time, it also says that God wants you to live a life that is more than abundant. (Eph 3:20) Many times throughout the Bible it tells of how very important you are to God, and how His Word is life and health to your body and His plans for you are for good and not evil, so the question in your mind should be "Where does sickness come from?" It definitely does not come from God.

One of the benefits of accepting Christ Jesus as your Savior is that you are a new creature, now able to perceive the unseen realms. This goes way beyond Mind/Body Medicine concepts; you are now Body, Soul and Spirit...Holy Spirit, that is.

So many churches preach salvation messages every Sunday, and yet fail to tell you what salvation has gained you, other than eternal life. This is like getting a life-time membership to the YMCA. Great, now you are a member, but that doesn't mean that you take advantage of all that is available to you.

Part of your membership in God's family is the awesome ability for all of this to make sense. The Bible says that this entire unseen world is nonsense to anyone outside, without a membership. (I Cor 2:14) Do you have to participate and learn new abilities? No, the bare minimum membership requirement is outlined in Romans 10: 9-10 "...If you will confess with your mouth, 'Jesus is Lord', and believe in your heart that God raised him from the dead, you will be saved." That's all!

Even now if you will stop and consider this verse and can speak it out loud, even if no one is around, and if you can believe in your heart that God did indeed raise Jesus from the dead, then congratulations, you are now a member of God's family with full rights to take advantage of all the power that comes with being a King's kid.

Chapter 45

The Better Perspective of Reality

You must recognize and address all areas of dysfunction in your life. God designed our bodies to give us all manner of signs and symptoms to help us realize when we have a problem. Without pain we would never know when a leg is broken until we collapse. In order to have sickness there must be something interfering with the perfect design of our body. As Christians we need to understand what God's Word says concerning the realities of our world, and what He has made available to us to ensure that we can live a "more than abundant life."

First, we must acknowledge that all that we can perceive with our five senses (see, touch, hear, smell, taste) is not all that is there. God's Word tells us that "we struggle not against flesh and blood, but against principalities and powers and spirits of darkness." What does this mean to us? It means that we should consider the source of our troubles. "The thief (dark spirits) comes not but to steal, kill, and destroy." (John 10:10) These are the attributes of the dark unseen side of reality. Jesus Christ said "I have come so that you might have life, and that you might have it more than abundantly." So, in order to be totally healed of any illness you must recognize its true origin. "God is light and love and in Him is no darkness at all." (I John 1:5)

I sometimes hear patients say that God is trying to teach them something by making them suffer. Many times the patients saying this have been suffering the same illness for 15-20 years! I try to help these patients understand how that God could spend all his time fixing every problem for everyone, but then we would never grow, we would simply grow lazy since we know that whatever happens "God will fix it." He is simply waiting for us to use our Sonship rights and be healed.

He set up the rules so that we can have what we need, whenever we need, by simply using our God-given authority. So if you think God is "doing this to you", or "trying you", you need to recognize that the truth is He already gave you the key to release yourself from your "prisons." You allowed yourself to be put there; He did too, only by default, since He will never "possess" you and force you to do the right thing. He is simply waiting for you to let yourself out. He has done His part. To learn is to grow and vice versa. Eventually you will learn how not to allow yourself to be in any "prison."

The concept of "needing to grow" is unclear to many people. What part of us needs to grow? It is our need to grow to a greater spiritual maturity. For example, how many of us walk around recognizing the "accidents, insults, and adversities" in life are often caused by our lack of understanding of how to stay in physical, mental, and spiritual Light? Not many, I'd say.

1 John tells us that "God is light and in Him is no darkness at all" and that we are to "walk in the light as He is in the light". To "walk" is an action word meaning we must actively do it all the time. In other words, one cannot just "be" in the light. Our Heavenly Father has set it up so that we can appreciate His incredible goodness towards us. He has made everything available to us (ask, knock, seek). He is waiting for you to access it. (Matthew 7: 7)

This is a good place to talk about love. The word "love" is used way too much in our society, i.e. "I love roller coasters" and such. I have raised my children to know when using the word "love" is appropriate by saying "You can only love something that loves you back," so instead they say, "I really like roller coasters."

So, what exactly is love? Is it extreme like? Is it just a warm fuzzy feeling? Is it sexual attraction? As a basic human emotion and from a scientific view, love creates a specific energetic frequency felt all over the body. Just like emotional depression causes a specific energetic frequency and a subsequent hypo-function of every cell, love creates the energetic frequencies that optimize the function of all aspects of the body. **Love at its purest form is the point wherein all things physically, mentally, and spiritually, become possible.** This may be a new thought for many of you. I know it is only recently that it became so real to me. Perfect love can only be realized by first accepting Christ as the Lord and Savior of our life. Then as 1 John 4:15 says, "Whoever confesses Jesus is the Son of God, God abides in him, and he in God", since God is Love and Light, and He now abides in you, every cell in your body is energetically charged. 1 John 4:18 speaks about a "perfect love" saying, "Perfect love casts out all fear." Here we see the two polarities of the universe, love and fear. But what exactly is perfect love?

Is this perfect love simply a matter of salvation through receiving Christ as your personal savior. No, when we go back to the original texts for more clarity, perfect love is a specific kind of love. The word "perfect" is the word teleios in the Greek, which is defined as "that which has reached its highest level of maturity, or achievement." This means this state of perfection is not an instantaneous development upon salvation. It is a level of achievement through constant reinforcement of the truths of God's Word through meditation and application.

The word "love" in the reference on "perfect love" is in the original Greek texts, the word agapê, a noun, indicating a specific type of love which is different than simply being fond of or regarding someone with favor; this kind of love is spontaneous love, irrespective of "rights". This love just is, no matter if it is deserved, justified, or warranted.

Perfect love is a state of being; a complete oneness with your heavenly Father: a total peace; a state where all of the gifts of the Holy Spirit are fully manifest in you. It need not take a lifetime to achieve, simply one must bring one's heart, mind, and body into alignment and agreement with God's Word. This necessitates that knowledge of God's Word must go from head knowledge to heart wisdom.

If perfect love were a gift given upon salvation then there would be no need to "meditate on God's Word" (Joshua 1:8) or "...put on the armor" (Eph 6)

Our responsibility is to keep our body, mind and spirit clean by staying in God's light and God's love. In doing this we keep our direct line of communication with God open and static-free. When we accepted Jesus Christ as our savior, (Romans 10: 9 & 10) we became a new creature, being made Sons of God, perfect and one with the Father.

There is only one thing God made us 100% responsible for – your thinking. It is always your free-will choice to do anything. God will never "possess" you. He could have made us robots, programmed to serve and love Him, but He wants you to always choose Him. If you choose to not use your Sonship rights of invincibility to the powers of darkness, He will not force you to. As you begin to exercise your spiritual authority you will grow to know that you are, as a child of God, invincible by birthright. You will begin to realize that the 'sudden knee pain that just came on you' is an attack from a dark energy, only via a lapse in your spiritual awareness. You can either get upset and grab the Tylenol, or you can recognize it for what it is and send it packing, using your God-given authority. It can be difficult at first to see that it is as easy as all this, when you see almost the entire world mired down in various illnesses. The preponderance of five-sense evidence suggests that illness is simply part of normal life. The reality is that all illness arises from the improperly maintained health and balance of body, mind, and spirit.

Some may say all of our problems are due to our lack of enlightenment, or are the result of our lack of individual consciousness - basically saying we create our own reality. I do not disagree. I simply take it further to say our problems arise from a lack of enlightenment and consciousness of universal truths set down from the beginning of time by God in heaven.

Some things seem to happen that are purely accident and are not related to "powers of darkness". Did you stubbing your toe on the way to the bathroom happen by chance? Did the deer jump in front of your car by chance? Was your body too weak to prevent actual Lyme disease from occuring once you got bit, just bad luck? Is it pure chance that you may have been born with deformity or illness? These and so many more examples have resulted in the belief in luck, fate and destiny. But are they really chance or are they a tendency you have acquired through yours or your ancestors free-will decisions and lack of consciousness in spiritual matters? Many "New Age" teachers teach their students that they control their own destiny, that positive affirmations direct the creation of their reality of the world. Guess what? This works! People the world over are speaking their new reality into being, without the knowledge of the Holy Bible. This is because it operates on one of God's universal laws – believing equals receiving, whether it is negative believing or positive believing! This is accessible by Christians and non-Christian alike. So if we all have this kind of control over our reality then is there really any chance or fate? No chance! Knowledge of the power of God in Christ in us takes this to greater enlightenment and greater consciousness. It is truly a matter of self consciousness and self awareness and a matter of spiritual consciousness and awareness.

Many people have told me they would rather not be responsible for knowing powers of darkness are behind the scenes screwing things up. Fear and anxiety are directly from lack of understanding of who has all the power here. The Bible says it is God in Christ in you, working in and through you, as you. *(1 John 4: 13, 15, 16).* There is no greater power in the universe! It's like the children's song, "Anything you can do, I can do better. I can do anything better than you." When you realize the power of positive affirmations combined with your power over all the power of the dark side through the God in Christ in you… then you will begin to realize true enlightenment and reach levels of consciousness not accessible to those who do not believe. Knowledge destroys fear.

Intellectual types often suffer from loss of believing. They believe that everything in the world can be explained without acknowledging spiritual matters and that the concept of God and the Holy Bible are for the weak-minded masses. The truth as I see it, being in the top 1/2 of 1% of the most educated people of the world is evident in this book. We live in a physical world that operates upon physical laws and embedded within this physical world is the unseen spiritual world that has its own spiritual laws. (2 Cor. 4:18) The physical world is temporal and the spirit world is eternal, both are interconnected. The physical world is full of opposites, such as hot/cold, light/dark, negative/positive. The spiritual world is made the same with opposites of light/dark, love/fear. Intellectuals often say we are all inherently good and that some people just have not evolved to goodness yet, thereby denying the existence of darkness and evil.

I on the other hand, the smarter I have become, the more clearly I see the spiritual nature of the universe as made up of two basic units, love and fear. God is love and although God made everything in heaven and earth, He allowed the dark spirits to be the counterweight of love…fear. God said, perfect love casts out all fear. (1 John 4:18) So, here we see that "walking in the light" is maintaining this perfect love, the love found and accessible only through having God in Christ in you!

What is always stronger? Light or darkness? Is there ever a darkness so dark that can even blot out the light of the smallest candle? Never! Luke 10:17-19 says that through the name of Jesus Christ all of the spirits of darkness are subject to us, and that He has given us power over all the power of the enemy, and <u>nothing</u> will hurt you! Now, either this is a blatant lie, or it is the absolute truth. There is no gray area here. It is the truth.

Recall that 1 John 1:7 tells us to "walk in the light as He is in the light." The word "walk" is a verb. This means that we are being instructed to take action to be in the light. We now as Sons of God have Christ within, so we are now a Holy Spirit-being occupying a physical body. We are now inherently invincible to the powers of darkness. So, why do we experience adversity? Because most of us have not learned, or been taught, to recognize the many varied methods and strategies used by the dark side to steal, kill, and destroy us. So, **how** do we "walk", or take action? God tells us how in Ephesians 6:11. We walk in the light by knowing and applying the truth of God's Word, by understanding your righteousness as His child, by walking with God's peacefulness, and by never allowing your faith to waiver. That no matter what it looks like that God's power in you is sufficient to shield you from any form of attack from the dark side.

The only time you have no power to resist the dark-side is when you try to do something yourself without operating within God's Word, and therefore you are not operating with "perfect love." (James 4:7) If you think you can do anything without being humble to the Word you will fail, because you have no strength or authority in the spirit world other than that granted you by the properly maintained Sonship rights. So, you begin to get the idea that you can avoid trouble only by walking in the light, since it is only from this position that you can see and render null and void the attacks of the dark side. There is no gray area here. You are either living in light or you are being manipulated by the dark.

Remember, before you accepted Jesus Christ as your Savior you had no ability to even perceive the spirit world, you were limited to your five senses. (1 Cor 2:14) It is always your free-will choice, or option, to live via your five senses even after you have the Holy Spirit within. It is your free will choice, since God does not possess you, to use or not use your Sonship rights. You can live inside or outside of God's protection He has made available to you.

God's Word says that "as a man thinks in his heart, so is he", (Prov 23:7. Prov 15:13) this means literally that if you think that you are weak and unworthy, then you definitely are (this is when you are operating from your five senses). This is not an example of walking in the light. When you are walking in the light it means you recognize that you are everything the Word says you are, and the Word says you are worthy and strong in Him. You cannot be lazy in guarding your thinking, since it is always going to be either right thinking or wrong thinking, and the consequences are either living a happy, more than abundant life, or living with fear, confusion, and disease.

If you don't get any other principle here, you need to know that absolutely every thought is every cell's command to make what you are thinking come true. Fifty trillion cells in your body are listening to everything you think and say and take it as a direct command, and set about to make it reality. Whether you are joking about yourself or just speaking without thinking, saying or thinking things that you don't mean, your cells take it as a command. This is the importance of why God's Word instructs us to 'take every thought captive'. You input the commands, your cells make it reality. Know now, with complete certainty, that you are the result of the sum total of your thoughts. This is a law of nature. It applies whether you are a Christian, or a "five-senses" person who does not agree that there is an unseen spirit world. As you learn to walk in the light every moment of every day, your reality will be the more than abundant life, with no illness and no need.

How exactly are we to maintain our thinking, so that we are only walking in the light? The following seven chapters are essential:

1. Living Only in This Moment-Healing Begins With Your Mind
2. Controlling your Thinking.
3. Who are You on the Inside?
4. Meditation Techniques
5. A Word about Moral Character
6. Realize the Truth of your Identity in Christ Jesus
7. Taking your Authority

Let's take each of these and make them real to you.

Chapter 46

Living Only in This Moment -
Healing Begins With Your Mind

A quiet mind is the most powerful mind of all. (Isa 26:3) All revelation and inspiration occurs most clearly when all intent and desire has been removed, and the mind is perfectly still and relaxed. You may have experienced this briefly at a time when you have been focusing all your mind on a problem, searching for a solution, without results, only to find that the solution comes to you later quite out of the blue.

All things become possible when the mind is still and you are living in the exact moment that you are in. Most people are more comfortable living in the past, or living in the hope that life will be better somehow in the future. If you would train yourself and master the concept of the first sentence in this paragraph, you would find that truly all things become possible. One of the prime benefits of living with a quiet mind and living in the moment is that true contentment follows.

Our society has trained us to be "Johnny on the spot" with a ready answer to any question, and to be a problem solver. In our down time we are taught to have a distraction going such as the radio or television, whether or not we are actually listening. It's "cool" to be a mover and shaker, living on the edge. Most of us unfortunately have also been trained in every way to never relax, especially our minds. I'm telling you now, it will take genuine effort and direction to unlearn the habits of your mind.

So just what is a "quiet mind"? To find out, try this simple exercise. Choose a time and place where you will have no distractions, and be in no hurry. Set a timer for one minute. Close your eyes and try not to allow any thoughts to enter your mind.

So, how did you do? If you had no thoughts cross your mind I applaud you. Most people performing this simple test fail miserably the first time. It just shows you how a quiet mind must be achieved through training and practice. It also shows you best what a quiet mind is, by showing you what it isn't. There are many techniques used to teach you how to reach a quiet mind. They are most often referred to as meditation. Now before you freak out with visions of mystic gurus and such, know now that the concept of meditation is a directive in God's Word. He tells us to meditate on His word night and day. Like everything in life there is a right way and a wrong way of doing things.

Is it possible to have a completely quiet mind all day long? I don't know, but the first time I personally achieved a quiet mind, it felt so good that I wanted to maintain that feeling all day. Does this mean that we should all be walking around with a totally blank mind? No, but it does mean that whatever task you put your mind to will be much more focused and the solutions will be much more clear. You see, living only in the moment that you are in, with a quiet mind, means that all the magnificent brain power is not cluttered by static energy created by thinking and living in many different places at the same time.

We have all been conditioned to fit the mold of society. To break this mold and find out who you truly are is another benefit of living every moment in that moment and finding new realizations through living with a quiet mind.

Remember, every thought is every cell's command to make reality. And if most of your thoughts are jumbled and cluttered with static, then what reality is being created? By changing and quieting your mind in this way you can change your reality.

This sounds all well and good from a conceptual point of view, you may be thinking, and you are correct to a certain extent. In order to achieve a new reality, you cannot be constantly flip-flopping back and forth between your old ways of thinking and these new ways.

Like everything in life, the better you get at this, the better the results you will get. It took your entire life to create the you of today. Start training your mind now with a long-term vision for a new and better you tomorrow and forever. The stakes are that you have everything to gain by making the change. If you will live only in the moment you are in, and approach it with a quiet mind, one with your Heavenly Father, all things become possible all the time. Reach out from death and mediocrity and find life and contentment.

Take a Moment, Every Moment
Reprinted with permission from the Hope Insight Newsletter

"Very few of us really live in the present. Very few of us ever really experience what God has for us in the right now. Very few of us ever learn to enjoy life the way God had intended.

Even right now as you read this letter chances are you are doing so in between something else. You are reading it in a spare moment while waiting on the kids to get home from school, before supper is ready, or during a commercial. Reading it as a way to wait for something else.

That's the way most of us live our daily lives. While God grants us the present moment, a moment full of blessings and wonder, much of the time we are somewhere else, either thinking about something that has already happened or looking ahead to future plans.

Instead of being grateful for and enjoying the meal set before us, we are thinking ahead to what we must get done. Instead of really paying attention to our children when they tell us about their day, we are off somewhere else thinking about other things. Instead of watching the sunset on the way home we are preoccupied with a thousand other things that have already happened or may never happen.

The problem is many of us can go through our entire lives and never really learning to appreciate and seize the present moment. We are too distracted to notice the many present blessings of God. We are too distracted to really enjoy the fleeting moments we have been given.

Study the life of Jesus and you will see He lived in the moment. He embraced what was presently happening around Him. Whether it was observing a woman drawing water from a well at noon, a widow giving all she had, or healing a man born blind, Jesus lived in and took advantage of the present moment.

I am afraid all too often we miss out on what God has for us because we are living in the past or future. What are your present surroundings? Look around and count your present blessings. Stop and take a deep breath and thank God for loving you. Stop and learn to experience life and be thankful for the present.

"Be still and know that I am God"   Psalms 46:10a

When was the last time you really enjoyed a piece of pizza? When was the last time you really studied the face of one of your children? When was the last time you stared in wonder at the stars? When was the last time you caught a snowflake on your tongue? When was the last time you praised God when you deposited your payroll check?

"Be still and know that I am God"

-written by: Pastor Steve Weldon,
Hope Community Church, Andover, Kansas, Feb. 6, 2001

Chapter 47

Controlling your Thinking

The Bible instructs us to "take every thought captive." (II Corinthians 10:5) Every word in the Bible is there because God knew it to be important. God said that we should take every thought captive, because every thought you think either lines up with the truth of your royal blood through Christ Jesus, or it is a thought that exalts itself above the truth of Christ in you – the hope of glory. (I Corinthians 1:27) You can never have power and health in your life if you are constantly "changing your mind." It is one way or the other, your thoughts either empower you or destroy you.

"Death and life are in the power of the tongue: and they that love it shall eat the fruit thereof." This is a proverb from King Solomon, one of the wisest men of all time. (Prov. 12:18, Prov 18:21) You must think before your tongue forms the words.

From scientific and clinical research we now know that life and death are truly in the power of the tongue. Every thought you think is every cell's command to make it come true. It was set up that way as part of God's design. Every cell in your body is eavesdropping on your thoughts. Every cell becomes programmed by your thinking, the programming is either temporary as in the case of a fleeting thought, or the programming is more long-term as is the case in a thought that is held and perpetuated overnight and beyond. It is because of this latter case that God tells us to not let the sun set upon our wrath or negative emotions. (Ephesians 4: 26) Perpetuating that negative thought pattern overnight is all that is required to program the cells to cease to function in a healthy manner.

This means that you need to be sure that you first know God, and serve Him with a perfect heart and with a willing mind; because God knows your heart, and understands all the imaginations of your thoughts. Without an intimate knowledge and relationship with God through Christ Jesus, and lining up your thoughts under His truths, your thoughts have no power to do anything but weaken and ultimately kill you. Conversely, when you reach full spiritual maturity following God's way, all things become possible, all the time.

Many stories come to mind that prove these principles to be true from patients I have seen, but one stands out as you will see. A lady came in with a prior history of breast cancer that had metastasized to the brain.

The doctors had already performed a double mastectomy (surgically removed both breasts), performed brain surgery, and exhausted chemotherapy and radiation. The cancer had recently returned in the brain, verified by various imaging techniques, and the tumor was pressing on the cranial nerves affecting the eyes. The tumor was causing her to be severely cross-eyed, and to have blurry vision.

On the day she received the news that the cancer had returned, she came to my office very upset. I immediately felt inspired to pray with her which she was fine with. After finishing the prayer, I told her to stand up. She stood up and gasped and said, "I can see! Oh my, I can see!" and as I looked at her, I could see that both of her eyes were in perfect alignment! She stood there weeping with joy in my treatment room and began to read with great emphasis outloud all of the printing on the various book covers and charts in the room to prove to herself and me that she could indeed see.

I had no idea this dramatic event would be the end result of my prayer, so I told her, "Let's go show my nurse what God has done for you!" So with three other patients in the waiting room watching and hearing of her miraculous event, she told my nurse the story afterwhich she finished it by saying in a very poignant voice, "And my doctor was going to do surgery on me!" Immediately upon saying this, she lost her eyesight again and her eyes were again severely crossed. I was standing not far away and she, now clutching the receptionists desk for support, said in a loud and desperate voice, "Doctor David, I can't see…help me!" It was a very dramatic and intense moment and I did the first thing that came to mind, I came up right behind her and spoke to her softly in her ear and told her to repeat after me as I recited what I call a "Cleaning Prayer", which is listed later, as she clutched the reception desk for support, and with the other patients watching in shock. The very moment we concluded with the words, "In Christ Jesus' name, Amen," her eyes once again were perfectly restored! Now she was so overcome by emotion that we had to lead her to another room to calm down. It was with great joy in the grace of my Heavenly Father that I turned to the next patient and said, "You're next!"

I learned many gems from this event. Primary to this discussion was the power of her own thinking; how that truly what you think is the command to your cells to make it come true. When she was rejoicing in the telling of her miraculous healing, all was fine, but when she went back in her mind to the past, being in her other medical doctor's office and being told he would have to do surgery, the old fear returned and the message her thoughts were sending to the cells was "I want you to function as you were in that other doctor's office." Her cells received the message loud and clear to instantly restore the tumor and symptoms back the way it was. What my "Cleaning Prayer" did was to bring her thinking back into alignment with the truth of God's way, apparently removing the effect of the tumor immediately. Another lesson learned was how we are to live in the moment we are in and never revisit the past as to rekindle all of the emotions and fear it holds.

Every visit this lady would return with the original symptoms back again, and every visit we would pray and every single time she would leave with perfect vision and eyes in perfect alignment. Try as I may I could not teach her to maintain her healing, because she refused to change her thinking. She would wear an eye patch to help her see when her eyes crossed. On each visit, she would have perfect alignment and perfect vision after I would pray for her, this was from no medicine and no treatment, but each time she would prepare to leave the clinic she would put the patch back on. She was a dramatic personality and liked the patch as part of a pirate outfit she'd wear. I'd tell her not to use it, and she would say "But I need it to drive" and I'd say "But you can see now". Regardless, she would return for her next visit wearing it and crosseyed.

She died several months later, leaving me to wonder at why God would allow this when He so obviously could and would restore her. So I asked God, and He told me that He had honored my believing and had used this to teach me many truths that I would be able to pass on to you here.

You cannot know what and how to think correctly without knowing God and His will, which is the Word of God, the Bible. However, once you know God, and His Word is in your mind, and your mind and heart agree, then you must choose through your free will thinking to maintain the correct orientation of truth and reality, even in the face of overwhelming symptoms.

Chapter 48

Who Are You on the Inside?

Out of the mouth come the issues of the heart. Nothing can come out of our mouth without first being a thought. Thoughts come from the heart. The King James Bible says in Prov. 4: 23 & 24, "Keep thy heart with all diligence; For out of it are the issues of life. Put away from thee a froward mouth, and perverse lips put far from thee." So, out of the mouth come the issues of the heart. Nothing can come out of our mouth without first being a thought from your heart.

In your heart of hearts, who are you? Do you see yourself as a victim? Are you who you let everyone else see? Is life just unfair? Do you feel that you are living a lie? Are you happy? Are you angry? Are you content? Has your illness become your identity?

Who you are on the inside, in your heart of hearts, makes all the difference in the world. All of the retraining of your mind to be quiet and live in the moment will enable you to reach new heights, but the you on the inside must line up, not with your past (Phil. 3:13 . . forgetting those things which are behind . . .), and not with who you hope to be someday, but to who and what the Word of God says you are now. (2 Ti 3:17). There can be no deceiving oneself. Recall that every thought is every cell's command to make it reality. This means that your body will do everything it can to support the view you have of yourself. Consider how you never see someone who is depressed acting hyper. Their body is sluggish and they have no desire to do anything. By your free will choice to be depressed you are sending the signal to all of your cells to not produce as much neurotransmitters, less brain chemicals, less hormones…after all you won't be needing them since you are not wanting to be alert, stimulated or actively living.

I hear patients tell me how relieved they were to find out that their other doctor finally figured out that their brain was not producing enough of this or that brain chemical required for them to not be depressed. Of course there is a deficiency of the brain chemicals! The cells responsible for producing "happy" brain chemicals received your thoughts which were stemming from your heart of hearts and sent a signal to produce less of it so that you can be depressed!

In the same manner there are those who have been told by a doctor that they only have a certain number of days or months to live, because of a terminal illness, say, six months. Sure as anything, they die in six months as predicted. They accepted the doctor's prediction as truth and the body created the reality. There are those people who live well beyond the predictions. The people who live the longest are those who refused to accept the prediction as their reality. Please do not place the responsibility for your illness and health on external sources.

We all physically manifest our heart of hearts. We must realize that our own actions are an integral part of all conflict and illness. As the Word says, out of the mouth come the issues of the heart, and out of the heart comes the issues of life and death. It also says that we are destroyed for a lack of knowledge (Hos. 4:6). Knowledge of what? Truth. What is the source of truth? God's Word. Of course, you can gain in knowledge by reading. Reading puts knowledge in your mind, meditation gets it from your mind into your heart. That is why God instructed us to "meditate on my Word night and day." To meditate is to focus all that you are to one task until it becomes part of you. The goal is to have your mind and heart agree. You can see why it becomes so very important *what* you put in your mind and ultimately into your heart. If you put in erroneous information, then that will create an unfavorable outcome in your mind, body, and spirit.

What are the only safe things to think and put in your heart? God tells us precisely – whatever things are true, whatever things are honest, whatever things are just, whatever things are pure, whatever things are lovely, whatever things are of good report; if there be any virtue, and if there be any praise, think on these things. Those things that you both learned, and received, and heard, and seen in me, do: and the God of peace shall be with you. (Phil. 4: 8-9)

Your heart will dictate the thoughts, which in turn are the commands to every cell. So thinking on these things produces health and a more abundant life. (Prov. 17:22 - A merry heart doeth good like a medicine: But a broken spirit drieth the bones.)

Believe it or not, your illness is a blessing. It is a signpost that can lead you on a journey and down a path that needs to be followed in order to find greater spiritual maturity. Through spiritual awakening, your outward journey is taken inward. With the illness as your guide, you can correct the imbalances in your body, mind, and spirit, the result being contentment and a long, healthy life. (Isa 26:3 & John 14:27)

All meditation techniques share a common goal, to help you achieve a quiet mind. From the very most basic, it should be clear to you that you would have a difficult time keeping a quiet mind with kids running around the house screaming and playing. Meditation techniques began just that simply. Someone determined that it was easier to meditate in a quiet environment, and so on.

Knowledge of God's Word, prayer and meditation are the foundation of a spiritual life. Prayer is the transmitter while meditation is the receiver, therefore prayer and meditation are part of the same process. From this perspective both can be practiced anywhere and anytime. Imagine all things, complete healing included, truly being possible all the time through God-designed living. (Psalms 103:3, 3 John 2, John 10:10, 2 Co 9:8, Eph 3:20)

Chapter 49

Meditation Techniques

You have spent your entire life training your brain to be busy. Now train it to be quiet. The results will amaze you. Meditation and prayer can be done anywhere, anytime. You can't go to the gym and workout a few times and be physically fit, and so it is with meditation. The more you practice, the better you become and the greater the results. The ultimate goal is to train your mind to be quiet, content, and focused no matter where you are, or what the circumstance.

Remember, if the mind is full of static energy, and jumbled thoughts, and songs, and random thoughts, then the body will do all it can to support the state of mind you are in. By quieting your mind you enable the body to heal.

There are many different techniques. The following are a few meditation techniques to get you started.

Relaxation Meditation

Relaxation meditation is one of the most fundamental techniques. It is the starting point for many of the other types of meditation which go on to more specific goals. This technique has been shown to activate the parasympathetic nervous system and create calming alpha brain waves. Tension and pain will be released through this healing meditation.

Lay or sit with your back straight, and completely tense every muscle in your body for five seconds, unless tension will cause pain. In this case, skip the tensing step. Take three deep breaths, breathing in through your nose and out through your mouth, letting the air exhale naturally. Close your eyes. Now breathe normally, but deeply exhale while you mentally concentrate on releasing the tension. Concentrate on relaxing all of the muscles in your face, head and neck. Now as you breathe consciously relax in the following order: your arms, chest, abdomen, legs, feet, and toes. Finally, relax from the base of your spine working up to the top of your head. Relax each part individually, as opposed to attempting to simply relax your entire body all at once.

Now with every muscle relaxed, continue to breathe in the same manner for 10-15 more minutes. Block out all negative thoughts and maintain a quiet mind. Focus your mind on the space between inhalation and exhalation.

Breath Meditation

This is a very simple and powerful meditation. In Breath Meditation you lay or sit with your back straight. You should breathe normally, but focus your mind on the breath itself. Feel it enter your nose and pass into your lungs. Simply watch your breathing. Block out all thought. The goal is to feel no separation between you and your breathing. It will begin to feel like you and your breathing are one. Observe every stage of breathing, the inhalation, the space between breaths, and the exhalation. Pay particular attention to the space between breaths. This space is very healing.

Focused Meditation

In a quiet environment, close your eyes and breathe regularly. Notice that your eyes may be flickering and moving about. This is common when the mind is not quiet. The eyes should be completely still with a quiet mind. This eye movement is caused many times by nervousness, and by thoughts running through your mind. It may also be due to external distractions as seen when someone thinks they are being observed.

Focused Meditation helps to calm your mind by directing the focus of your mind to a certain area of your body. When performed correctly, your eyes will be completely still and your mind will quiet, which is the goal of all meditation.

To perform focused meditation, concentrate your closed eyes and your entire mind to the area in the center of the forehead and between the eyebrows. With your eyes trained upon this area, you will find it easier to hold the eyes still.

Focused meditation may be the most effective way to slow the brain waves from beta all the way to theta waves.

Meditating on God's Word

We are directed to meditate on God's Word. In this type of meditation it is best to have already developed the ability to achieve a quiet mind through practicing the other methods outlined.

As with all meditation assume your preferred meditative position.

Select one verse from the Holy Bible that you need to get from your head knowledge into your heart. Focus your quiet mind upon the verse. Observe inwardly your heart. What does it say in regard to the verse? It may surprise you that your heart says that it is 'just words' and that it 'is not really true'. Conversely, it may ring true in your heart. Either way, with high intent and focus, contemplate the truth that is the verse without straying into side thoughts. Maintain the meditative quiet mind while repeating the verse. The goal is that your heart of hearts will accept the verse as absolute truth. At that point, the power of the Word of God is made manifest in you. Nothing, no meditation or power, is more healing.

Meditating, One with Nature

Meditating in nature can be very healing. If you live in a city there are still options that will allow you to get closer to nature. Botanical gardens and some zoos as well as city parks can suffice. To get out away from the sounds and smells of the city is most desirable. Find a spot where you don't have to be observed or distracted.

Bio-Scalar Meditation

While not taught by its developer as a meditation technique, I have found the Bioscalar work can be used in the same way and is really a powerful treatment in its own right. Many people have see a dramatic improvement in an unending list of illnesses and often report a complete disappearance of the disease. This meditation uses a technique developed by Valerie Hunt, a renowned researcher in the field of bioenergetic medicine. Bioscalar meditation is presented here exactly as she teaches it.

How to create bioscalar energy

"We can create the bioscalar energy inside our bodies by consciously manipulating the environmental electromagnetism in the air we breathe. This is done by focusing on the breathing; imagine each breath as coming from opposite sides (simultaneously) on a straight line into the body. The bioscalar is easier to create if we start our breathing concentration in the chest area.

Creating the bioscalar

- Lie down and stretch your arms straight out sideward from you body. On each breath imagine the same frequency (color) of energy coming through each hand into the middle of the body. To ensure the same energy in each hand pick a pure primary or secondary color (red, orange, yellow, green, blue, violet or white).
- Visualize that color of energy entering each hand at the same time and bring the energy into the body on inhalation
- On exhalation leave the energy inside your body and just decrease the air so you can take another breath. The same electromagnetic energy inside the body pools in space. The frequencies have canceled each other out, and what is left is a bioscalar stationary energy. The scalar is apparently a zero point in quantum energy.
- As you continue your scalar breathing you will become aware that your chest feels full – not of air but of standing scalar energy. Now stop concentrating on your inhalation and you will feel the bioscalar energy expanding outward in circles again, like a stone thrown into still water. This is the automatic action of the scalar wave. It separates the compacted tissue and cells, facilitating the healing phenomenon.
- As you create the bioscalar energy in the central part of the body you will establish an automatic pattern. Stop conscious creation of the scalar and use your mind to tell the energy what you want it to do as it spreads out: to heal the pain, regenerate the tissue, eliminate the bacteria or virus. Be intent here –"command" the energy, don't just give a passive suggestion.

How long should the bioscalar process take? In the beginning the process should take about 30 minutes, two times a day. As you become more skillful, 10 minutes several times a day should give excellent results. As you become more skillful in creating the scalar, you can try lying on your side and creating the bioscalar also between the back and front of the body, and between the sacrum and occiput.

Additional scalar information

Colors have different frequencies, but each (color) if used in both hands will cancel out all the frequencies creating the same bioscalar energy.

From my experience the red-orange frequency spectrum seems to have a faster build-up while the blue-violet spectrum seems to continue the expansion longer.   If you create the bioscalar energy to calm pain, the blue-violet energy works best. If your need is to heal damaged tissue start with the red spectrum, but shift back to the blue violet to calm the pain. With each session try using both at different times, and see which one works best for you.

Remember that healing is first healing the entire body, so do a central bioscalar first. If the problem is in one area of the body you can also create the scalar in a limb or local body area. Bring into the body energy that has the same frequency and that comes simultaneously from opposite sides; with practice bring it into the center from the back and the front of the body, and from the cervical to the tailbone. This later technique was one of the profound discoveries of John Upledger in his stunningly successful craniosacral therapy.

When you become very skillful in concentration you can bring energies from all directions simultaneously, like the sun's radiations, because each breath activates all vectors.

Chapter 50

A Word about Moral Character

It is difficult to discuss moral character. Each of us has been raised up experiencing a diverse mix of the good and bad of society. Some of us have suffered horrible events, while others have had it relatively easy. Having personally lived in thirty-two different places, I feel I have seen a wide section of the United States, and have experienced life overseas as well. In all of my travels I have come to the point or realization that I am responsible for and can only change myself. As a result, I am constantly under construction to improve myself. The journey truly is the prize.

Strife and malicious intent, bigotry and racism, greed and envy, hate and unforgiveness, condemnation and fear, lying and deception, jealousy and bitterness, worry and gossip - all are destructive forces. All negativity is destructive to you and leads to misery, illness, and death. The problem is that how we were raised is usually the most comfortable way to act. It is possibly the way of your family. You may be so comfortable with the negativity that you don't even realize it is poison.

In our attempts to reestablish the rhythm of healthy living, all could be for naught if you are poisoning yourself from a lack of moral character. All of the right medicines, all of the most clever thought out blends of therapies will not overcome this poison.

Consider what the Word of God says... be kind one to another... a soft word turneth away wrath…bless those who persecute you...work as unto the Lord...be tenderhearted... give more than asked of you...don't let the sun set on your wrath...do not be weary of welldoing...do not think better of yourself than you aught...be angry but sin not. Can you see that we are called to be the counterweight of darkness. We are called to live in the rhythm of light. God's word also says that we are to "walk in the light, as He is in the light." Doing so will bring health and long life to you.

It would be the greatest medicine for you to drop your life's training of poison, which is negativity in all of its forms.

Forgive and forget. We have all heard this quip. Some may say it is easier said than done. True atrocities may be in your past. We are no longer in the administration of "an eye for an eye." The only way to move on without them is to live only in the moment you are in. You are not to live in the past, however you are most definitely defined by the past. The life you have led has created the reality of today. The past is "road-kill." God tells us to "put away the things of the past, pressing onward toward the prize."

Every day is a blank slate, a new beginning. If you want a new, better reality, you need to eliminate the negative aspects of your life today and every day. In your healthy future, you should be able to look over your past and see a healthy reality as a result of focusing on all things pure, just, true, and of good report.

You will find that your life is like a dirty garbage pail. If you will study God's Word and practice simple truths like living in the moment, controlling your thinking, and meditating, you will find that these actions are like putting clean water in that dirty garbage pail. At first a bunch of garbage will run out of the pail and it will be unnerving to let go of that garbage. But as you continue to put water in that dirty garbage pail that pail will become cleaner and cleaner and the next thing you know, all the issues of the past and present will just disappear. All your old issues will not be in your pail anymore, only clean water and you will truly be free to practice God Designed Living and God Designed Healing on a moment to moment basis.

Chapter 51

Realize the Truth of Your Identity in Christ Jesus

According to the Bible it says in 2 Tim 2:15, "Study to shew thyself approved unto God, a workman that needeth not to be ashamed, rightly dividing the word of truth." So, this chapter is designed for you to write. Many Christian patients that I see, have not studied these scriptures or have not been taught these verses. I have prepared topics that will give you the "I can do" attitude, and also verses that will show God's point of view of things not to be ignorant on in actions, attitudes, emotions, thoughts, or words. This is your chance, to have God talk to you and to put into your mind, body, soul, and spirit, pure living energy. So, don't skip this chapter, this will be the most important chapter in your healing process. But before you pull out your Bible, I must help you with your new foundation. As I heard from Dr. Tony Evans, senior pastor of Oak Cliff Bible Fellowship, and author of twenty books, when one tries to build a skyscraper, one must dig a very, very, very, deep foundation before one could build a tall skyscraper. Same principle goes when one is building a life on God-designed living. The first step one must realize is to understand that we are in the Grace Administration. We are no longer in the Law, therefore, are no longer servants of God and no longer sheep that need a shepherd. Once, one believes in Romans 10: 9 & 10, they are now sons of God, athletes, more than conquerors, but one must realize that to be born again or to be born with the seed of God in you, that seed can never be removed. Just like you will always have the seed of your earthly father in you, you will always have the seed of God in you. Just like you were first born from your mother, you had a lot to learn. It is the same principle of being born with the seed of God in you. You will always have a lot to learn. Now accept what the Word says, and start your journey by realizing you are no longer a sheep that needs a shepherd but a joint-heir with Christ and that you are no longer a servant of God but a son of God with His seed in you that you will never lose.

Athlete: 1 Co 9:24, Eph 6:12, Phil 3:14, Heb 12:1

_____

_____

_____

_____

_____

Born- Again: John 3:5, Rom 10:9, 1 Pe 1:23, 1 Jo 3:9

_____

_____

_____

_____

_____

Chosen: Eph 1:4, 2 Th 2:13

_____

_____

_____

_____

Christ in You: Col 1:27

_____

_____

_____

_____

Complete: Col 2:10

_____

_____

_____

_____

_____

Condemnation: Rom 8:1, 1 Jo 3:20

_____

_____

_____

_____

Conquerors: Rom 8:37

_____

_____

_____

_____

Delivered: Col 1:13, 1 Th 1:10, 2 Ti 4:18

_____

_____

_____

_____

Doers: 1 Co 2:4, Phm 21, Jas 1:22

_____

_____

_____

_____

_____

Not Ignorant: Rom 1:13, Rom 11:25, 1 Co 10:1, 1 Co 12:1, 2 Co 1:8, 2 Co 2:11, 1 Th 4:13

_____

_____

_____

_____

_____

Ignorant: 2 Ti 3:7, Hos 4:6, Matt 22:29

_____

_____

_____

_____

_____

Wrong Actions: Rom 12:11, Rom 13:11 1 Co 7:2, 2 Co 6:14, Eph 4:28

_____

_____

_____

_____

_____

Wrong Attitudes: Rom 8:1, Gal 5:16, Eph 4:32, Col 3:15, Heb 3:8

_____

_____

_____

_____

_____

Wrong Emotions: Psa 37:8, Rom 12:10, Eph 1:4, Heb 13:5, 1 Jo 2:16

_____

_____

_____

_____

Wrong Thoughts: Luke 12:29, John 14:27, Phil 3:13, Col 3:2 2 Ti 1:7

_____

_____

_____

_____

Wrong Words: Prov 29:11, Rom 12:21, Eph 4:25, Eph 4:29, 1 Jo 1:6

_____

_____

_____

_____

Eternal Life: John 3:15, Rom 6:23, 1 Jo 2:25, 1 Jo 5:11

_____

_____

_____

_____

_____

Grace: Rom 3:24, Rom 5:2, Rom 6:14, 1 Co 6:12, 2 Co 9:8, Eph 2:8, Eph 3:2, 1 Pe 1:10

_____

_____

_____

_____

_____

Greater: John 14:12, 1 Jo 4:4

_____

_____

_____

_____

_____

Habitation: 1 Co 3:16, Eph 2:22

_____

_____

_____

_____

_____

Heirs: 8:17, Gal 4:1, Eph 1:11, Titus 3:7

_____

_____

_____

_____

_____

I Can Do: Phil 4:13

_____

_____

_____

_____

Law: Rom 3:20, Rom 7:4, 1 Co 6:12, Gal 2:16, Gal 5:1, Gal 5:14

_____

_____

_____

_____

Light: Matt 5:16, Eph 5:8, Phil 2:15, 1 Jo 1:5

_____

_____

_____

_____

Love: Matt 22:37, John 3:16, Rom 13:8, 1 Co 13, Gal 5:6, Gal, 5:14, Eph 3:17, Eph 5:2, Eph 5:25, 2 Ti 1:7, 1 Pe 1:22, 1 Jo 4:18, 1 Jo 5:2

_____

_____

_____

_____

_____

Mystery: Rom 16:25, 1 Co 2:8, Eph 3:6, Eph 3:9, Eph 5:32, Col 1:26, Col 1:27, 1 Pe 1:10

_____

_____

_____

_____

_____

Power: Luke 24:49, Eph 1:19, 2 Ti 1:7, Heb 4:12

_____

_____

_____

_____

Prosperity: Matt 6:33, 2 Co 9:6, 2 Co 9:8, Phil 4:19, 1 Ti 6:17, 3 Jo 2

_____

_____

_____

_____

_____

SONSHIP RIGHTS: *Justified, Reconciled, Redeemed, Righteousness, Sanctified*

Justified: Rom 3:20, Rom 3:24, Rom 3:28, Rom 4:25, Gal 2:16

_____

_____

_____

_____

_____

Reconciliation: Rom 5:10, 2 Co 5:18, Col 1:21, 1 Ti 2:4, Heb 2:17

_____

_____

_____

_____

_____

Redemption: Rom 3:24, Gal 3:13, Eph 1:7, Titus 2:14, 1 Pe 1:18

_____

_____

_____

_____

_____

Righteousness: Rom 3:21 & 3:22, Rom 4:3, Rom 5:17, 2 Co 5:21, Phil 3:9

_____

_____

_____

_____

_____

Sanctified: John 17:17, 1 Co 6:11, Heb 2:11, Heb 10:14

_____

_____

_____

_____

_____

Renewed Mind: Rom 12:2, Rom 13:14, 2 Co 10:5, Gal 5:24, Eph 4:22, Eph 4:23, Eph 4:24, Phil 3:13, Col 3:10

_____

_____

_____

_____

_____

Rest: Psa 37:7, Phil 4:6, 1 Pe 5:7

_____

_____

_____

_____

_____

Thanks: Psa 100, 1 Co 14:17, 2 Co 2:14, 2 Co 9:15, Phil 4:6, Col 3:17

_____

_____

_____

_____

_____

Walk: Rom 6:4, Gal 5:16, Eph 4:1, Col 1:10, 1 Ti 4:12

_____

_____

_____

_____

_____

Working of God: Eph 1:19, Phil 2:13

_____

_____

_____

_____

Wrestle: Eph 6:12

_____

_____

_____

_____

For more reading material, I highly recommend, *"The Rest of the Gospel When the Partial Gospel has Worn You Out"* written by Dan Stone and Greg Smith (800- 915-8771) One Press, P.O. Box 832442, Richardson, Texas 75083

Chapter 52

Taking Your Authority

The following are a few of examples of prayers that you may use anytime you feel the need. Once you realize in your heart, who exactly you are... a child of God... joint heirs with Christ... higher than the angels... with full Sonship rights over all that God has created, including the adversary and legions of darkness, you will be able to use these prayers as basic templates, to be changed as the need arises, and realize the true power over your symptoms and diseases, indeed your entire life.

I have used these and similar prayers in my own life on innumerable occasions. From a symptom perspective, the symptoms are usually gone within 5 seconds of completing the prayer.

This chapter on "Taking Your Authority" is what we referred to earlier as using your "First Aid", in the chapter called "Get the Hurt and the Dirt Out of Your Life."

You must realize that you absolutely get what your heart believes. You must pray with the power of believing, just like you believe the Statue of Liberty is in New York, even if you have never actually seen it personally. If you think you are believing, or hoping you believe, then you likely are not believing effectively. When you truly believe, it is a non-issue... it just is true in your mind and heart.

This believing in your God-given authority to control your circumstances must be understood as to where the power comes from... from the God in Christ in you, working within you as you. (1 John 4:15)

Sometimes I feel as though I am "in the zone" spiritually, kind of like very much in power. These are the times when I am most effective with these prayers. Being in the zone comes from the continual need to be "walking" and "living" and "putting on the whole power available to us all the time". This zone level is achieved by continually putting the truth of God's Word in front of you, starting each morning with prayer, meditating on and reading the Word, speaking the Word, living the Word, and being very spiritually aware of the adversary's wiles and barbs aimed at you, and immediately shielding and blocking these dark forces.

These prayers are true power given to you by your heavenly Father for your own use. Use them!

Don't get caught up in the ineffectual prayers of "Dear God, please fix this problem." (fig. 1) God said, "I give you power over all the power of the adversary and nothing shall hurt you, through the power of Christ within you." (fig. 2) You are invincible by birthright through Christ... use your power! NOW!

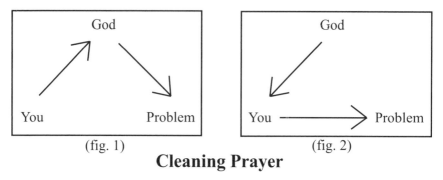

(fig. 1)   (fig. 2)

Cleaning Prayer

"Dear Heavenly Father, I acknowledge you in and commit to you in all that I do and say now.[1] I now clean my <u>vessel</u>* and make it sacred (pure) with your love and light.[2] I am thoroughly perfect by the God in Christ in me.[3] In Jesus Christ's name, I remove and bind all that is not of God's light and love.[4] Be gone from my <u>vessel</u>* now, and do not return." "I thank you that it is done, now, Father, in Christ Jesus name, amen."

<u>An Alternate Cleaning-type prayer</u>:
"Dear God, I acknowledge you in and commit to you in all that I do and say now.[1] I now clean my <u>vessel</u>* and make it sacred (pure) with your love and light.[2] Creators of all darkness and disease (or their exact names if you know them), I now command you to restore any damage you have caused in my vessel. I renounce any right you may have had to be affecting me. I now command you and all of your dark spirits, beings, forms, entities, or anything in this or any other dimension, inside or outside of my consciousness or awareness to be cast into the abyss. And not harm another sentient being, nor tag-team, or reaccess through any means. And make it so NOW! I speak it NOW through the God in Christ in me, who gave me power over all of the power of the adversary! I now clean my <u>vessel</u>* and make it sacred (pure) with God's light and love."[2]

Notice in this last prayer we are requiring the dark spirits to clean up the mess they have caused in your body. I was inspired to do this when I realized that sometimes you may tell a demon to leave and he basically says "sure I'll leave now… the damage is done, my work here is done, and this person is going to die anyway as a result of my work." It's kind of like being a parent, coming home to find your kids and their friends had a party and the house is a wreck. Just telling everyone to go home leaves you with the job of cleaning up the mess! I think every parent would want the kids that made the mess actually to clean up the mess!

*Vessel meaning "all that I am, not just my physical body." (Substitute whatever you are wanting to clean, such as food, people, areas, houses, medicines, etc.)

You can know that when you bless (clean) your food and medicines that it will taste better, digestion is improved, and only the beneficial components will be optimally utilized by the body.

When to use the cleaning prayer:

Use it when you feel under attack from sudden or chronic symptoms, also before and after sleeping. Another good time to use it is before you go into what you know will be a troublesome meeting or situation, and again afterwards. Recognize that any sneeze, cough, or irritation is a sign of some energy attempting to attach itself to your energy. Learn to observe yourself on a moment by moment basis, so that you are always aware of energy changes. It may come from a phone call, a person you are around, an environment you are in, or even from a distant unknown source. You cannot afford to be lazy in this. It will always be easiest to recognize and remove as soon as it tries to attach to you. Look at it as "energy parasites from the dark side." Parasites feed off of you while you gain nothing. Be a victor, not a victim.

Scriptural References:

1. Prov. 16:3, Prov. 3:5, 1 Chronicles 29:11-12

2. 1 John 1:5, Phil. 4:13, Rom. 6:12-14

3. Col. 1:27 The great mystery that was hid for all the generations, it is "**Christ in you the hope of glory**" Because the devil would have never crucified Jesus Christ if he knew that after the day of

Pentecost all born again believers (i.e. the saints) would now have Christ within them and now would be joint heirs with Christ and have all the power that Christ had. So, now instead of one powerful man that could resist the devil, now there are millions of people who have the power over the devil. This was not available until the day of the Pentecost. Therefore, if a born again believer spends all his time studying the Word prior to the day of Pentecost (Acts 2:4) he would be walking in the ways of people who did not have the power of having Christ within them (Romans 15:4). This is why it is important to study the Epistles heavily because they are specifically addressed to the saints which are the born again believers. The Epistles shift from being servants of God to being adopted sons of God and joint heirs with Christ, therefore the saints are athletes of the Spirit with power.

4. Luke 10:17, 1 John 1:10, whatever is bound on earth is bound in heaven. Resist the devil and he will flee from thee.

The bible repeatedly says that God has given us the authority through the God in Christ in us, and power over the adversary. When we receive salvation, all things are made new, and we are a new creature filled with God's Holy Spirit. We now are Holy Spirit-beings occupying a physical body. It is only through the God in Christ in us that we have any authority, but we being spirit Children of God have the right to speak outright to the spiritual powers of darkness. The Word tells us that "In my name, YOU will...," and "I give YOU power over all the adversary..." "These things and more shall YOU do in my name" Therefore, God has made it already available to us through salvation to speak our deliverance. We then are not to pray as many of us have been taught saying "Dear God, please fix this problem", rather, we should pray "I claim healing, or I bind and remove this spirit of infirmity from my body, in Jesus Christ's name"

God made all available to us through Christ. Therefore, I can do all things through Christ which strengthens me.

I clean my vessel, medicine, area, food, by the power of the Spirit within me, provided me by Christ Jesus

Clearing Inherited or Acquired Negative Conditions

I Am What God's Word says I Am; I cancel, nullify and dissolve all vows or agreements that I have made or my ancestors have made that keep me from realizing my Sonship rights, and from accessing all God's power promised to His children.

I Am What God's Word says I Am; I cancel and nullify all vows or agreements that I may have made with any and all entities that may be attempting to keep me from realizing my Sonship rights, and from accessing all God's power promised to His children.

I Am What God's Word says I Am; I release any and all entities that may be attempting to keep me from realizing my Sonship rights, and from accessing all God's power promised to His children.

I Am What God's Word says I Am; I dissolve any bonds or connections that I may have to any and all entities that may be attempting to keep me from realizing my Sonship rights, and from accessing all God's power promised to His children.

I Am What God's Word says I Am; In the name of Jesus Christ, I de-curse myself, I de-hex myself, I de-haunt myself...Now!

I do demand in Jesus Christ's name that any and all entities that may be attempting to control me, or use my energy, or are attached to me in any way, leave me now and do not return. And I demand that you do not attach yourselves to any other sentient being.

In the name of Jesus Christ I demand this and make it so…now.

Clearing Negative Conditions

Dear God, I commit all that I do to you, now.

It is for my highest good to dissolve all blockages and distortions that keep me from accessing my Sonship rights of accessing God's more than abundant life.

It is to my highest good to release all sin, guilt and fear.

I invoke the Light of God's Love; cleanse me.

I invoke the Light of God's Truth; inform me.

I invoke God's Infinite Power; make me strong.

I invoke God's Wisdom and Understanding.

Through the power of the God in Christ in me:

I Am What the Word of God Says I Am,

I heal all things that have caused me pain,

I heal all wounds that I have received in this life.

I forgive those who have hurt me or wronged me in any way, and I ask that all those who have hurt me or wronged me to forgive me for my part in creating the circumstances that led to our conflict.

I give thanks to God our heavenly Father for all the blessings I have received and all blessings I am to receive.

I ask for, and now invoke, the healing power of God.

In the name of Christ Jesus I demand this and make it so, now, amen.

Section 10

Advance Diagnostic Considerations

Chapter 53

Laboratory Testing for Lyme Microbes

I don't trust any run of the mill hospital lab to perform Lyme testing accurately. Labs do not get paid any more or less to find it or not find it. Lyme testing is a touchy matter at best, and if the lab is not used to handling Lyme tests then I have a hard time trusting their results.

I recommend if one desires to be tested then use the top Lyme and Lyme-associated microbe lab in the country – IGENEX, in Palo Alto, California. This lab has, due to the political incorrectness of Lyme disease diagnosis, had to jump through numerous hoops, and have been analyzed under the microscope themselves, always passing these governmental tests of efficiency and compliance. I'm not saying you can't get a good test from any other lab, only that I believe IGENEX to be more reliable.

Don't let one negative blood or urine test convince you that you don't have Lyme disease. Repeat the test at least three times and use both blood and urine tests. I like combining the Lyme IgG/IgM Western Blot and Lyme PCR blood tests with the Lyme Urine Antigen Test (LUAT) or Lyme Urine Dot Blot test.

If desiring to do the blood tests, it is best to do these before starting any treatment since they are antibody tests. The LUAT or Lyme Urine Dot Blot test should be done shortly after starting treatment, i.e., in the first 1-3 weeks AFTER starting treatment. You should catch your first morning urine, as it is most concentrated, for a minimum of three days and up to seven days. Understand, any one day that is positive confirms your urine on that day contained dead Lyme spirochetes in it.

Another favorite lab is the Bowen Research Lab, run by Dr. Barbara Whittaker, M.D. This may be my favorite lab in that they will actually send you a color picture of the microbes they find in your blood. This lab uses completely different methods than IGENEX and other conventional labs.

We order these tests to confirm what we already have found during our physical exam using the adjunctive diagnostic technique, Bio-Resonance Scanning.

While we do not treat microbes directly, it helps to know what the body is up against and how to support the body.

Chapter 54

Bio-Resonance Scanning™

Bio-Resonance Scanning™ is a term I coined to describe the advancements I developed upon other established manual (non-computerized), dynamic, sensitive testing techniques for the purpose of improving the diagnosis and treatment of real people in my first clinic. I developed it during a period of 3 years, right after I graduated from Chiropractic College that I call my period of "original thought". I didn't want to read anyone else's work, or seek out others ideas.

I came out of my period of original thought, only to realize that there must be no such thing. I found pieces of what I came up with "originally" were already known and published, sometimes by Einstein or some other notable characters, but rarely were the ideas put together in the same manner or sequence. So, I became convinced that there is no such thing as completely original thought, only original arrangements of thought. BRS is a combination of the world's best healing techniques integrating CPK, Biological Medicine, Quantum Physics, Energy Medicine, and the principles of what has evolved into Circuit Healing™. BRS operates on the God-designed laws of the universe. It is not a psychic phenomenon, nor is the testing metaphysical or spiritual in nature.

BRS is defined as the utilization of a live human test brain as a bio-computer to identify and isolate specific never before known frequencies of various pathological specimen in various suspensions, for the purpose of future adjunctive diagnosis. BRS also incorporates the knowledge of frequency matching these pathological frequencies to develop new medicinal botanical or otherwise corrective substances. The theoretical foundation behind Bio-Resonance Scanning™ hinges upon the theory that the microbial or pathological substance's molecular structure resonance dictates its specific bio-resonance frequency signatures. The result is ultimately a much faster diagnosis through more accurate ordering of conventional laboratory testing.

History is full of people working on new technologies at the same time. The telephone, internal combustion engine and even calculus were developed at virtually the same time, independently of each other.

I mention all of this to answer people who might question if this is like some other technique they have heard of... I don't know all the other techniques, only the form of testing I created. Admittedly BRS is like all technology – advances are made by one person leaping off of the back of someone else's life work, who jumped off of someone's work, who never imagined the twist someone would put on his work to create something different. At the time, Einstein had no idea his brainchild, $E= MC^2$ would eventually result in the development of the atomic bomb.

My BRS work jumps primarily off of a technique called CPK (Chiro Plus Kinesiology), developed by Dr. Milton Dowty, D.C., to whom I am eternally grateful for the training I received under his tutelage, and whose insight and knowledge continues to know no bounds.

Today when I train other younger doctors I always tell them that I totally expect them to take what I have done and advance upon it and improve upon it... it is the natural order of things. No two doctors approach any problem in the same manner because we all draw from completely different experiences and knowledge and are only limited by our vision of what might be, and what might work.

Why Bio-Resonance Scanning™ Works

Every substance in the universe is made out of the same "stuff". Everything fits somewhere on the electromagnetic spectrum, color, sound, radio waves, ultraviolet waves, x-rays, microwaves, gamma rays – everything. In order to understand Bio-Resonance Scanning™, these facts must be understood. Every substance – your shirt, skin, tissues, organs, the table, and even bacteria, viruses and fungi all are made up of the same stuff – electrons, protons, neutrons, and smaller and smaller particles. To remind you of basic chemistry, we have atoms, such as carbon, hydrogen and oxygen. You combine atoms, which connect through electrical bonds to form molecules. Combine a bunch of molecules and you may have a piece of nylon, or bacteria, or virus, or any substance. Everything, at its core, is electrical, therefore everything has its own unique electrical frequency (electrical signature) determined by its unique electrical bonds in its molecular structure.

It is the type of atoms and the unique electrical bonds that give a virus a generalized electrical frequency range. How the atoms are arranged in the molecule is completely unique to the virus. Nothing else can emit or create the viral frequency, because nothing else has that unique atomic and molecular structure. Bacteria, fungi, and even cancer all have a unique frequency that follows this principle.

For those of you who took Organic Chemistry, you will remember that the only difference between an alcohol, a benzoic acid, an aldehyde and a jillion other molecules is the unique arrangement of the same three atoms… carbon, hydrogen and oxygen. Each one of these substances contains nothing more than these three types of atoms. You can spend years simply rearranging these three elements in longer or more complex arrangements. How atoms bind together makes all the difference.

Understanding these concepts allows you to go the next step – frequency matching of pathogens.

Microbes and pathologies have their own individual and unique electrical frequencies, therefore, once one knows what those frequencies are then bio-electrical frequency matching becomes possible.

Going back now, remember everything fits somewhere on the electromagnetic spectrum of frequencies. So, when a piano tuner goes to tune the piano, since nobody hears the note of "C" exactly the same, the tuner will use a tuning fork, precision-made to the exact frequency for the note of "C". He will strike the tuning fork as he tightens the string with a wrench. He knows the "C" string is perfectly tuned when the string begins to vibrate harmonically with the "C" tuning fork. This is an example of frequency matching.

Bio-Resonance Scanning™, I believe, works in a similar manner. The doctor creates the electrical frequency for say a virus over certain access points on the body. The only way that a frequency match is possible is if the patient does indeed have a virus operating within the test frequency range. The only way the doctor knows if it is a positive frequency match is by the electromagnetic change on the Resonator.

Bio-Resonance Scanning™ (BRS) and the resonator can be likened to a radio. As you search the dial, you are scanning through various electrical frequencies looking for a certain radio station within your area. Now the only way you know that you even have found the frequency for let's say Lite 99.1 is because you hear the music through the speaker of your radio.

In the above analogy, the radio station generating a frequency can be likened to the frequency of a virus within the patient's body. The doctor, using Bio-Resonance Scanning™, is turning the dial on the radio station looking for a match. The speaker, in this scenario, is the resonator that picks up the frequency match. BRS is not to be confused with the Electro-dermal computerized devices. First of all, it does not utilize a computer, and second, these computerized devices at present are testing the body's reaction to a frequency instead of frequency matching as in BRS. The difference is that BRS should detect the frequency of pathologies whether the body is reacting to the pathologies or not at the time.

I have had patients argue and say, "How can we get a frequency match for a virus, when it is deeply embedded and surrounded by the body's tissues, and fluids, which also have their own unique frequency?" The answer is simple. One must first understand that the body, from an electrical point of view, is almost not even here. We are not very dense. Consider for a moment, the smallest particle found is a quark. A quark is so small that it is said to be able to pass through an I-beam of steel and never touch or run into anything. How much denser is steel than our body?

So, the body is a cloud of energy, and even though everything is floating around in blood and lymph and is in close proximity to each other, each has and emits its own unique frequency...unique to its molecular structure. In the same way, you can isolate just one radio station frequency, even though the room is bathed in 50 or so different radio frequencies that have penetrated the walls.

Another example is that we live in an electromagnetic soup. Our eyes are electromagnetic filters. If we could visually see the entire electromagnetic spectrum, such as all the radio waves, television waves, gamma rays, microwaves, etc. we would not see anything. BRS is like our eyes; it can filter out certain frequencies.

Not only can BRS "see" different frequencies, it can also frequency match the exact remedies that you would need.

If you are still with me, and comprehend what I just said, then you can see the logic in frequency matching to medicines. Every medicine is made out of differing molecular combinations. Therefore, every medicine, whether pure substance or crude plant extract, is emitting its own unique frequency as dictated by its molecular structure. This frequency is no more contained or blocked by the plastic or glass of the bottle the medicine is in than the radio frequency is blocked by the walls and windows of your house.

Not only can BRS help find the appropriate medicine, but it can also help determine the compatibility of the medicine to the patient. How many times have you heard of someone dying from an allergic reaction to a medicine? BRS can determine if you are allergic or toxic to a substance prior to you taking it.

How precise is Bio-Resonance Scanning™? In some applications and perhaps to a degree, all applications, clinical findings have lead to the belief that it is 100% accurate. However, like many new technologies, mainstream, conventional medicine does not acknowledge BRS as viable. Various State Healing Arts Boards have reviewed the research and okayed doctors to use this technique only after alerting patients to the fact that they consider the technique to be an **"equivocal" technique.**

After a staggering amount of money, time and tears becoming a doctor, the only reason I would choose to use an unusual technique such as BRS is my desire to eliminate cookbook doctoring that treats symptoms instead of people with real diseases. Conventional lab testing has verified about 86% of the microbes previously detected via BRS frequency matching. Understanding that labs are not very sensitive much of the time, 86% represents phenomenal results.

Frequency matching may make all blood drawing obsolete someday. More research is needed before BRS can be relied upon 100% with no conventional backup testing. However, it is the most tremendous diagnostic and treatment tool I have ever known.

Bio-Resonance Scanning™, and the treatment concepts of Circuit Healing™ and Biological Medicine, is truly the secret of our great success at facilitating the restoration of the quality of life for many people who were sent home with no hope. These people are affectionately called our "Humpty Dumpty Bunch" – people whom all the king's horses and all the king's men could not put back together again.

Armed with this technique, our favorite patients are the lost causes of the world, the people that most doctors do not want to see walk through their door, because every test and every treatment in the cookbook had already been tried.

Chapter 55

Computerized Regulation Thermograpy™

Through powerful computerized thermodiagnostics your physician can finally see the multiple functional problems that lead to disease. When one realizes that Lyme Disease is an infection affecting multiple organ systems and even the teeth, then one can understand how computerized regulation thermodiagnostics can help physicians stop the treatment of symptoms.

Chronic Lyme disease indicates a total dysregulation of every organ circuit and tissue in the body. Multiple areas of dysfunction in predictable patterns can be easily seen using the Computerized Regulation Thermography, giving the physician a way to see the body beyond the symptoms.

There is a reason for our poor treatment record in chronic Lyme disease, cancer, and chronic illness; a doctor cannot fix what he does not know is broken. Doctors rely on blood tests to monitor illness. Many people suffering from Lyme, cancer and other chronic degenerative illnesses will attest to the fact that blood testing can be a very poor way of identifying illness and tracking progress. Many people are diagnosed with Lyme disease and/or cancer only after exhaustive lab testing, which most of the time showed no dysfunction in the body.

Computerized Regulation Thermodiagnostics (CRT) is not to be confused with the colorful imaging thermographic devices, which are also coming of age after three decades of research. CRT displays multiple graphs revealing to a certified thermologist or trained physician specific information as to how fifteen different organs and related systems regulate themselves in response to a cold stimulus.

With over 1500 CRT units in the hospitals and physicians' offices in Europe, and over 20 years of correlative research, it is about time the people in the U.S. benefit from this technology.

CRT is a relative newcomer to the United States, as it was only three years ago that it received its FDA approval as a Class 1, adjunctive diagnostic device. The CRT is scientifically reliable, provides reproducible results, is totally non-invasive, and is completely safe, with absolutely no side-effects. It truly is the "ultimate early warning system" and premier Preventive and Longevity Medicine tool of this century.

Does the CRT do away with the need for conventional lab testing? No, your physician will still need to use other tests that can monitor specific aspects of your health, but it is amazing the amount of information the physician can see even on totally asymptomatic patients.

The CRT is an awesome tool for the early diagnosis of dysfunctional aspects of a person. It also may provide the doctors with the following information:
- Where the primary problem resides.
- It enables the doctor to give tailored-made protocols for individual patients instead of the same treatment plan for the same diagnosis for each patient.
- The CRT clearly shows a patient if they can handle an aggressive treatment, since an aggressive treatment may kill them before the illness kills them.
- The CRT also shows the physician and the patient if the treatment protocols are working and improving the functional capacity of the patient's body and it also shows if the prescribed protocols are actually creating more problems and doing more harm than good.

Who is Using the CRT?

Primary care physicians, Oncologists, Radiologists, Biological Dentists, and the full spectrum of healthcare professionals are beginning to use this effective new tool. When a CRT test is performed, your physician will provide the you with a computer-generated graph of the test. This allows easy tracking of any progress. This is not to be confused with the Electrodermal computerized testing devices.

The CRT supports what is called Functional Medicine, or Biological Medicine, whose philosophy is that if every tissue were functioning correctly then your body would have no disease. These doctors seek to remove any interference and provide your body with the building blocks it needs to heal completely. From this functional perspective, patient quality of life and lifespan is maximized.

As of yet it is not cleared to be a primary diagnostic device, but who cares? History has proven that putting a label on a disease does nothing to help us see the disease outside of its symptoms. For example, fibromyalgia, chronic fatigue syndrome, multiple sclerosis, and indeed cancer are all basically a non-diagnosis. These terms all simply describe a set of symptoms. A true diagnosis identifies the cause of a disease. Since we can't identify the cause of these diseases, your physician will treat the only thing he can see…the symptoms. Even in cancer, the tumor is truly nothing more than the symptom created by dysfunction in multiple tissues of the body. The CRT provides the doctor with so much relevant information, that he can finally stop the "cookbook" doctoring and start treating with a sense of where the primary causes lie and how to strategically tailor a treatment plan, from a total body functional perspective.

Why wait until you have an irreversible problem?

Who Should be Tested with the CRT?

Every person over 5 years of age should be CRT tested annually, at the minimum. Prevention of serious illness is made more realistic via periodic CRT testing, and subsequent preventive medicine.

The Center for Disease Control's (CDC) tracking of diseases are revealing ever increasing occurrence of childhood and adult asthma, ADD, dermatitis, cancer, chronic fatigue, fibromyalgia and other chronic illnesses. There is no one who shouldn't be tested. We all know that prevention is best, but how do you prevent what you do not know is about to happen. Should everyone be taking fistfuls of remedies to prevent every conceivable illness? Or, should you strategically support those areas you know need help? Definitely the latter.

Occasionally people will say, "I'm afraid of what it may find." It should be recognized that this comment stems from fear created by the poor treatment record of most serious diseases. Doing nothing will not change the future. The CRT is not about "putting nails in people's coffins" as some people like to think. It is actually all about "taking nails out of their coffin," and prolonging their quality of life.

The CRT offers <u>reproducible</u> and scientifically valid information that can be crucial to the development and tracking of a successful treatment strategy.

What to Expect in a CRT Exam

A professional Thermodiagnostic technician will perform the CRT testing. You will be asked to sit in a fairly cool, but not uncomfortable room for 10 to 15 minutes.

We will then take the first skin temperature measurements of the head, teeth, and neck. This is performed by a gentle touch of the probe to the surface of the skin. You are then asked to remove your clothes to your underwear, thereby subjecting your whole body to a controlled cold air "stress." The room is not excessively cold, only about 68° F. The remaining measurements on the chest, breast, abdomen and back are made rather quickly.

You are then asked to sit as you are, exposed to the room air for 10 minutes to complete the stress effect. According to clinical research, it takes 10 minutes for your body to stabilize and acclimate to the regulatory changes from the internal organs onto the skin. After this period, all 112 measurements are then repeated and the test is concluded.

The results are shown by a computerized printout, which reveal the reactions of the body and the functional health of various organs and their associated systems.

How does the Skin Temperature Reveal Organ Dysfunction in a CRT Test?

How well the body maintains an optimum skin temperature is determined by the integrity or health of the organ or tissue directly beneath the point of the skin being measured by the CRT temperature probe.

A healthy body, in reaction to cold weather, will cause a constriction of the superficial blood vessels of the skin and organs. This constriction shunts blood away from the skin and organs, and sends it to the head to keep the brain from getting too cold.

The diverting of blood from the skin causes the skin to cool in the absence of the warm circulating blood. The normal amount of blood left in the skin in response to the 68 degree cold stimulus of a CRT test is enough blood to maintain a 0.3-1.0 degree cooler temperature after ten minutes of exposure.

When the organ underlying the point being tested is not functioning correctly, your skin temperature will show the type of dysfunction by the difference in the first and second CRT temperature readings. Correlations can then be made to all of the other temperature readings. Your CRT test will reveal much about your state of health.

Chapter 56

Lyme Disease Meets Biological Dentistry

Get a Biological Dentist to Check Your Dental Work…

Biological Dentists are all previously conventional dentists who became aware that the teeth play an important role in the overall health of the body. One of the leaders in Biological Medicine, Dr. Thomas Rau, M.D., stated that if he could have only one other doctor to work with him, it would be a biological dentist. This is because of increasing amount of research showing a connection between cancer, degenerative diseases, and infectious diseases and the heavy metals and toxins leaching out of dental materials, appliances, and root canals.

You have read earlier in this book about Circuit Healing™ (Chapter 11). These circuits are electrical/energetic organ circuits in the body that have been identified through thousands of years of research and only recently verified by technology. Each tooth has been determined to share the same electrical pathway as a specific organ, gland, spinal segment, joint, and muscle group. Anything goes wrong in the circuit and they all share the same fate. The entire circuit can be poisoned by toxins leaking into the circuit. For example, a "silver" or more accurately called mercury amalgam in a wisdom tooth will steadily release small amounts of the mercury, tin, silver and nickel that the amalgam is made up of into the heart and brain specifically, because the wisdom teeth and these organs share the same circuitry. Hidden infections and cavitations in the jawbones will leak bacterial toxins throughout the entire circuit wreaking havoc as well.

Teeth are hiding places for Lyme spirochetes that must be resolved, because they are a major interference to the body's efforts to heal. Research reported in the book, Root Canal Cover-Up Exposed, by Dr. George E. Meinig, D.D.S., F.A.C.D., stated that Dr. Weston Price, a renowned dental researcher performed thousands of tests on people with chronic degenerative diseases – those that did not respond to treatment. He found root canals harbored bacteria inside the microscopic dental tubules of the dead tooth. He found that most often the bacteria to be pleomorphic, as described earlier, and that most often the bacteria were streptococcus, staphylococcus, and spirochetes! People, how important is it to recognize that Lyme spirochetes can be hiding in your old root canals and jaw infections?

The next finding of Dr. Price's is monumental – he found that even when the root canalled tooth is extracted and heat sterilized it did not stay sterile. Dr. Price found that within 24-48 hours the disinfecting medications lost their disinfecting ability. People, this is when they are trying to kill all the bacteria specifically in the teeth, not like typical Lyme disease antibiotic treatments, which attempt to kill bacteria everywhere in the body! So, one can see further evidence of the extreme limitations of antibiotics against most microbes.

In some amazing research he found that he could surgically implant the old root canal tooth under the skin of a rabbit and the rabbit would develop the same disease as the person the tooth belonged to! Very often, once the root canal tooth was removed, a large percentage of the patients recovered.

Even though many dentists believe the methods they are using to seal and sterilize root canals are efficient, Dr. Price found that the bacteria remain within the microscopic tubules of the teeth and even in the rare occasion where they cannot escape from these tubules, their toxins can still leach out through the cementum sealers. Most often however, he found a disturbing fact, that these bacteria are almost always found in the first few millimeters of the adjacent bone in the jaw.

Dr. Price's findings have been confirmed by many bacteriologists. What this means to you is that if heat sterilization does not ensure the killing of the Lyme spirochetes inside of your teeth, that antibiotics, which you now understand are not that effective in the first place, have little chance of reaching these hiding places. This may be why so many people seem to mysteriously get "reinfected" or suffer a relapse of the Lyme disease.

"Dental factors have been associated not only with the cause but also with the cure of chronic disease." Also, research has demonstrated that "factors contributing to chronic degenerative diseases include energy blockages and toxicity from mercury amalgam dental fillings. Symptoms ascribed to mercury toxicity include fatigue, depression, anorexia, insomnia, arthritis, moodiness, irritability, memory loss, nausea, diarrhea, gum disease, swollen glands, and headaches, among others." Published studies have reported reversal of illness in such cases as Multiple Sclerosis, Alzheimer's, Cancer, Arthritis, and Parkinson's. Read: *The Key to Ultimate Health*, by Ellen Hodgson-Brown and Richard T. Hansen, DDS.

Research performed by Dr. Harold Hawkins, D.D.S., Melvin Page,

D.D.S., and Emanuel Cheraskin, M.D., D.M.D. and many others found that people with tooth decay are more susceptible to degenerative disease. Understand now that each tooth effects every tissue and organ on its electro-energetic circuit, so decay from the tooth could be from poor dental hygiene, but it could also be the tooth is having problems due to problems in the organ, gland, muscle, or joints that share the same circuit with that tooth. One begins to see even more clearly why doctors must specialize in addressing the entire body, including the teeth, instead of specializing in "pieces and parts" doctoring.

Get on the internet and use the keywords "Biological Dentistry" to find a local doctor. Only a dentist who has been trained this way will know what to do for you and have the correct tools and knowledge to undo the damage.

The political environment is such that at this time no claims for treating organic disturbances can be made by a Biological Dentist. So please respect this and come to him having already done your homework, i.e., reading the above book and others. That way you can simply request a Biological Dental Assessment and removal of potentially harmful filling materials for cosmetic reasons.

Section 11

No Doctors Practicing Biological Medicine In Your Area? Then Come See Us.

Chapter 57

The Somerleyton Center
For
Biological Medicine

Everyone is looking for good doctors…
We are looking for good patients

Good Doctors… Forever Learning and Improving

Our Doctors are all nationally and State Board certified and licensed to treat the whole person. They are trained in the latest advances of European and American scientific healing methods. Truly, aspects of the best healing methods from around the world have been melded into a functional method of healing we call Circuit Healing™. Circuit Healing™ was created right here at the Somerleyton Center, by Dr. David A. Jernigan D.C., and is now taught to other healing centers around the world.

Our doctors are trained to facilitate and work with the body's own efforts to heal, instead of forcing the body to do something. Our doctors believe the true definition of doctor is…One who guides, teaches, and facilitates life-balance and healing through natural means, and God-designed living.

Our passion is helping those people with chronic illness of any type. We want those people whose doctors have thrown up their hands in resignation, or told them that "it is all in your head." Armed with phenomenal adjunctive diagnostic and treatment tools, such as Bio-Resonance Scanning™ (BRS) and Computerized Regulation Thermodiagnostics (CRT), along with approximately 5,000 of the world's best natural remedies at our disposal and over 56 different tools and healing techniques to facilitate the body's ability to heal itself, our doctors favorite patients are what we affectionately call our "Humpty-Dumpty Bunch," whom all the king's horses and all the king's men couldn't put back together again.

Not every patient can be saved, but almost every patient can be helped. There is only one thing we can guarantee, if you continue doing the same thing, you will continue getting the same result. It would be very surprising to hear someone say we are doing more of the same in our Circuit Healing™ program. Even people who think they have tried everything are surprised at our diversity of healing.

Our doctors do not want to be just "another doctor" to be added to the long list of doctors you have seen. We want everyone to say, "I am a better, healthier person because of the Somerleyton Center for Biological Medicine."

Good Patients...Our Expectations of You

At the Somerleyton Center for Biological Medicine, we are looking for certain types of patients. Regardless to the type of illness, the only patients accepted are those people desiring to participate in their healing. Our happiest patients are those who came seeking healing and enlightenment in Body, Mind, and Spirit in a Christian Environment.

One cannot come with the mindset of "Okay, I'm here...now heal me!" We expect you to be teachable, guidable, and follow through with our process of transformation and healing.

In this Information Age we now live in, patients are more educated than ever. However, much of the information is based upon mainstream medicine's "pieces and parts" mentality and pharmacology. There will be much required reading and accountability for the information read, so that you understand the science behind Circuit Healing™, why we are using the many different therapies, and so that you will be able to share your new found health knowledge with all you come in contact with.

During your time at Somerleyton Center you will be empowered by knowledge to make lasting change in your life, and the lives of those you care about.

Take a quiz to see if you qualify:

Y/N   Do you seek to improve every aspect of your life?

Y/N   Are you a chronic learner?

Y/N   Are you humble enough to receive instruction and act on it?

Y/N   Can you commit to a program requiring a large commitment of time?

(Initially 3-4 hours per week in clinic, plus homework)

Y/N   Are you willing to change your lifestyle for the better?

Y/N   Do you see yourself as on a journey?

Y/N   Do you seek to be healed as a result of and through your journey?

Y/N   Do you want to be taught to be responsible for your health?

Y/N   Are you interested in learning how your body works and what must happen to maintain health?

Y/N   Do you seek to expand your perceptions of reality?

Y/N   Would you want to help others learn from your journey?

If you answered "Yes" to these questions we believe you will fit well into our family of patients at the Somerleyton Center for Biological Medicine.

Time for Restoration and Transformation

I tell every new patient that the biggest commitment in our program of care is TIME... not money. Your time is precious, however, you must decide to bend your life's schedule to allow the necessary time to follow through with your healing program. To ensure maximum results we cannot bend our program around your life. We will make all efforts to provide you with the most convenient appointment times for your life's schedule.

Your time here should be viewed much the same as attending College, where you must attend whenever class is actually in session, and a good grade for the class is the result of receiving all of the instructor's knowledge. Each office visit may take an hour or more to complete the treatments, therapies, and educational materials. One should also plan on time spent at home for lifestyle changes and home therapies.

The orchestration of your time with us has been given much forethought and consideration to ensure that you receive maximum restoration of your quality of life, and that you are transformed to a higher level of existence.

Throughout history, the two primary responsibilities of the patient were to simply show up for their appointments and to take their medicines. This "health in a bottle" mentality has unquestionably been shown to be a myth. Americans suffer some of the worst health in the world, even though we take more prescription medicines and more dietary supplements and even eat the widest range of foods than any other country. Health in a bottle does not work!

The truth is that illness is always the result of an imbalanced life. Illness is the result of extremes in life…too much stress, too little exercise, too much mental activity, too little relaxation, too much of a food, too little of other foods, too much accumulated toxins, and the list goes on…all of which can be passed on to the next generation causing inborn predispositions and tendencies to illness.

This concept can be seen in another way. The habits and ruts we have been living with for years have created the reality of today. The very process of changing and getting out of the ruts of your life will necessarily cause an entirely new reality. Spending the time and effort on treatments, therapies and lifestyle choices will breed the improvements in life quality.

The Programs of Care

It must be understood that healing takes time. Our patients are those who have been chronically ill. By definition this means that they have been growing sicker for a long time. It also should be clear that it will take a long time before full correction is realized. Our Programs of Care are based upon an initial two-week program with a view of up to a year-long estimation of what will be necessary to truly begin the healing process.

Does anyone really believe that they are miraculously healed when Tylenol immediately relieves a painful headache? There is no healing going on here! The causes of the headaches remain untouched. This is symptom relief only. True healing can never occur by simply masking the symptoms.

If you cut yourself, I hope you have a Band-Aid, because I cannot heal your cut. Most people do not get very concerned over a small cut, because it is totally expected that their body will heal that cut in time. But what if the cut didn't heal? Would you go to the doctor so that he could put stitches in it to close it up? If you did, what would happen the next time you cut yourself? This may sound ridiculous, but this is basically what the standard of treatment is for chronic problems. It only makes sense that the ideal thing to do is seek a doctor who can identify and help remove whatever is interfering with the body's ability to heal the cut.

The goal of your year long program of care is to, through Circuit Healing™; provide the maximum care, leaving no aspect of your being unaddressed. If every tissue and aspect of the body is brought back into healthy balance, and every interference is removed…there can be no illness.

Since only your body can truly heal itself, our goal is to keep it functioning at peak efficiency long enough and consistently enough that the body can finally get the job done.

Through years of dealing with the chronically ill people, our doctors have developed programs of care, since we know what needs to happen to achieve maximum results. Our doctors determine which program is best for you after completing the case history, in the case of out-of-state or out-of-country patients, and for those in town after the completed physical exam. This way, out-of-towners can have some idea of expected costs and time for planning their schedule.

It is usually a surprise to people that they may be required to come in three to six times per week, and our doctors are doing something different on almost every visit. Some people feel somewhat off-balance initially because of this. They are so used to the doctors generally just talking to them a little, possibly doing some testing, and writing a prescription – and definitely not seeing their doctor two to three to six times per week!

We see your initial three months of care as being an Intensive Care of sorts. During this phase of care we are being very aggressive, yet gentle enough so that you do not go into a crisis. Since our doctors specialize in the entire human organism instead of specializing in just one body system, there is much more work to be done.

Circuit Healing involves keeping all of the electrical organ circuits up and running at maximum efficiency for the entire year! Seeing how the body and illness is dynamic and constantly changing, all the treatments must be dynamic and change to adjust to the way the body and illness have changed between visits. This concept of dynamic change can be easily seen in the way some bacteria can mutate and become resistant to an antibiotic within 20 minutes of taking it! Would your doctor be able to detect when the medicine is no longer working and needs to be changed? This is the challenge to all doctors, and also why we used adjunctive testing methods like Bio-Resonance Scanning™ (BRS). BRS allows our doctors to know when the treatments need to be modified.

One of the biggest surprises to most patients is that you are immediately placed into our Educational Program, which is a part of every extended Program of Care. In the Educational Program you are given required reading of short topics to enhance your healing experience. This is not an "elective"; it is required reading and yes there will be quizzes. Remember that the definition of doctor is "Teacher". We are teaching you to live a balanced life and to demystify how your body works and heals itself. There are videos and lectures all of which lead to Certificates of Completion, and Recognitions of Achievement, all leading to diploma status (unaccredited) and Mentoring Programs where you may be able to assist with incoming new patients education. We desire to empower you through health and knowledge.

All of the programs are designed to achieve four basic goals, which are to result in Happy, Healthy, Drug-Free, Well-Educated patients.

Chapter 58

Statement of My Faith

To Whom It May Concern,

Thank you for this opportunity to share with you what I believe and where my faith comes from. From time to time patients ask me what religious orientation I come from and if the methods of healing I use are based upon God's Word, so this letter should help set the basic foundation of this clinic.

I am a Christian by faith, and I believe with all that I am in the accuracy and truth of God's Word – The Holy Bible.

I believe in and do confess with my mouth the Lord Jesus Christ, and I do believe in my heart that God raised Jesus Christ from the dead, and am therefore saved. Romans 10:10 says, "For with the heart man believeth unto righteousness; and with the mouth confession is made unto salvation." I believe it is the God in Christ in me that works to will and do of His good pleasure.

Most of the people that ask me about my faith are also wanting to know if what we do at the clinic is "New Age". To answer this, first and foremost, I have not made a study of the "New Age" philosophy. As a child of God, I have the responsibility of separating truth from error on a moment by moment basis. Therefore, when I desire to be able to identify counterfeits, I do not study the many ways of counterfeiting, I only have to study the original and genuine. God's Word is THE ORIGINAL. From this perspective, with the Word of God as my foundation for truth, counterfeits are easily identified.

I will say that the closer to the original, the greater the counterfeit. With this in mind, I can see that one must not allow themselves to robbed of the heavenly power promised to God's children in an attempt to avoid "New Age" principles. Remember, the adversary cannot create anything (Only God can create something from nothingness) – the adversary can work only within the laws of this universe. The adversary can only manipulate the laws of the universe to bring glory to himself. My goal is to bring glory to God in heaven.

Many Christians recognize the work of the adversary in the New Age movement. Instead of being fearful, Christians should say, "Hey, if the adversary can do signs, miracles, and wonders and he understands the energy of the universe, just think what signs, miracles, and wonders I can do through God's power that works within and through me, to glorify God, by having God the original and only Creator on my side." (John 14:12) (Philippians 2:13) (Colossians 1:27)

Sincerity is no guarantee of truth. History is full of very sincere people labeling new things as "of the devil", only to find out later that it was based upon fact. For example, for hundreds of years it was believed by all of the wise men of the world that blood did not circulate throughout the human body. Along came a scientist who proposed and demonstrated that it did indeed circulate. This was not well received by the wise men at first. Today, many very sincere people are propagating fear in the Christian community about the New Age. From what I can tell, many of the principles of the New Age are close to what the Bible says is available to the children of God. Miraculous things are promised to be available to believers and yet the churches for the most part are not teaching how to access and utilize all the power promised to God's kids.

I believe it when John 10:10 states that "The thief cometh not but to steal, kill, and destroy: I (Jesus) am come that they may have life, and that they might have it more abundantly."

I believe my first concern is to keep myself lined up with God's Word.

I believe that as a child of God, we are joint heirs with Christ. (Rom 8:18)

Luke 10: 17-19 says that even the demons are subject to us through the power of the Christ in us – In My name I give you power, and power over all the power of the enemy (dark side), and nothing shall hurt you. In my mind, God's Word is either all truth or all a lie. I know God's Word is true.

As a doctor, I feel that I am in a unique position to destroy the works of the adversary, i.e., stealing your ability to work for a living through illness, killing you physically, destroying your fellowship with God through his destroying your health, breaking your spirit.

I have a different view than most on the realities of Somerleyton Center, which is based upon 1 Chronicles 29: 11-12. I belong to God. This is God's clinic. God brings who He wants to be here. The techniques and natural medicines belong to Him. I work as unto God. God our Heavenly Father heals.

We have not advertised our clinic for 8+years. There is no big sign out in front of our office. If you are here it is because God wanted you here.

I pray that I will always manifest the heart of a servant, and my God given ability to help those He sends in need.

Yours in Health and Healing,

Drs. David & Sara Jernigan, D.C., B.S.

Chapter 59

It is Your Body.

It is Your Decision.

**(The following is written to help you handle those who may
oppose your decision to heal naturally.)**

Someone you know has decided to heal, live or die their way… using
Biological Medicine. This decision is easy for some and not so easy to
make for others. One way or the other we will all have to decide for
ourselves how we want to heal, live, and die. It is a very personal decision,
although friends, family, doctors, and "Joe at the pub" all seem to know
exactly what someone else should do. Try to put yourself in this person's
position and understand that they have arrived at their decision in an
intelligent manner.

Biological Medicine is a well-documented and well-researched method
of healing that was first developed in Switzerland and is now practiced in
countries all over the world. The doctors who now practice Biological
Medicine, were all board certified in conventional medicine. All of the
biological doctors saw the short comings of conventional medicine and
through great courage spent many extra years of training in Biological
Medicine.

Leading edge research is being published in this type of medicine at the
rate of about 1000 peer-reviewed articles per month. The success of
Biological Medicine is so overwhelming in some types of cases that new
hospitals around the world are being set up to specifically provide these
services.

The methods and treatments in Biological Medicine are not conventional.
However, they can be incredibly effective. The basic premise is that for
every illness, there is a cause, which is, an interference to the body's ability
to heal itself. Keep in mind that the most astute and celebrated physicians
cannot even heal the simplest paper cut. The body must and always must
do the healing. This is true for a cut and it is also true in the worst illnesses
of our time. Biological Medicine seeks to identify and remove any

interference to the body's ability to heal itself, while providing the building blocks and information necessary to restore balance in all aspects of life.

The winds of change are upon us, no place more obvious than in health care. There is a generational gap between those who were raised to accept the word of their Conventional Medical Doctor without question, and those who have become disillusioned to the entire pharmaceutical path chosen by most doctors.

Every doctor practices in the most conscientious manner, based upon their training. All doctors sincerely believe what they are advising you to do is best. The very nature of the business requires a doctor to believe that they do all that should be done, so that when real people die the doctor can go on knowing they did everything they thought was needed. But, sincerity is no guarantee of truth.

I have often heard people say, "My conventional doctor is so nice, and he goes to my church, and has taken care of my family for years." They go on to say, "I don't want to hurt his feelings and not do the conventional drugs that he recommends." My point here is that you must do what you know to be true for yourself. You should not relinquish your health to the responsibility of someone else just to be nice. It is your body, and it is your decision to make, as to how you want to be treated. You are smart enough to determine your own way.

Illnesses of life or death:

It is not popular to discuss the potential of death. However, I have seen too many people who desperately wanted to choose Biological Medicine as their way to live or die, only to be badgered and harassed into conventional medicine where they died a miserable death. Try to understand the one you care for is not wanting to die, but if death comes they want to face it their own way.

One woman's story communicates this well. Having been diagnosed with a terminal relapse of cancer in 21 different places in her body. The lady told her family that she was going to a Biological Medicine clinic not expecting to get "cured", she was going so that she could be as completely balanced physically, mentally, emotionally, and spiritually for herself and her family in her last days. We see death as a transition only… many do not want to be drugged-up and incoherent when they go. At the Somerleyton

Center for Biological Medicine we strive to maximize LIFE, whether that life lasts two weeks or 100 years... right up to the last minute.

A Word to Our Patients:

Doctors, friends and family may oppose natural medicine, and the philosophy of "do no harm," but ultimately the choice is completely yours to make. It is your body. Be true to yourself. Don't let their fear poison you. It may even be necessary to separate yourself from these negative influences while you heal. Their fear and negativity will definitely upset the balance that you are striving to achieve. In the Bible it says,

"Behold, we put bits in the horses' mouths, that they may obey us, and we turn about their whole body. Behold, also the ships, which though they be so great, and are driven of fierce winds, yet are they turned about with a very small helm, whithersoever the governor listeth. Even so the tongue is a little member, and boasted great things. Behold, how great a matter a little fire kindleth! And the tongue is a fire, a world of iniquity: so is the tongue among our members, that it defileth the whole body, and setteth on fire the course of nature; and it is set on fire of hell. For every kind of beast, and of birds, and of serpents, and of things in the sea, is tamed, and hath been tamed of mankind: But the tongue can no man tame; it is an unruly evil, full of deadly poison." James 3: 3-8

You also should be at peace with your decision to follow this path. In your heart of hearts you need to be committed to this path. In healing as in photography, if you are constantly losing focus then your end result will be blurry. You are to be as committed to the path of wellness as an athlete training for the Olympics. It is no one else's decision to make. You must decide to become a Spiritual Athlete, a Physical Athlete, and an Athlete of the Mind.

Consider chemotherapy for a moment. It is the dominant cancer treatment at this time. If your body is constantly sending you signals to let you know where you are out of balance, what message is being sent when all of your hair falls out, organs shutdown from toxicity, and your immune system is greatly reduced? I choose to view all illness as signs of imbalance, and I consider true healing to be those treatments and methods that restore balance.

At Somerleyton Center for Biological Medicine, we are here to attract those patients who have chosen to have circuit healing, to get their bodies to heal itself. We are not a cancer clinic, a Lyme disease clinic, nor do we try to cure any chronic illness. Our primary function, is just this simple; true healing cannot occur by simply masking the symptoms or by pushing around bacteria. True healing comes from within your body. Therefore, our goal is to maximize your body's ability to heal itself.

References

All references are listed either in the text where they occur or are provided below.

Chapter 3

1. Mattman, L., Cell Wall Deficient Forms, Stealth Pathogens, 2nd Ed. 1992.

2. Per telephone conversation with Dr. Lida Mattman Ph.D., July, 1999.

3. Mattman, L., Cell Wall Deficient Forms, Stealth Pathogens, 2nd Ed. 1992.

4. Cotran, Kumar, Robbins. Robbins Pathological Basis of Disease. 4th Edition

5. Mattman, L., Cell Wall Deficient Forms, Stealth Pathogens, 2nd Ed. 1992.

6. Murphy R. Lotus Materia Medica, Lotus Star Academy Publishing,

Chapter 7

1. Mattman, L., Cell Wall Deficient Forms, Stealth Pathogens, 2nd Ed., p 13, 1992.

2. Popular Science, April 1999

3. Donta, S.T., Fibromyalgia, Lyme Disease, and Gulf War Syndrome, 12th International Conference on Lyme Disease, New York, 1999.

4. Nicolson, G.L., Nasralla, M. Hier, J. and Nicolson, N.L. Mycoplasmal infections in chronic illnesses: Fibromyalgia and Chronic Fatigue Syndromes, Gulf War Illness, HIV-AIDS and Rheumatoid Arthritis. Med. Sentinel 1999.

5. Nicolson, G.L., The Institute for Molecular Medicine, 1999.

Chapter 8

1. A Novel Toxin (Bb Tox 1) of Borrelia burgdorferi, Mark J. Cartwright, Ph.D.

2. Martin, S.E., Donita, S.T., International Conference on Lyme Disease, New York, April, 1999.

Chapter 9

1. Coyle, P.K., Neurologic Lyme Disease Update, International Conference on Lyme Disease, New York, 1999.

Chapter 23

1. Chaitow, 1987

2. Morton MA, Doulhy C 1989 Energy Fields in Medicine. John E. Fetzer Foundation, Kalamazoo MI

3. Oschman JL, 2000 Energy Medicine, The Scientific Basis, Churchill Livingstone

4. Chien CH, Tseui JJ, et al. 1991 Effect of emitted bioenergy on biochemical function of cells. American Journal of Chinese Medicine 19:285-292

5. Adolf EF, 1982 Physiological Integrations in Action. Physiologist 25 (2) (April) Supplement

6. Kobayashi A, Kirschvink JL 1995 Magnetoreception and electromagnetic field effects: sensory perception of the geomagnetic fields in animals and humans. In Blank M (ed) Electromagnetic fields: biological American Chemical Society, Washington DC pp 367-394

7. Baule GM, McFee R 1963 Detection of the magnetic field of the heart. American Heart Journal 66: 95-96

8. Cohen D 1967 Magnetic fields around the torso: production by electrical activity of the human heart. Science 156:652-654

Marinellli R, van der Furst, 1995 The heart is not a pump: a refutation of the pressure propulsion premise of heart function. Frontier Perspectives 5:15-24

9. Oschman JL, 2000 Energy Medicine, The Scientific Basis, Churchill Livingstone

10. Oschman JL, 2000 Energy Medicine, The Scientific Basis, Churchill Livingstone

For additional reading on Electromagnetic Pollution on your Body: Becker RO 1990 Crosscurrents: The perils of electropollution, the promise of electromedicine. Los Angeles, CA Wolff M 1993 Fundamental laws, microphysics, and cosmology. Physics Essays 6:181-203

Chapter 26

1. Murphy, R., Lotus Materia Medica, Lotus Star Academy Publishing, 1995.

2. Davidson, J., Subtle Energy, p. 222-28, C W Daniel Co, 1993.

Appendix A

Recommended Reading

-*Nourishing Traditions*, Sally Fallon

-*Energy Medicine, The Scientific Basis*, Oschman

-*Reference Guide for Essential Oils*, Connie and Alan Higley

-*Eat Right for Your Type*, Dr. Peter J. D'Adamo, N.M.D.

-*Excitotoxins, The Taste that Kills*, Russell L. Blaylock, M.D.

-*What Your Doctor May Not Tell You About Menopause*, John R. Lee, M.D.

-*Cell-Wall Deficient Bacteria, Stealth Pathogen,* 2nd edition, Lida Mattman, Ph.D.

- *Prozac; Panacea or Pandora*, Dr. Ann Blake Tracy, Ph.D.

- *The Rest of the Gospel; When the Partial Gospel has Worn You Out*, Dan Stone and Greg Smith (800- 915-8771)

Appendix B

Internet Resources

Lyme Disease Foundation
    www.lyme.org
Lyme Disease Network
    www.lymenet.org
American Lyme Disease Foundation
    www.aldf.com
Center for Disease Control - Lyme Disease Site
    www.cdc.gov/ncidod/diseases/lyme
Lyme Alliance
    www.lymealliance.org
Lyme Disease in the United States & useful links
    www.geocities.com/HotSprings/Spa/6772/
        lyme.html
National Center for Homeopathy
    www.healthy.net/nch
Eat Right For Your Type - Dr. D'Adamo
    www.dadamo.com
Alternative Medicine Practitioners Directory
    www.altmedweb.com
IGENEX Reference Laboratory
    www.igenex.com
HealthWorld Online - Free Medline
    www.healthy.net
alternativemedicine.com

Appendix C

For Doctors Only

Biological Medicine Training for Doctors is available.

Call for more details at 316-686-5900.

Doctor discounts are available on certain products. One must provide the name of the clinic, the name of the doctor, address and phone number and the tax ID number in order to receive doctor prices.

Appendix D

Research On Borrelogen™

Acute Oral Toxicity Test – ISO

Borrelogen has been found to be essentially non-toxic at 150 times the maximum recommended dosage.

ISO is designed to assess the acute oral toxicity of the test substance, Borrelogen, occurring within 14 days of the oral administration of a single dose or multiple doses of the test substance administered within 24 hours.

The test substance, Borrelogen, was evaluated for its potential to produce death following oral administration at a dose of 2 grams/ kilogram of body weight in male and female Sprague-Dawley rats. Based on the absence of mortality and the criteria of the study protocol, *the test substance is defined as nontoxic.* This study was conducted in compliance with the U.S. Food and Drug Administration (FDA) regulations set forth in 21 CFR, Part 58 and OECD GLPs, current version. The sections of the regulations not performed by or under the direction of Toxikon Corp, exempt from this Good Laboratory Practice statement, include characterization and stability of the test and its mixture with carriers, 21 CFR, Part 58.105, and 58.113. The assessment of an LD_{50} was not necessary. No toxicity was observed in post study necropsy of the different organ systems[1].

Why Borrelogen™ is considered effective

Borrelia burgdorferi antigen release stimulation by nutraceutical formula as determined by Lyme Urine Antigen Testing (LUAT)

It is understood that antigens are the cause of numerous sensitivities resulting in much of the symptomology experienced in chronic illness.

This clinical study was restricted to determining whether Borrelia burgdorferi specific antigen could be purged from circulation by the use of a nutraceutical formula called Borrelogen. The results are very preliminary as more research is needed to rule out physiological interference. LUAT assay was utilized to determine antigen release after 68 subjects used the nutraceutical for one week. Results revealed 73% of the subjects released specific antigen to the degree of being considered positive or highly positive by LUAT. (Only seventeen of the 68 subjects were tested by Lyme Western Blot IgM/IgG prior to starting Borrelogen. All seventeen subjects were either Equivocal or Positive via this serological assay.) This study in itself cannot be used to make definitive statements about the efficacy of Borrelogen, only that an antigen was released from whatever mechanism. Note: IGeneX is not in any way endorsing this nutraceutical, nor is IGeneX associated in any way with Jernigan Nutraceuticals, Inc. IGeneX was blinded to the use of the nutraceutical and only performed the testing procedure. True research seeks to find the truth in an unbiased manner for the betterment of mankind.

Introduction

Bacteria contain many particulate and soluble antigens that evoke strong, often lasting immune responses, both humoral and cellular.[2] According to Stedman's Medical Dictionary, an antigen (allergen); is any substance that, as a result of coming into contact with appropriate tissues induces a state of sensitivity.[3] Antigens are understood to cause many of the symptoms experienced by LD sufferers. It would stand to reason that decreasing the antigen load on the body would correspondingly decrease the number and severity of symptoms. A proprietary nutraceutical formulation was developed in 1998 to specifically target the functional release of spirochetal antigen from the tissues of the body. The historical and pharmacognostic data of the individual plant-based extracts reveal very low toxicity, while being functionally beneficial in many ways to the body. The research presented here was performed as a clinical study to aid in our understanding of the potential effectiveness of the nutraceutical formula, Borrelogen™. Lyme Urine Antigen Testing

(LUAT) was chosen as a viable determinant due to its specificity to Borrelia burgdorferi antigens seen as a result of a release of antigen from an appropriately applied therapy. Because the body will as a natural process release Lyme specific antigen in about 30% of untreated cases, the nutraceutical formula was tested to see if the body could be stimulated to release a greater amount of antigen, with a higher percentage of positive LUATs. A nutraceutical is defined as a plant-based remedy that is specifically formulated to target specific body dysfunctions.[4]

Methods

Participants in this study were pre-selected based on positive Borrelia burgdorferi screening using, Bio-Resonance Scanning™ assay. The group consisted of 68 people residing in a non-endemic area of the United States. All were suffering from a range of 3 to 44 chronic problems based on a 55 question Lyme disease symptom questionnaire. Lyme Urine Antigen Testing (LUAT) was utilized to monitor the release of antigen. LUAT testing is an antigen capture assay specific to detection of low levels of antigen, in spite of the presence of other proteins. The antibody being used in this antigen capture is a unique polyclonal antibody that is specific for the 31 kDa (OpsA), 34 kDa (OpsB), 39 kDa, and 93 kDa antigens of Borrelia burgdorferi. This assay appears to be very specific to these antigens with a reported false positive rate of less than 1% in a study of 408 controls.[4] The reference range of a LUAT is based on P-values or confidence levels. Antigen levels reported as ⊕32 ng/ml have a 95% confidence level of being positive and distinguishable from a negative population.[4] A LUAT is a highly controlled and reproducible assay which is used in conjunction with patient history, symptoms and serumpanels. The nice thing about LUAT assay is that it is positive throughout all three stages of infection: early, which is said to be <60 days (which is before you normally can get a seropositive result); second stage, which is defined as 60 – 360 days; and the third stage >360 days.[5]

Result

Reporting only the highest score of the three-day urine collection the majority of positive LUATs scored over 100 ng/ml. Out of the 68 LUATs performed 44 were reported as positive or highly positive, while there were 4 borderline, and 18 negative results. The total percentage of positive scores was 73%. When the nutraceutical formula was used instead of prescription antibiotics the majority of positive LUATs were reported over 100 ng/ml, and as high as >400 ng/ml. Although a score of >400 does not indicate that a patient is more highly infected than a score of >45, it does indicate a high rate of antigen release which can only benefit the patient. An interesting side-note, only seventeen of these 68 cases were also tested by Lyme Western Blot IgM/IgG prior to taking the Borrelogen. All seventeen subjects tested as positive or equivocal by Lyme Western Blot.

Conclusion

Based on this study, it appears that this nutraceutical formula does indeed stimulate the purging of Borrelia burgdorferi antigens from the body. This antigen-detox can only be seen as a good thing as these antigens when circulating throughout the body cause a multitude of systemic sensitivities, which in turn causes increased suffering in the patient. An infected person does not release antigens daily or uniformly.[6] The fact that in this study, 73% of the time when using this nutraceutical a high release of antigen was stimulated is significant.

Further research must be performed to determine if a negative control group on the same protocol would yield a similar effect. However, based on positive patient symptomatic response and clinical observations we are encouraged that this botanical formula may effectively stimulate and increase the tissue elimination of deleterious antigen via the urine. Further research may also result in increased probability of highly positive Lyme Urine Antigen Test confirmations.

Interference studies performed by IGeneX lab confirmed that Borrelogen does not cause a false positive LUAT when negative patient urines were spiked in various concentrations. This *in vitro* assay does not, however, effectively rule out the possibility of *in vivo* interference.[7]

References - Appendix D

1. Glenn T. Shawaery, G. TPH.D., 99G -09-05, 1999 Toxikon Corp. Sponsored by International Nutraceutical Research Group

2. Cotran, Kumar, Robbins. Robbins Pathological Basis of Disease.

3. Stedman's Mediacl Dictionary. 25th ed. Williams & Wilkins

4. Journal of Neutraceuticals and Functional Foods, 1994

5. Callister SM, Schell RF. Laboratory Serodiagnosis of Lyme Borreliosis. J. Spirochetal Tick-borne Inf 1998;1:21.

6. Harris NS. IgeneX Reference Laboratory Guide. 1998;4.

7. Harris NS, Stephens BG. Detection of Borrelia burgdorferi Antigen in Urine from patients with Lyme Burreliosis. Journal of Spirochetal Tick-borne Inf. 1995;2:41.

Glossary

Applied Kinesiology- A treatment technique used primarily by Doctors of Chiropractic, but also by some Medical Doctors, which uses a patient's neuro-muscular system to identify problem areas in the body to determine the most effective treatment. This type of treatment is very individualized to the patient and helps to eliminate guesswork on the part of the doctor.

Auto-suggestion- a condition where an unconscious reaction to news suggesting that something may happen causes fear that leads to weakening of the body's energetic defenses, setting one up for illness. An example would be the news on T.V. that "Flu season is here. Reports are coming in that many people are experiencing a scratchy throat and fatigue, with body aches" Upon hearing this report many start remembering past flus and may "hope" they don't come down with this one.

Clinical Kinesiology- the offspring of Applied Kinesiology which is even more precise in determining not only what the patient's brain thinks is most important, but also uses the patient's brain as a bio-computer to determine the most effective treatments.

Electro-dermal Testing- this encompasses many different types of machines, which are usually computerized. Through meridian contact points, doctors can determine which systems of the body are being most stressed, what specific problems the body has, and which remedies will correct the problems.

Excitotoxins- a substance added to foods and beverages that literally stimulates neurons to death, causing brain damage of varying degrees. Can be found in such ingredients as monosodium glutamate (MSG), aspartame (NutraSweet), cysteine, hydrolyzed protein, and aspartic acid.

Homeopathy- a form of medicine in which the "electrical signature" of a substance is harnessed and imprinted upon a carrier substance such as distilled water or milk sugar crystals. Most homeopathic remedies contain no molecules of the original substance, but only carry the homeopathically modified electrical signature of that substance. *"Homeo,"* meaning similar, and *"pathy"*, meaning symptoms. By definition, a homeopathic remedy is a remedy which will create "symptoms" when repeated doses are given to a healthy individual. Conversely, for an unhealthy individual, it will cure the symptoms.

Meridians - These are superficial electro-energetic pathways that do not follow nerves. Meridians have been the subject of much controversy in western medicine for hundreds of years, even being called "of the devil" by well-meaning churches. However, the National Institute of Health recently announced that these meridians have been found to be a naturally occurring phenomenon verified by MRI. The controversy was due to the fact that up until recently no one could physically dissect out or see these meridians. A Korean scientist has been reported as having actually dissected these meridians, further documenting their existence. Meridian therapies include low-level lasers, microcurrent therapies, bio-electrical treatments, acupuncture and acupressure. These meridian therapies, as well as Electro-dermal Testing, seek to facilitate healing by stimulating and/or balancing the many meridians of the body.

Mycoplasma - A class of organism which is normally non-pathogenic. Its size is said to be in between that of a virus and a bacteria. Interestingly, the Gulf War Syndrome is causing many of the same symptoms as Lyme Disease and is now said to be caused by Mycoplasma fermentans incognitus.

Number Credulous Medicine - The practice of medicine that focuses on the microscopic view of the blood. This type of medicine reduces the importance of the human as an interdependent, interconnected, fully integrated organism and sees the patient from a strictly numerical basis. Focus is placed primarily upon numbers and percentages on a laboratory blood test and the response of those numbers to the treatments applied.

Nutraceuticals- complex plant based medicines.

Pleomorphic- the ability of an organism to change shapes at different stages of its life. *"pleo"*, meaning "many", and *"morph"*, meaning "shapes". A butterfly is said to be pleomorphic in that it is a caterpillar, then a butterfly.

Preamble- immediately preceding an event, such as signs and symptoms that come before the actual disease.

Spirochete- a class of pathogenic bacteria typified by its spiral or corkscrew shape. Lyme disease is caused by a spirochete called Borrelia burgdorferi.

Suppressive Therapies- medicines and therapies that suppress or weaken the body's natural reactions and mechanisms of bio-regulation. Any time you take a medicine that performs a task that the body should do for itself, the body becomes weak from disuse. Antibiotics are a suppressive treatment in that they weaken the immune system and disturb the normal fluid transportation mechanisms of the body. They also kill the friendly bacteria that help us digest foods correctly and provide us with essential nutrients as a byproduct of their life.

Synergism- when two or more remedies complement the action of each other, achieving a greater effect than using either one by itself.

ORDER FORM

Jernigan Nutraceuticals
13150 SW 41st, Benton, KS 67017
Order line…Toll Free 877-456-8872
(877-4JNUTRA)
www.jnutra.com

(Due to the nature of book printing all prices are subject to change without notice and in most cases reflect the manufacturers suggested retail price at the time of this printing.)

Products for the Lyme Disease Program

Quantity	PRICE	TOTAL
Nutraceutical Products		
_____Borrelogen 4 oz.	$ 48.00	_____
_____Microbojen 4oz.	$ 48.00	_____
_____Neuro-Antitox – Cardio (240 capsules	$ 84.00	_____
_____Neuro-Antitox – Musculo-Skeletal (240 capsules)		
	$ 84.00	_____
_____Neuro-Antitox – CNS/PNS (240 cap)	$ 84.00	_____
_____Neuro-Antitox – Basic (240 capsules	$ 84.00	_____
_____VCS Test Device (Neurotoxin Testing)		
	$310.00	_____
_____Wobenzym-N -800 count	$150.00	_____
_____Pleo-Alkala	$ 13.00	_____
_____Alkala Urine pH strips	$ 7.00	_____
_____Molybdemum	$ 15.00	_____
_____Beyond Chelation	$ 50.00	_____
Essential Oil Support		
_____Clarity oil blend – 15ml.	$ 27.00	_____
_____Joy oil blend - 15ml.	$ 36.00	_____
_____RC oil blend – 15ml.	$ 22.00	_____

_____Sacred Mountain oil blend – 15ml. $ 25.00   _____
_____Thieves oil blend – 15ml. $ 36.00   _____
_____White Angelica oil blend – 15ml. $ 51.00   _____
_____Aconite Nerve oil- 4oz. (Wala/Raphael$18.00   _____
_____Solum Uliginsoum oil 4oz.(Wala/Raphael)
                    $ 18.00   _____

All of the oils listed as 15ml or less are from Young Living Essential Oils, Company and may be ordered directly from the company. You will receive a discount on all their products if you call and enroll at 1-800-763-9963 then when prompted, key #497019.

Magnetic Resonance Bio-Oxidative Therapy
Comfort Covered Ceramic Bio-Oxidative Magnets
_____ 2- 4" x 6" x 1/2" Magnets $ 98.00   _____
_____ 2- 4" x 52" Elastic Strap (To hold magnet in place)
                    $ 22.00   _____

_____ 1 1/2" x 1/2" Bitemporal Soother Magnets w/strap
                    $ 22.00   _____
_____ Super Head Unit $629.00   _____
_____ Super Magnetic Bed (400 lbs.) $2,895.00   _____

Products as listed for
Low Body Temperature Program

Quantity	**PRICE**	**TOTAL**

_____ Iscar® injections (Weleda) $64.00 - Requires a doctor's prescription

_____ Women: Iscar-Mali® series-0

_____ Men: Iscar-Quercus® series-0

_____ Equisetum Oil (Wala/Raphael) $ 18.00   _____

_____ Solum Uliginsoum Oil (Wala/Raphael) $18.00   _____

_____ Solum Uliginosum Bath Essence (Wala/Raphael) $ 14.00   _____

_____ Cuprum/Nicotiana Ointment (Wala/Raphael) $ 15.00   _____

_____ Iodine Tincture (for skin stain testing) $ 3.00   _____

_____ Liquid Iodine… (for oral supplementation) $ 10.00   _____

_____ Thermometer, Digital… any reliable brand is fine

_____ Dry skin brush… $ 10.00   _____

_____ Silica Powder… $ 16.00   _____

_____ Dry Mustard for foot baths… any grocery or health food brand is fine.

_____ Ground Cayenne… any grocery or health food brand is fine

_____ Teslar Watches   Between $150-$250   _____

_____ Peat/wool blend products: Must be ordered directly from the company at www.ForTheLoveOfPeat.com

_____ Peat/wool socks

_____ Peat/wool shoe insoles

_____ Peat/wool kidney wrap

_____ Peat/wool hat/cap

_____ Peat/wool bedding...mattress pad
    •Full •Queen •King
_____ Peat/wool bedding... Comforter
    •Full •Queen •King
_____ Peat/wool apron computer shield
_____ Peat/wool seat cover
_____ Color Therapy Glasses $120.00 _____
_____ Chi Oxygen Exerciser®   call for price_____
_____ Home Infrared Sauna: Two person $2,995.00 _____
    Three person $3,295.00 _____

Products For Lyme-Related Conditions As listed in the section on "Adjunctive Therapies for Lyme-related Conditions" (Chapter 13)

Quantity	PRICE	TOTAL
_____ Belladonna 6x	$ 17.00	_____
_____ Silver 30x (Argentum)	$ 17.00	_____
_____ Sulphur 6x	$ 14.50	_____
_____ Hepar sulphuris 6x	$ 17.00	_____
_____ Solum Uliginosum oil 100ml	$ 18.00	_____
_____ Solum Uliginosum Bath Essence 100ml		
	$ 14.00	_____
_____ Homeopathic Solum Uliginosum	$ 14.50	_____
_____ Echinacea augustafolia	$ 20.00	_____
_____ Quartz 3x	$ 17.00	_____
_____ Aconite 30c	$ 17.00	_____
_____ Total Enzymes	$ 43.00	_____

_____ Neogen-4 (4oz.)	$ 80.00	_____
_____ Wobenzym-N (800 pills)	$150.00	_____
_____ Silphium lac. Capsules (90/375mg)	$ 30.00	_____
_____ Total Heart – 90 tabs.	$ 28.00	_____
_____ DSF – Formula – 120 tabs.	$ 35.00	_____
_____ Total Mitochondria – 90 tabs.	$ 49.50	_____
_____ Melatonin 5 mg	$ 17.50	_____
_____ Progesterone Cream	$ 30.00	_____
_____ Vitamin B-6 – 200 mg 90 tabs	$ 12.00	_____
_____ Rescue Remedy	$ 15.00	_____
_____ Palladium Cord	$ 17.00	_____
_____ Liquid Iodine (oral)	$ 10.00	_____
_____ Total Thyroid 90 tabs.	$ 26.00	_____
_____ Endoflex oil 15ml.	$ 28.00	_____
_____ Thyme oil – 4 oz. (Wala)	$ 18.00	_____
_____ Shower Head filter	$ 41.00	_____
_____ 2-4"x 6" x 1/2" ceramic magnets	$ 98.00	_____
_____ 4" x 52" elastic strap (holds magnet)	$ 22.00	_____
_____ Super Magnetic Head Unit	$629.00	_____
_____ Super Magnet bed	$2,895.00	_____
_____ Eucalyptus oil - 4oz. (Wala)	$ 18.00	_____
_____ Pleo-Reb (4x potency) 20 caps.	$ 40.00	_____
_____ Melaleuca Oil (Tea tree oil)	$ 22.00	_____
_____ Aconite Nerve Oil	$ 18.00	_____
_____ Rhus Toxicodendron Cord	$ 15.00	_____
_____ SF-734 – 90 caps.	$ 17.50	_____
_____ Gather Vitality	$ 16.00	_____
_____ Homocystiene Redux – 60 tabs	$ 17.50	_____
_____ Rheuma Comp Oil – 4 oz.	$ 30.00	_____
_____ Joint-Aide 90 caps.	$ 35.00	_____
_____ Marjoram oil 15 ml.	$ 35.00	_____
_____ Neuro-Plus	$ 17.00	_____
_____ Eyelights	$150.00	_____
_____ Molybdenum 90 caps.	$ 15.00	_____
_____ Yeast Ease 4 oz.	$ 40.00	_____

_____Total Probiotics 90 tabs.	$ 27.00	_____
_____Helichrysum oil – 5ml	$165.00	_____
_____Strengthen Kidneys	$ 15.00	_____
_____Quiet Contemplative	$ 15.00	_____
_____Vitamin B-complex - 90 tabs.	$ 17.00	_____
_____Cypress oil – 15ml	$ 20.00	_____
_____Pleo-Alkala	$ 13.00	_____
_____Alkala pH urine strips	$ 7.00	_____
_____Cocculus comp. tabs	$ 23.00	_____
_____Juvaflex oil – 15ml	$ 48.00	_____
_____Ledum oil – 5ml	$ 43.00	_____
_____Champion Juicer	$call	_____
_____Primula Oil	$ 18.00	_____
_____Valor oil – 15ml	$ 25.00	_____
_____Total Brain	$ 36.00	_____
_____Brain Power oil – 5ml	$ 48.00	_____
_____F-Complex	$ 15.00	_____
_____Ozone Air Purifiers	$669.00	_____

All of the oils listed as 15ml or less are from Young Living Essential Oils, Company and may be ordered at a discount by calling and enrolling at 1-800-763-9963 then when prompted, key #497019.

The Progesterone Cream is from the Arbonne Company and may be ordered at a discount by calling and enrolling at 1-800-Arbonne then when prompted, key 10433061.

Jernigan Nutraceuticals
Order line…Toll Free 877-456-8872
(877-4JNUTRA)
www.jnutra.com

Non-toxic Personal Care Products

After all of the years of searching and trying all kinds of products, these personal care products are my favorites.

Soaps: **All of these soaps use essential oils and contain no toxic ingredients.**

Quantity   **Price**   **Total**

_____ **Rose Soap** (Weleda)   Body Tonic
$7.95   _____

Rose oil in this soap has the highest energy of all plant oils and enhances the frequency of every cell. It helps maintain emotional balance. It is beneficial in convalescence and when recovering from illness.

_____ **Rosemary Soap** (Weleda) Invigorating
$4.95   _____

Rosemary is invigorating and improves vascular and lymphatic circulation. It is especially good for when you feel tired and worn out.

_____ **Iris Soap** (Weleda) Balancing of Skin
$4.95   _____

Iris soap is especially healing and balancing to the skin.

_____ **Morning Start Soap** (YLO) Invigorating
$8.00   _____

The essential oils in this soap are uplifting and energizing to the body and mind. A great choice to improve your outlook on life. Contains: essential oils of lemongrass, rosemary cineol, peppermint and juniper.

_____ **Thieves Soap** (YLO) Immune stimulating
$8.00   _____

Thieves soap contains an essential oil blend that was used by thieves in England robbing the homes of victims of the Bubonic plague. Its antimicrobial effect kept them frombecoming infected. Contains: essential oils of clove, lemon, cinnamon bark, eucalyptus radiata and rosemary cineol.

_____ **Melaleuca-Geranium Soap** (YLO) Antimicrobial
$8.00   _____

Melaleuca ericifolia is a very gentle form of melaleuca that is known to kill bacteria, fungi, and viruses on contact. This soap is suitable for children or those individuals who are more sensitive to oils. It is revitalizing to the body while calming in effect. Contains essential oils of melaleuca, geranium and vetiver.

Vetiver in this soap is good for Lyme sufferers since it is warming to the body, good for arthritis, muscular rheumatism and is anti-spasmodic.

_____ **Valor Soap** (YLO) Strengthening/Balancing
$8.00   _____

The oils in this soap are what I consider almost miraculous. They seem to cause the spinal muscles to align the spine, eases pain, and at the same time brings courage, emotional balance, self-esteem and calmness. It is also beneficial in hyper-activity and ADD. Contains: essential oils of spruce, rosewood, blue tansy and frankincense.

Shampoos: Each of these shampoos use non-toxic ingredients and do not contain chemical dyes or toxic additives.
Quantity   **Price**   **Total**

_____ **Lavender Volume Hair and Scalp Wash** (YLO)
$21.00   _____

This shampoo is very gentle and therefore good for fine hair and babies.

_____ **Lemon Sage Clarifying Hair + Scalp Wash** (YLO)
$21.00 _____

Good for removing chemical residues and the buildup of hair styling products from the hair and scalp.

_____ **Rosemary Shampoo (Weleda)**
$8.75 _____

Rosemary is invigorating and improves vascular and lymphatic circulation. It is especially good for when you feel tired and worn out.

_____ **Rosemary Conditioner (Weleda)**
$8.75 _____

_____ **Chamomile Shampoo (Weleda)**
$8.75 _____

Chamomile has a calming effect on the body. It is good for when one needs to relax. Well suited for irritable types.

_____ **Chamomile Conditioner (Weleda)**
$8.75 _____

All of the soaps and shampoos listed as (YLO) are from Young Living Essential Oils, Company and may be ordered at a discount by calling and enrolling at 1-800-763-9963 then when prompted, key #497019.

Jernigan Nutraceuticals
Order line…Toll Free 877-456-8872
(877-4JNUTRA)
www.jnutra.com

Deodorants: It is best not to use antiperspirants due to the fact that all efforts should be made to allow the skin to breath and perspire in the armpits. The armpits contain many lymph nodes that must not be clogged from the blocking of detoxifying perspiration by antiperspirants. Many antiperspirants contain toxic aluminum.

Quantity	Price	Total
_____ **Citrus Deodorant** (spray) 4 oz. (Weleda)	$8.50	_____
_____ **Sage Deodorant** (spray) 4 oz. (Weleda)	$8.50	_____

Toothpaste: Lyme is said to have specific areas of the body in which it likes to hide and grow. According to research the teeth are one of these areas. It is imperative to use toothpastes that are not sugar-based, that do not contain formaldehyde as a preservative, and that have no "warning" as to its toxic nature on the label, such as every toothpaste in the grocery stores.

Quantity	Price	Total
_____ **Dentarome Toothpaste, Extra-strength (YLO)**	$6.00	_____

This toothpaste is always my first choice for anyone suffering with Lyme disease. The essential oils kill bacteria and viruses on contact and promote healing of the bones, and gums while protecting and energizing the electrical circuits that the teeth share. This toothpaste is sweetened with stevia and contains extra amounts of the essential oils of wintergreen, peppermint, and the oil blend from the "Thieves" formula – clove, lemon, cinnamon bark, eucalyptus radiata, and rosemary cineol.

Young Living Water Purifier-

_____Whole House Water Filtration System

$1,323.00 _____

_____ UV Filtration System

$997.00 _____

The toothpaste and water purifier are from Young Living Essential Oils Company and may be ordered at a discount by calling and enrolling at 1-800-763-9963 then when prompted, key #497019.

Jernigan Nutraceuticals
**Order line…Toll Free 877-456-8872
(877-4JNUTRA)**
www.jnutra.com

Notes

Notes

Notes